The Fern Pharmacy

"For years I have wanted a reference on the medicinal uses of ferns on my herbalist bookshelf. The old books have a few lines but pass on archaic traditions. It is clear that ancient people thought very highly of fern medicine. Their accounts are full of mysterious, magical, and fairy references. I have only ever used one fern for one thing—*Osmunda regalis*, a specific remedy for lumbago—but wow does it work! I wanted more. The fairies delivered this wonderful, comprehensive, detailed book by Robert Dale Rogers, who is not just an 'armchair herbalist,' but a practitioner with many years of experience."

Matthew Wood, author of *Holistic Medicine and the Extracellular Matrix* and *A Shamanic Herbal*

"As some of the most ancient and successful plants of Earth, ferns have long been integrated into traditional healing practices across the globe to treat a wide range of maladies. In *The Fern Pharmacy*, we find many practical ways to connect with these powerful plant allies. With its exhaustive survey of the bioactive compounds, ecological roles, agricultural applications, and health benefits of the world's ferns—all interwoven with illuminating insights into the cultural impacts of these subtler plants—this tome provides an engaging and comprehensive survey of this overlooked corner of nature's pharmacopeia. It is an excellent addition to the bookshelf of any herbalist, naturalist, or ethnologist wanting to integrate the powerful offerings of these understory elders into their practice or paradigm."

Peter McCoy, mycologist and author of *Radical Mycology*

"This book is a treasure! A comprehensive collection of the medicinal virtues of ferns that can't be found anywhere else. Bravo to Robert Dale Rogers for gifting us this compendium of often forgotten botanical medicine."

ROSALEE DE LA FORÊT, AUTHOR OF
ALCHEMY OF HERBS AND *WILD REMEDIES*

"It is a rare thing these days to find a book filled from cover to cover with knowledge conveyed by almost no other source, but *The Fern Pharmacy* is just that. This collection of history, lore, and science is made all the more valuable by the addition of Robert's own understanding and insight."

JIM MCDONALD, HERBALIST

The Fern Pharmacy

Indigenous Wisdom & Modern Pharmacology

A Sacred Planet Book

Robert Dale Rogers

Healing Arts Press
Rochester, Vermont

Healing Arts Press
One Park Street
Rochester, Vermont 05767
www.HealingArtsPress.com

Healing Arts Press is a division of Inner Traditions International

Sacred Planet Books are curated by Richard Grossinger, Inner Traditions editorial board member and cofounder and former publisher of North Atlantic Books. The Sacred Planet collection, published under the umbrella of the Inner Traditions family of imprints, includes works on the themes of consciousness, cosmology, alternative medicine, dreams, climate, permaculture, alchemy, shamanic studies, oracles, astrology, crystals, hyperobjects, locutions, and subtle bodies.

Note to the reader: *This book is intended to be an informational guide. The remedies, approaches, and techniques described herein are meant to supplement, and not to be a substitute for, professional medical care or treatment. They should not be used to treat a serious ailment without prior consultation with a qualified health care professional.*

Cataloging-in-Publication Data for this title is available from the Library of Congress

ISBN 979-8-88850-180-1 (print)
ISBN 979-8-88850-181-8 (ebook)

Printed and bound in India by Nutech Print Services

10 9 8 7 6 5 4 3 2 1

Text design by Virginia Scott Bowman and layout by Kenleigh Manseau
This book was typeset in Garamond Premier Pro with Acumin Pro Wide, Frutiger LT Std, and Minion Pro used as the display typeface.

Images not otherwise credited are Adobe Stock Images.

To send correspondence to the author of this book, mail a first-class letter to the author c/o Inner Traditions • Bear & Company, One Park Street, Rochester, VT 05767, and we will forward the communication, or contact the author directly at **SelfHealDistributing.com**.

To my father, Robert Erwin Rogers (1926–1982).
He was born in North Sydney, Nova Scotia, where coal mining
was a way of life. He encouraged my deep appreciation
and love of nature and wild foods, including
dandelion greens and fiddleheads.

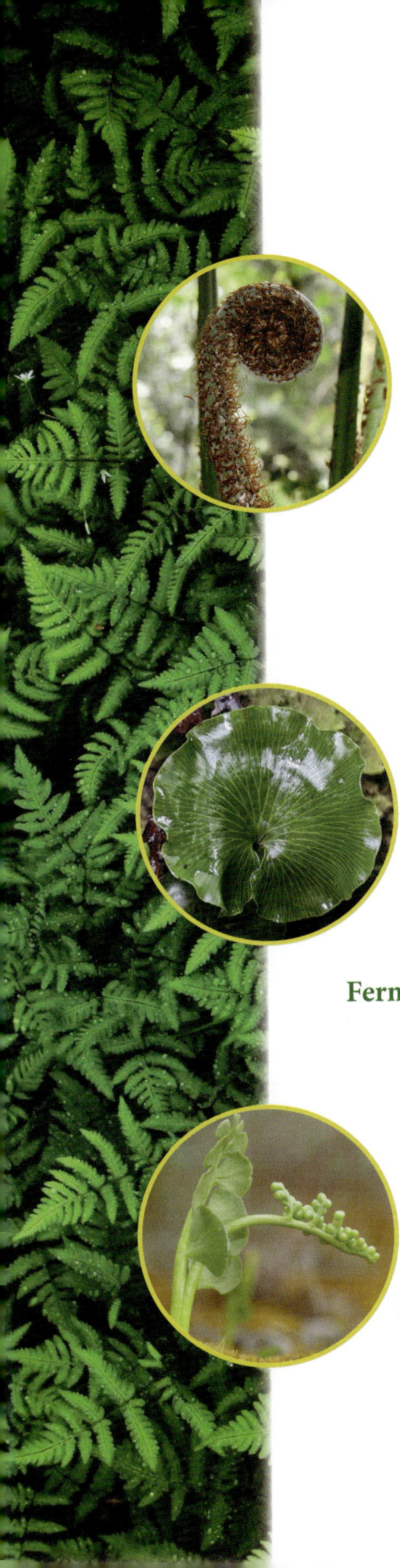

Contents

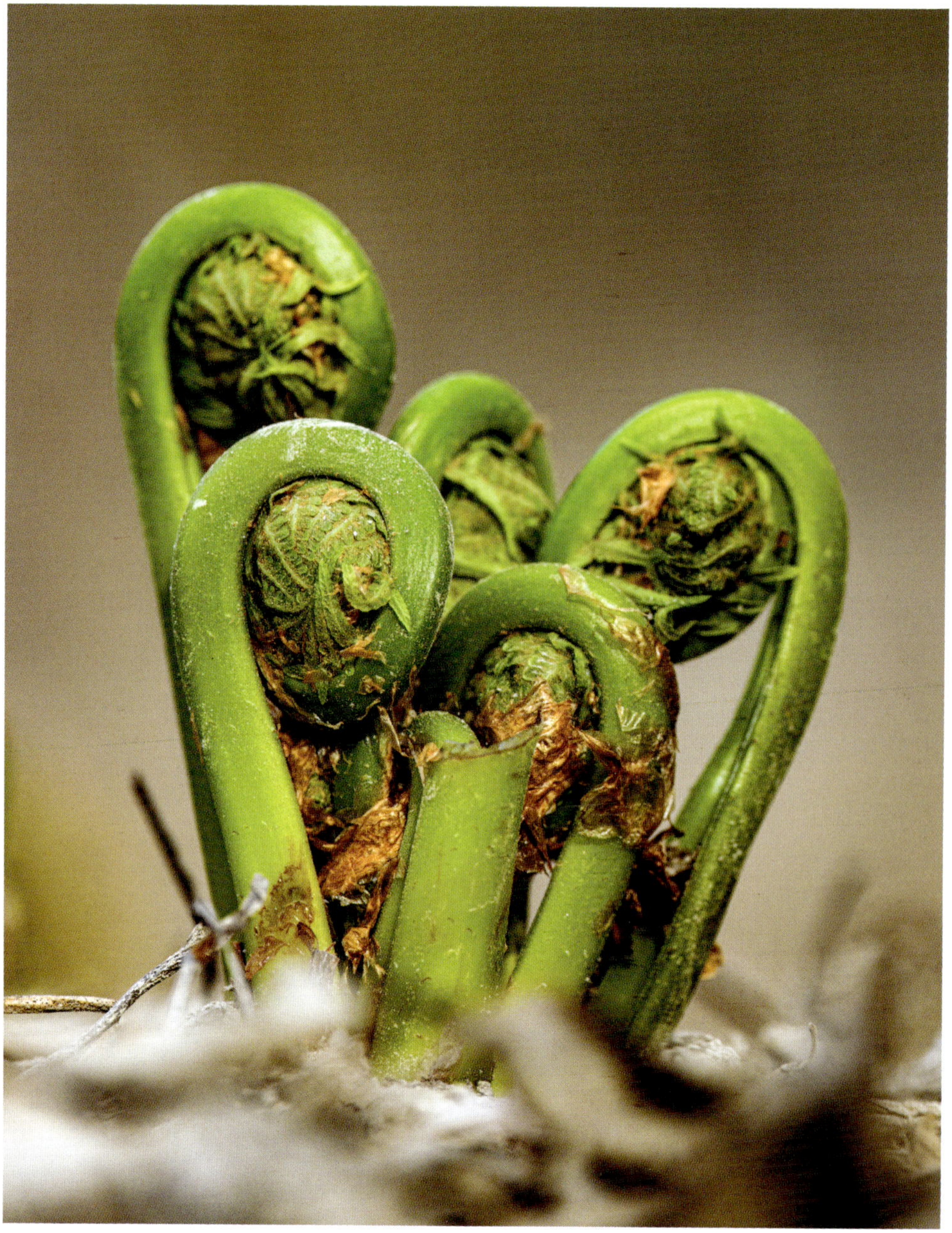

Ostrich Fern Fiddleheads
(*Matteuccia struthiopteris*)

Preface

Beneath the forest emerald veil,
Ferns whisper of an ancient grail.
Unfurling fronds, a spiral delight!
In the woods they dance at night.
They whirl and swirl with wind's gentle push,
create a ballet in the evening's hush.
Next time you wander down your woody trail,
listen, as ferns tell their verdant tale.

Robert Dale Rogers

When a youngster, I lived in Saint John, New Brunswick. Each spring, my father would take me upriver to pick fiddleheads (crosiers). The unfurled treble clef-shaped ostrich fern greens were fun to pick, take home, steam, and eat with butter and salt.

One May, many years later in the mid 1970s, I was walking through a swampy area of Northern Alberta and came upon a patch of unfurled fiddleheads that I just knew were the prized ostrich ferns (*Matteuccia struthiopteris*).

I took some home to enjoy and then realized a cash income could be possible for an unemployed young man living in a log cabin without electricity or running water. I teamed up with a neighbor and we started Fiddlehead Farms. The next spring, with help, we gathered and sold 600 pounds to a food store chain in Edmonton for one dollar per pound. We thought we were doing well! During those years, I wrote a fiddlehead cookbook and was later interviewed on CBC radio about the edible greens (see figure on page x).

The government then got involved, as they did not believe ostrich ferns grew in the province. This turned into a song and dance with a University of Alberta professor eventually correctly identifying the fern. To this day, I still enjoy a meal of wildcrafted fiddleheads every spring to remind me of early

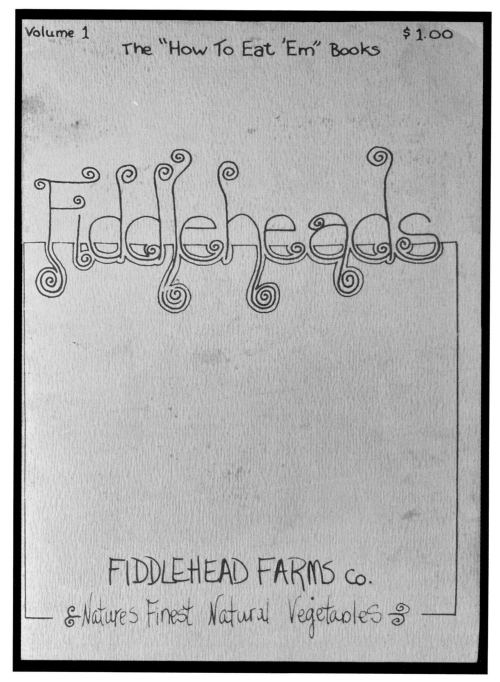

Fiddlehead Farms Company Cookbook Cover

wilderness adventures. A small industry in Northern Saskatchewan and British Columbia started up in 1993.

I first became aware of the healing power of ferns when I ventured out to Alert Bay, British Columbia, in July 1974. I was taking an online herbal course at Greenvale College, taught by noted herbalist Norma Myers, and years later became aware of her summer seminar.

I hitchhiked from Northern Alberta to Vancouver Island and then north to catch the ferry to Alert Bay. Outside of Nanaimo I stuck out my thumb and a car pulled over and gave me a lift. It was the well-known ethnobotanist Nancy Turner and her husband Robert! I had no idea at the time of her stature and brilliant work. Later, I myself became an ethnobotanist on medicinal plants of Northern Alberta. In October 2024, fifty years later, I spoke at the Olympic Peninsula Fungi Festival, and Nancy was lodged in the same house. We had a wonderful time recalling our ethnobotanical ventures over the past half century.

There were some excellent herbal teachers at the event. I remember attending a class with James Green on Bach flower remedies, which I worked with for the next forty years. My wife, Laurie, and I later researched and created Prairie Deva Flower Essences (Szott-Rogers and Rogers 1997) and later Mushroom Essences (Rogers 2016).

One day I badly sprained my ankle and renowned herbalist Norma Myers suggested I apply a fern poultice. It worked like a miracle, helping reduce the swelling within a few hours.

Years later, I read a fairy tale by Hans Christian Anderson (1835), called "The Traveling Companion." A young orphan boy has the ability to see fairies and sets out to seek his fortune. He soon meets a fellow traveler, and they join up. One morning, an old woman passes by, carrying a huge load of willow twigs and three fern stipes.* As she turns, she slips and breaks her leg. The young traveler's companion takes from his pocket a salve that knits her bone like magic. In return he asks for the three ferns. As the story unfolds, the kindly traveler uses the ferns to become invisible, and chases a killer witch, beating her with ferns until she bleeds. In the end, an evil spell is broken, and the witch reverts to her kind-hearted and beautiful self.

*Stipes are the long stems, separate from the fronds.

Since that day, nearly fifty years ago, I have researched and found that these "primitive" plants possess incredible healing potential.

A small booklet originally published in German in 1911, titled *The Herbs and Weeds of Fr. Johannes Künzle*, was republished in 1975 under the new title *Herbs and Weeds: A Useful Booklet on Medicinal Herbs* (Künzle, 1975).

> Which is the best bed for people suffering from cramps, pains in the joints, rheumatism, rheumatic tooth ache, rheumatic headache? A sack filled with dried ferns. The fern absorbs all these complaints and gives the sufferer complete rest. Moreover, fleas and bedbugs run away from this bed to a great distance, they move out immediately. . . . All kinds of ferns, even the smallest, used internally (in very small doses, however and mixed with wine, three quarters of wine to one quarter of ferns) drive away all kinds of worms.
>
> Foot baths of this fern root, taken for a week or two, cure the worst spasmodic and gouty diseases. . . . Fern root boiled in vinegar, and used as a compress cures gangrene of the feet, even though they may have turned black and blue already.

One of my early Indigenous mentors was the Cree healer, Russell Willier. We lived near each other on the south shore of Lesser Slave Lake, Alberta, for several decades.

He passed a few years ago but left all of us a legacy of plant wisdom and knowledge in *A Cree Healer and His Medicine Bundle* (Young et al. 2015). His favorite fern was narrow wood fern (*Dryopteris carthusiana*, see page 135).

Acknowledgments

This project would not have been possible without the support of the wonderful people at Inner Traditions including Richard Grossinger, Courtney B. Jenkins Mesquita, Lisa P. Allen, Erica Robinson, Tessa Cappelle, and numerous others. I would like to thank Alan Rockefeller and Drew T. Henderson for sharing their amazing photography with you and me. I am so grateful.

Thank you as well to Dr. Christopher Hobbs, Matthew Wood, Jim Mcdonald, Peter McCoy, Nancy Turner, and Rosalee de la Forêt for their support and kind words. It is especially gratifying when herbal and fungal colleagues recognize your work. And a special thanks to Franchelle Ofsoské-Wyber for permission to include her vibrational fern essences from New Zealand. Similar to flower, lichen, and mushroom essences, they facilitate healing, peace, and stillness at the soul level.

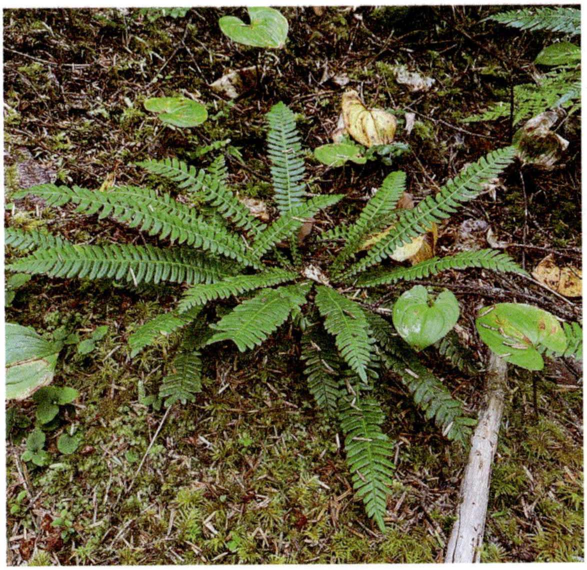

Blechnum spicantum (Deer Fern)
Photo by Drew T. Henderson

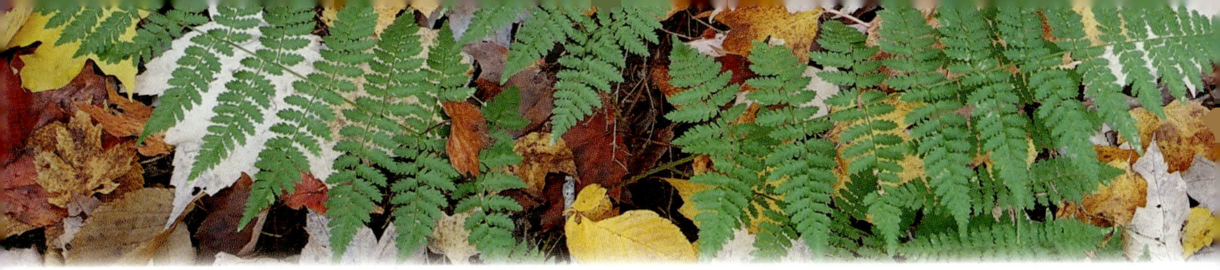

INTRODUCTION

Unfurling the Fronds

Nature made ferns for pure leaves to see what she could do in that line.

HENRY DAVID THOREAU

The term *fern* is often misused. Examples of this are the unrelated asparagus fern (a flowering plant) and sweet fern (a flowering shrub of the *Comptonia* genus). Even a group of animals called hydrozoans, distantly related to jellyfish and coral, are named air ferns. Their skeletons are dried, dyed green, and falsely sold as a plant that lives on air.

Ferns are ancient plants, with fossils dating back to the Middle Devonian era, about 390 million years ago—several hundred million years before the emergence of flowering plants. The true ferns *Polypodiales* making up 80% of today's ferns, arose about 180 million years ago.

The word *fern* may derive from the Anglo-Saxon contraction *fepern* or German *Farn*, both derived from Sanskrit *parna*, meaning "feather" or "wing." Some authors suggest it derives from *farr* (a bullock), from its use as livestock bedding. These words ultimately trace back to Proto-Germanic "farną," which is also related to the Latin "fērnum" and Ancient Greek "péron" or "pterón," all of which refer to ferns or fern-like plants.

THE LIFE OF FERNS

Fern ancestry is traced to the green algae that moved from water to land, similar to mosses. However, unlike mosses, ferns developed vascular tissue to transport water and nutrients, providing them with greater adaptability. Ferns consist mainly of a leaf stalk, with the real stems being underground rhizomes.

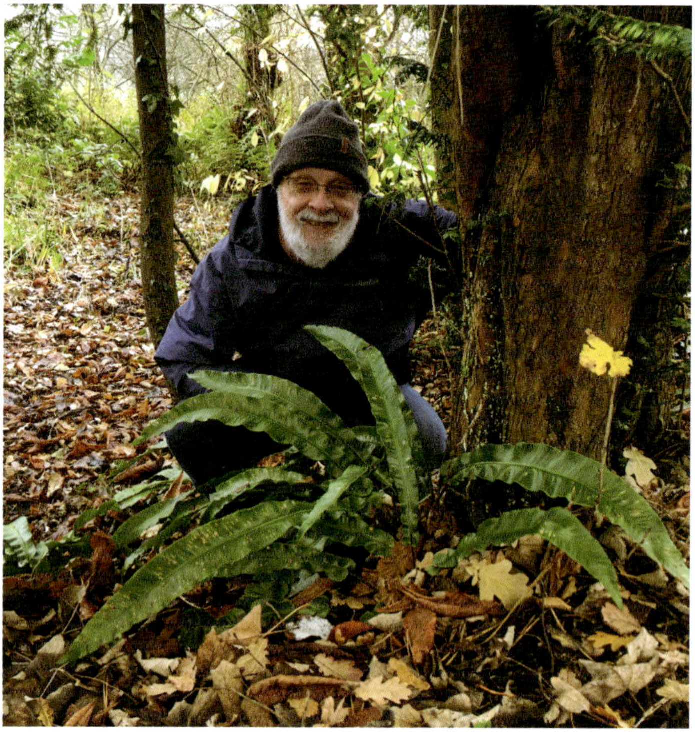

Myself with Hart's Tongue Ferns (*Asplenium scolopendrium*)
Photo by Robert Dale Rogers

They are the intermediate between mosses and flowering plants.

Forty-meter-tall tree ferns with five-meter fronds existed on Earth before animals evolved. Today, a tree fern on Norfolk Island in the South Pacific reaches a spectacular twenty-two meters in height.

Ferns are vascular plants that access water and nutrients from the soil and produce spores. They are found in forest shade, cracks in rocks in deserts, floating in water, in acidic swamps, or twining up fifty-foot tree trunks. The scaly tree ferns of the *Cyathea* species can reach up to twenty meters (sixty-six feet) tall.

It is estimated that North American and European Stephanian-era coals may be composed of up to 75% ancient tree ferns. Many ferns associate with mycorrhizal fungi and can grow in a wide range of pH, from intensely acidic soils to those found on limestone.

Besides vascular tissue that allows ferns to draw up water and nutrients, they possess another unique property: thanks to horizontal gene transfer from hornworts (to be covered in my book on *Moss Medicine*), they possess a special

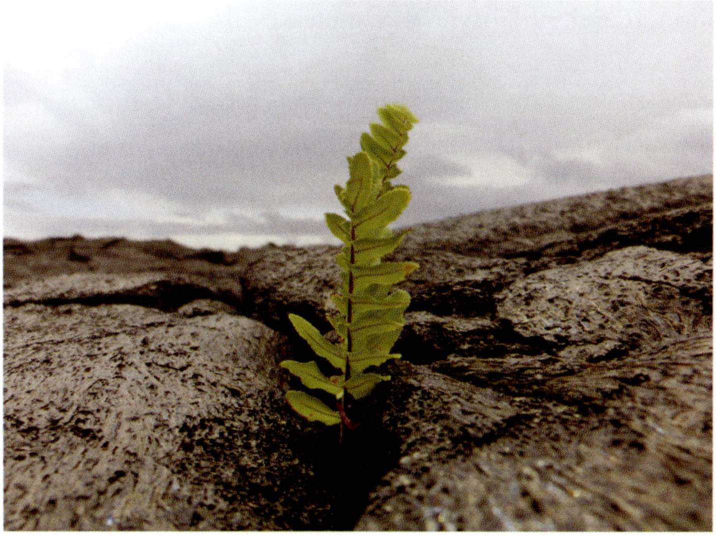

A Growing Fern

red light-sensing protein called neochrome. Most plants can only detect blue light, but due to their shaded environment ferns can use the "leftover" lower-energy red light for photosynthesis. This was possible due to germinating spores of hornworts and ferns picking up DNA, facilitating the leap from the bryophyte to modern ferns (Li et al. 2014).

Ferns don't produce pollen, and are therefore not reliant on insects, birds, or bats for reproduction.

The life cycle of ferns is fascinating. When a spore lands in the right mixture of temperature, light, and moisture, it begins to germinate, forming a small green, heart-shaped leaf that looks nothing like a fern. This is called a prothallium and contains the sex organs of both male and female on its underside. An egg is fertilized by sperm (which has a whip-like flagellum) and grows into an embryo with roots, stems, and leaves. It takes three generations for a fern to create another fern. Note that flowering plants have sperm that lack flagella, making ferns more like humans in this respect.

Ferns associate with mycorrhizal fungi, sharing carbon and sugars in exchange for the transport of nutrients to their offspring (gametophytes) growing underground.

Grape fern (*Botrychium* sp.) and adder's-tongue (*Ophioglossum*) produce gametophytes that develop underground without chlorophyll and depend upon exchange of nutrients from fungal networks. Spores released by adult ferns germinate into gametophytes living securely underground, preventing drying out, and then produce above-ground, photosynthesizing leaves after emerging from the soil.

Adult ferns nurture the "children" of neighboring ferns via fungal networks, suggesting cooperative breeding (Beerling 2019).

> Because of sporulation, it is often believed that the sex life of ferns is simple. But consider this. The mobile and independent sex cell of a fern is attracted by malic acid and makes towards it when it "scents" it. Only 0.00000008th of a milligram is enough, a figure that even the most sophisticated scientific equipment would be hard pressed to identify. (Rogers 2014a)

There is another difference between ferns and flowering plants. The latter push out of the soil, with the leaf developing its tip first and parts of stem follow as the leaf grows larger. The frond, however, develops in the opposite direction. Rather than growing from below upward, it grows downward or from the inside out, as the part providing tissue is inside the center of the curled frond. If you watch carefully as it uncurls, it appears to be pushed down on the earth from above (Grohmann 1989).

Being a student of anthroposophy, Grohmann noted how Rudolf Steiner

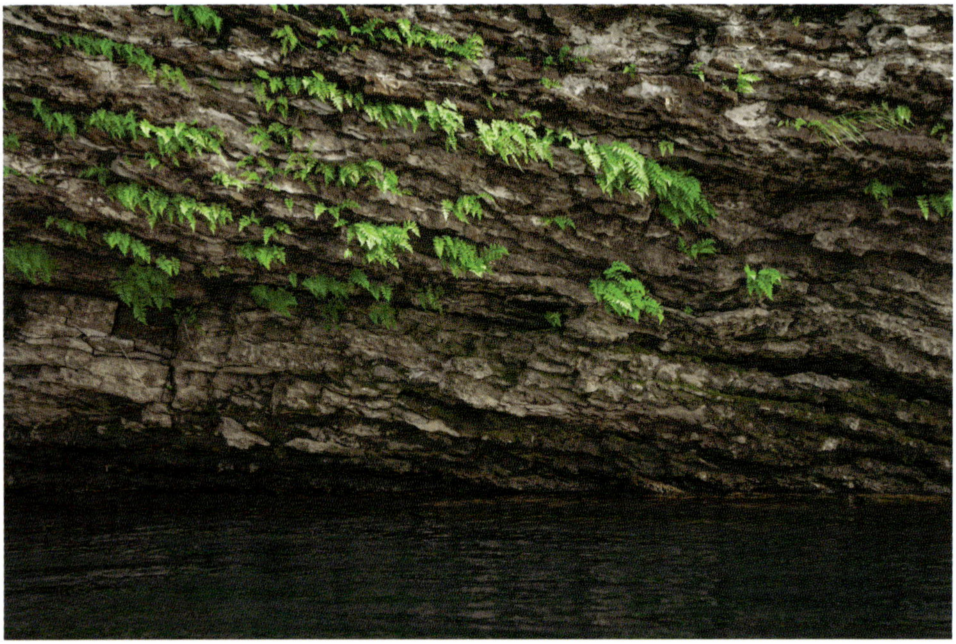

Ferns Growing Downward

compared ferns with the first stage of a child's development, when they say "I" for the first time. The frond is nature's image of the "I" felt by children.

I am a huge fan of Steiner and his unique contributions to agriculture, education, and medicine. However, his statement suggests he believed ferns to be less developed or immature. In my opinion ferns developed their own evolutionary path and have been so successful that they continued along it. Why fix something that is not broken?

HISTORICAL POPULARITY

During the 1840s, pteridomania, or the Victorian fern craze, was popular. The name pteridomania is derived from the Greek *pterido*, meaning fern. The British botanical journal *The Phytologist* (1841) published newly discovered ferns, and the race was on.

John Smith (1868) documented 560 fern species in his *Catalogue of the Ferns and Their Allies Cultivated in the Royal Gardens of Kew*.

Charles Kingsley, in his book *Glaucus; or, The Wonders of the Shore*, coined the term *pteridomania*. The craze led people, particularly women, to collect unusual varieties of ferns, recording their sightings, and pressing them in their herbariums (or *fernariums* to be precise).

During this time in the United Kingdom, images of ferns were found on wallpaper, clothing, ironworks, printed paper, textiles, pottery, glass, metals, wood, ceramic sculptures, gravestones, and memorials. The obsession abated in the 1890s.

Kingsley (1890) wrote, "Since the 'Lady-ferns' and 'Venus hair' appeared; and that you could not help yourself looking now and then at the said 'Venus's hair' and agreeing that Nature's real beauties were somewhat superior to the ghastly woollen caricatures which they had superseded." After all, it was Victorian times of suppressed sexuality and female nether regions were not openly discussed.

Early terrariums, known as Wardian cases, were very popular at the time, resembling miniature greenhouses for indoor fern cultivation. Dr. Nathaniel Ward collected and observed moth cocoons in sealed glass bottles and noted that a male fern in one bottle lived for over four years until the seal broke and allowed toxic air pollution to enter. He continued to experiment and, in 1842, published *On the Growth of Plants in Closely Glazed Cases*.

His "discovery" led to the transplantation of live plants in British households and on long sea voyages. This enabled the transport of tea plants from China into India and the movement of rubber trees from Brazil to plantations in Sri Lanka (formerly Ceylon).

This historical practice of cultivating plants in controlled environments inspired my own interest, and I cultivated a moss/fern terrarium for a number of years when I was in my twenties.

FERN FOLKLORE

We have receipt of fern-seed, we walk invisible.

WILLIAM SHAKESPEARE, *HENRY IV*

Ferns do not produce seeds; they reproduce via spores. Because ferns do not have seeds, the idea of a fern seed was purely mythical. This rarity of the so-called fern seed led to the belief that it had magical properties, specifically the power of invisibility. The logic follows that something so rare and unseen (since it doesn't actually exist) would grant the power to become unseen or invisible.

Ben Ionson got into the act with his comedy *The Nevv Inne, or The Light Heart* (1631). A servant ordered to stay hidden explains to his master, "Because indeed I had no med'cine, Sir, to go invisible: No fern-seed in my pocket" (Act I, Scene VI).

Fern folklore also involves restoring sight. *A Description of the Western Islands of Scotland* by Martin Martin (1703) notes a remedy for "eyes that are blood-shot or become blind for some days." The recipe involved applying the blades of fern fronds mixed with egg whites to the face and brows of a patient lying on their back.

Other myths involved summoning the fairy Puck, a character from William Shakespeare's play *A Midsummer Night's Dream* written between 1590–96, entering a fairy world by stepping on a fern.

In Slavic folklore, it is believed that ferns blossom once a year during Kupala, at midnight on the summer solstice. Finding a fern flower is said to give one the understanding of animals and birds. Weaving ferns into one's hair was believed to protect those bathing or swimming in a lake from *rusalki*, the freshwater sirens.

In the Middle Ages in England, harvesting fern seed was thought to be a complicated procedure. Twelve pewter plates were stacked in a bed of ferns. At the stroke of midnight, a blue blossom was believed to open and drop a single golden seed that passed through eleven plates and landed on the last one. If pewter plates were not available, the wide leaves of mullein were used.

In other myths, the red fern flower was snatched by the devil before anyone else could claim it. St. John's Eve (the shortest night of the year) was believed to be the best time to catch a fern seed, as St. John the Baptist was believed to be born at precisely midnight.

But on St. John's mysterious night
Sacred to many a wizard spell,
The hour when first to human sight
Confest, the mystic Fern seed fell.

The Ukrainian/Russian writer Nikolai Gogol (1809–1852) tells a story of a young man who plucks a red fern "flower" shining like a flame as it opens. The old man who told the story to the youngster turns out to be the devil, who appears with Baba Yaga, a prominent figure in Slavic folklore, often depicted as a witch. Jewels appear but before the youngster can access them, the witch tells him she requires human blood. It does not end well.

Many fern myths suggest that if you see a fern flower at midnight, it is better not to touch it.

In Finland, the seed from a fern bloom was believed to enable the holder to become invisible and travel to a spot holding treasure. Will o' the wisps, or ghostly vapors over swamps, called *aarnivalkea*, marked the spot, but were protected by a magical spell that prevented anyone but those holding a fern seed from ever finding the location.

A Russian folktale involved a cattle rancher who lost his herd. As he walks through ferns, a seed accidently fell into his boot. He immediately sensed the location of his lost cattle and fetched them. While traveling home, he had a vision of treasure and its location. After taking the cattle home, he changed his boots and forgets the location. In Bohemia, holding fern seeds was believed to bring prosperity.

In *The Wonders in the Spessart*, a magpie calls out to a traveling teacher, saying he should spread fern seeds onto the breast of a magic princess to make her invisible.

König von Sion tells the story of an older soldier who gives advice to a new recruit: "Put a packet of fern seeds next to your chest and you'll be invisible to the enemy."

In another anecdotal observation, carnin (an extract from meat) was mixed with fern spore powder to make fingerprints visible.

In Styria, Southeastern Austria, it was believed that the devil appeared on January 6th (Bertha's Night). A magic circle was formed, and one stood in the middle with elderberries gathered on St. John's Eve in hopes of obtaining fern seeds. The seeds were said to give one the power of thirty to forty men or help discover hidden treasures.

Other myths involved shooting at the Sun. If the shot hit, three drops would fall to Earth and turn into fern seeds. In Wiccan magic, tossing dried fern into a fire was believed to banish evil spirits.

Hildegard von Bingen (1098–1179), a visionary 12th-century Benedictine Abbess, was noted for her contributions to herbal wisdom. Her book *Subtleties of the Diverse Qualities of Created Things* was published as *Physica* in 1533 and later translated from Latin into English by Priscilla Throop (1998). "Fern (*Farn*) is very hot and dry and has a little bit of juice in it. It holds within itself great power, namely such a power that the devil flees from it. . . . In the place where it grows, the devil rarely practices his deceptions."

PRACTICAL USES

Ferns have been used by Indigenous people around the world for food and medicine. Over 300 ferns are used in Traditional Chinese Medicine (TCM) to treat a wide range of conditions (Ding et al. 2008). Notably, Ding and colleagues conducted a study examining the antioxidant activity of thirty-one species.

The fiddleheads of bracken (*Pteridium aquilinum*), ostrich (*Matteuccia struthiopteris*), and cinnamon ferns (*Omundastrum cinnamomeum*) have long been consumed. At least thirty-three fern species are consumed in Nepal, with twenty genera used as cooked vegetables.

The tubers were used for food in Europe thirty-thousand years ago, according to Van Gilder Cooke (2010). The Guanche of the Canary Islands turn fern tubers into *gofio*, a starchy flour.

The Cree of Northern Canada used wood ferns (*Dryopteris* sp.) for food and medicine, calling it "fat root."

Licorice fern (*Polypodium glycyrrhiza*) rhizomes were chewed by Indigenous people of the Pacific Northwest for flavor.

Generally, allergic response to fern spores is not significant in many parts of the world. Because of this, there are numerous medicinal applications for ferns.

HOMEOPATHY

Modern homeopathic provings of ferns are few and far between. Several accounts describe difficulties in expressing oneself verbally or physically, which is metaphorically linked to the retention of stool and the sensation of constipation.

Some common symptoms associated with fern remedies are frequent and copious urination, weak libido, partial loss of vision or visual disturbances, and difficulties with concentration, depression or lack of joy alternating with periods of hot temper and violent outbursts.

Common symptoms associated with fern remedies include burning pain in the eyes and stomach, dry mucous membranes including the mouth, with the tendency to not perspire easily (see *Mosses and Ferns: Spectrum of Homeopathy* 2021).

MEDICINAL APPLICATIONS

Fiddleheads from various ferns are a rich source of omega-3 and omega-6 fatty acids with a beneficial ratio, high antioxidant activity, and good source of lutein comparable to that of spinach.

Ferns are generally rich in essential fatty acids. Twenty-three fern species from twelve families were tested for their content and variability.

However, ferns contain thiaminase, an enzyme that destroys thiamine (vitamin B1), which is essential for good health.

Severe thiamine deficiency causes beriberi, resulting in mental depression, poor memory, fatigue, insomnia, difficulty walking, and cardiovascular issues.

Thiamine deficiency has been observed in cancer patients with quickly growing tumors. Cell cultures and in vivo animal models suggest rapidly dividing tumors require high levels of thiamine.

John R. Swanton (1905) recorded Haida mythology around ferns. The Haida are an Indigenous people native to the Haida Gwaii archipelago in British Columbia, Canada, and parts of southeastern Alaska. "A long time after that they began to starve. . . . Then they gathered edible fern stumps right behind them. Those they ate. They hunted outward and inward. Finally, after the hero Big-tail performed shamanistic rituals all night, Supernatural-Being-Looking-Landward promised to feed his people if they would 'stop making the little supernatural being living along the shore cry.' He was referring to the fern spirit woman, who cried because the ferns were being eaten."

Ferns have potential for removing heavy metals, especially arsenic, from contaminated soil. They also contain high levels of tin, up to 30 ppm.

Around the world, ferns have been used to stuff mattresses to repel fleas and bedbugs. In early England, the poor would mix the fern ashes with water and form round masses known as fern balls. These were heated by the fire and made into lye for washing flax linen. In Sweden, the fern ashes were mixed with strong lye, and then formed into balls.

Fern dyes were once popular and are discussed in their respective sections.

The ash from burnt ferns was used in France to manufacture glass, due to its almost pure alkali residue.

AUTHOR'S NOTE ON HOW THIS BOOK IS ORGANIZED

As you read ahead, you'll notice that the ferns are organized by genus. Each genus has a list of common ferns found in that species (such as "Hart's Tongue Fern") as well as names for groups of ferns in plural (such as "Maidenhair Ferns"). For more prominent genera, a green box contains descriptions of the geographic range, habitat, practical uses, and medicinal applications of a number of species in that particular genus. Each species does not necessarily have every attribute presented in the summary, but collectively the species in that genus share these characteristics.

In each blue box is a description of a notable essence from that particular genus, including its emotional gifts and guidance bestowed. A recommendation of where to find the essence is also given.

At the end of the book you will see a comprehensive list of ferns by their common names. If you happen to know a particular fern in your area by its common name, you can look up the common name in the list to see the fern's Latin binomial. Then use the first part of the binomial, the fern's genus, to flip to that section in this book. And if you are as passionate about ferns as I am, you may review this list frequently to become familiar with the names. Enjoy!

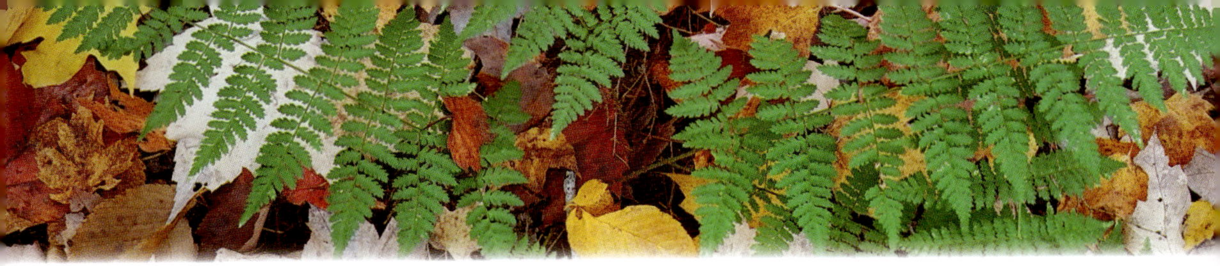

Medicinal Ferns

Abacopteris to Woodwardia

If you would make acquaintance with the ferns, you must forget your botany.

HENRY DAVID THOREAU

As of the latest count, there were 319 genera of ferns, with an estimated 10,578 species or more. Here are a few species, categorized by genus, with known medicinal benefits.

ABACOPTERIS

Chinese Peng Fern — River Fern

Geographic Range: Asia
Medicinal Applications: antioxidant, anti-inflammatory, blood circulation, cancer, cytotoxic, edema, dampness (TCM), hypoglycemic, hypolipidemic, memory, metabolic syndrome, neuroprotective, prostate protection

A water extract of *Abacopteris multilineata* syn. *Thelypteris nudata rhizome* is given in India to patients suffering from stomach pain. The rhizome of Chinese peng fern (*Abacopteris penangiana*) is known as *san xue lian* in Traditional Chinese Medicine and promotes blood circulation, removes blood stasis, treats inflammation, edema, and dampness, a condition characterized by an excess accumulation of fluids in the body. Today, it is additionally used to reduce symptoms associated with metabolic syndrome.

Abaco may derive from Greek *apax* meaning "board," and the Latin *abacus*, "counting board." Penang may refer to the Malaysian island.

The fern rhizome of *Abacopteris penangiana* contains eruberin B and C, as well as the anthocyanidin glycosides abacopterins A through D and abacopterin J. *Abacopteris* combines a flavan and an anthocyanidin moiety (Zhao et al. 2010). Earlier work identified the flavan glycosides 4'-hydroxy-pneumatopterin B and 6'-O-acetyl triphyllin A.

Abacopterin A is a flavonoid isolated from the fern that exhibits hypolipidemic and anti-inflammatory properties by inhibiting NF-κB expression. Work by Lei and colleagues (2011a) found that the ill effects of a high-fat diet on mice were reduced by daily supplementation of the flavonoid.

Total flavanol glycosides were tested on diabetic vascular impairment by measuring oxidative stress and inflammation in mice fed a high-fat diet and then induced with diabetes using streptozotocin. Results found that the flavanol glycosides exhibited hypolipidemic, hypoglycemic, and vascular protection effects, all suggestive of treating aortic pathology associated with metabolic syndrome (Chen et al. 2011b).

Abacopterins A through D, as well as triphyllin and 6,8-dimethyl-7-hydroxy-4'-methoxyanthocyanidin-5-O-β-glucopyranoside were identified in the rhizome. The four abacopterins and triphyllin were shown to be cytotoxic against HepG2 (human hepatoma) cell lines (Zhao et al. 2006).

Two flavan-4-ol glycosides, isolated from the rhizome, show significant anticancer activity against HeLa (cervical) and L929 (fibrosarcoma) cancer cell lines (Fang et al. 2010).

Abacopterin E lowered hydrogen peroxide-induced cytotoxicity and improved learning and memory abilities in a neurotoxicity mouse study. In vitro, the compound protected PC12 cells, prompting the authors to move on to animal trials. In the mouse brain, the compound also restored activities of superoxide dismutase and glutathione peroxidase and attenuated the increase in malondialdehyde. These findings suggest that abacopterin E offers neuroprotection against oxidative stress-induced neurotoxicity (Lei et al. 2011b).

A flavone and flavanone showed significant antioxidant activity in vitro and an in vivo protective effect on dopamine-induced neurotoxicity in PC12 (neuroblastoma) cells. In a mouse study, these compounds were found to upregulate the level of brain-derived neurotrophic factor (BDNF) (Wei et al. 2011c; 2013a).

A caffeic acid derivative, named 7'Z-3-O-(3,4-dihydroxyphenylethenyl)-caffeic acid (CADP) was extracted from the *Abacopteris penangiana* rhizome, and showed significant neuroprotection in mice treated with CADP (Fu et al. 2013).

Eruberin B, also found in rhizomes, exhibits moderate activity against various cancer cell lines (Shen et al. 2020).

Research by Yang and colleagues (2014c) found flavanol glycosides and their acid hydrolysate inhibit chronic non-bacterial prostatitis in rats via various pathways.

The fern exerts testosterone-induced benign prostatic hyperplasia protection by regulating inflammatory responses, reducing oxidative stress, and having antiproliferative effects on prostate cells in an animal study (Yang et al. 2014b).

ACROSTICHUM

Golden Leather Fern   Mangrove Fern   Swamp Fern

Golden leather fern (*Acrostichum aureum*), found in mangrove swamps, has long been a traditional medicine in Bangladesh for various conditions, including peptic ulcers. The genus name, given by Linnaeus, relates to the felt-like sori appearing acrostichoid, meaning distributed uniformly across the back of the frond.

In India, the fern is commonly known as swamp, or mangrove fern. Tea extracts of the fronds were taken to promote a healthy pregnancy (Goswani et al. 2016). The fronds were traditionally used in the Philippines as a

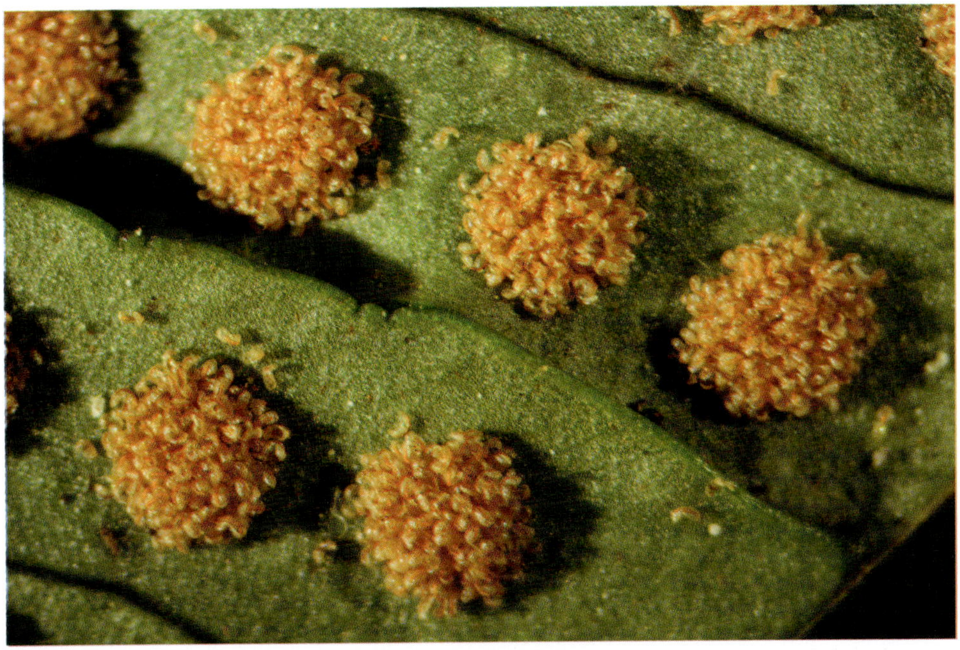

The Felt-like Sori

topical emollient, and the rhizomes as a vulnerary for obstinate skin ulcers. In Malaya, a historical region that now forms part of Malaysia, the rhizomes were prepared into a paste to treat wounds and boils, while in Egypt a frond paste is used to treat headaches. The tender leaves are eaten either raw or cooked as a vegetable, made into brooms for sweeping, or as a fish attractor (Bandyopadhyay and Dey 2022).

The fertile frond was applied to syphilitic ulcers in Borneo (Quisumbing 1951).

The rhizome was used for intestinal worms and bladder complaints in China (Usher 1971). In Bangkok, Thailand, fern spores are the third most common type of airborne spores. Among 226 patients with allergic rhinitis, 61.5% had reactions attributed to these fern spores (Scevkova et al. 2022).

The golden leather fern exhibits the potential for phytoremediation of antibiotic-contaminated sediment, especially fluoroquinolones, widely used in Vietnam shrimp farming (Hoang et al. 2013). In 2005, the Food and Drug Administration (FDA) banned the use of these antibiotics in the poultry industry in the United States, due to the presence of fluoroquinolone-resistant bacterium *Campylobacter jejuni*, one of the most common causes of bacterial gastroenteritis. The Centers for Disease Control and Prevention (CDC) estimates that the bacteria yearly cause infections in 1.5 million residents of the United States. Although Australia never legalized the use of fluoroquinolones in commercial chickens, drug-resistant bacteria have appeared in the country, likely introduced by humans, pest species, or wild birds.

Methanol extracts of the fronds yield pterosin sesquiterpenes. One sulphated pterosin-induced apoptosis on AGS (gastric cancer) cell lines, and methanol extracts showed selective cytotoxicity against different cancer cell lines (Uddin et al. 2011a; 2011b).

Patriscabratine is moderately cytotoxic against AGS (gastric cancer), and the breast cancer cell lines MDA-MB-231 and MCF-7. Tetracosane exhibited some cytotoxicity against gastric, breast, HT-29 (colon), and NIH 3T3 (mouse fibroblast) cancer cell lines. Both patriscabratine and tetracosane displayed apoptotic effect comparable to, if not greater than, the positive control cycloheximide (Uddin et al. 2012). Patriscabratine down-regulates nitric oxide production and pro-inflammatory cytokines and upregulates NQO1, nuclear NRF2 and heme oxygenase. The compound is stable in animals and human liver microsomes (Mak et al. 2022).

Water extracts show benefits in gastric ulceration, induced in a rat study.

The fern prevented damage from ethanol-induced injury, increased the levels of glutathione, superoxide dismutase, and catalase, and decreased malondialdehyde. The extract also decreased the expression of pro-inflammatory cytokines and protein expressions of p65 (Wu et al. 2018c).

Early work by Prakash et al. (1985) found that golden leather fern extracts exhibit anti-implantation activity in female albino rats, suggesting possible inhibition of pregnancy.

ACTINIOPTERIS

Peacock's Tail Fern   Ray Fern

Geographic Range: Africa, Afghanistan, Australia, Botswana, India, Nepal, Southeast Asia, West Indies

Habitat: deep soil, shady areas, hot and dry climates

Practical Uses: phytoremediation (selenium)

Medicinal Applications: analgesic, allergies, aphrodisiac, anti-biofilm, antimicrobial, asthma, birth control, bronchitis, cancer, chronic cough, cooling agent, dandruff, diabetes, diarrhea, diuretic, dysentery, female reproductive problems, fertility stimulant, fever, gallstones, gastrointestinal conditions, Hansen's disease, hemorrhoids, hyperglycemia, hyperthermia, hypertension, infections, inflammation, intestinal worms, irregular menstruation, leucorrhea, liver protection, malaria, parasites, rickets, skin conditions, skin disease, sore throat, tuberculosis

Ray fern (*Actiniopteris radiata* syn. *Actiniopteris dictotoma*) enjoys deep soil in shady areas, but is equally at home in hot, dry climates in parts of Africa, India, Nepal, Afghanistan, Southeast Asia, and Australia. The genus name derives from *actino*, meaning ray or radiate; and *pteris* "wing." A popular English name is peacock's tail fern. In Botswana, the popularity of the fern led to a postal stamp issued in 1992.

These ferns known as *mayursikha* or *morpankhi* have been used in traditional ayurvedic medicine for parasites, skin disease, fertility issues, diarrhea, and dysentery. Their rhizomes are used to treat a variety of conditions, including chronic cough, gallstones, gastrointestinal issues, infections, Hansen's disease, skin conditions, hyperglycemia, and hyperthermia. The rhizomes are decocted, and when cooled, the water is used as hair rinse for dandruff. Additionally, the fronds are chewed to alleviate sore throat (Singh et al. 2005).

Ray fern rhizomes have been traditionally used to treat asthma and female reproductive problems. Watery stools and fever are treated with juice derived from the stem, ingested twice daily (Karthik et al. 2011).

A sugary rhizome is given to kill intestinal worms, twice daily for three consecutive days, and is also used as a cooling agent for syphilis. The fern is mixed with cow's milk for leucorrhea and hemorrhoids. The fresh fronds are consumed with honey several times daily for bronchitis or are soaked in water overnight and taken orally in the morning for hypertension. A paste made from two fronds, administered twice daily, was used for children with rickets. For irregular menstruation, a paste of five to six fronds is combined with 200 ml of fresh cow's milk and taken for a week and a powder of eight to ten fronds is mixed with curd as a supposed measure for birth control. The decoction is taken for tuberculosis (Singh et al. 2016).

The fresh fronds are mixed with sugar and taken twice a day to increase and strengthen women, stimulate fertility, and supposedly act as an aphrodisiac (Parihar and Parihar 2006). In the West Indies, the fronds are chewed for sore throat, and the rhizome is decocted to treat dandruff (Lloyd 1964).

The main compounds of the ray fern are hentriacontane, hentriacontanol, β-sitosterolpalmitate, β-sitosterol-D-glucoside and rutin (quercetin-3-rutinoside). Hentriacontane possesses anti-inflammatory, antitumor and antimicrobial activities.

An initial in vitro study, followed by an in vivo mouse trial, identified the compound as a potent suppressor of inflammatory cytokines, and a regulatory effect on NF-κB (Khajuria et al. 2017). Hentriacontane exhibits biofilm inhibition of tuberculosis-causing mycobacteria (Akande et al. 2022). A study by Kim et al. (2011) found that hentriacontane attenuated weight loss, colon shortening, and levels of IL-6 in mice with dextran sulphate sodium-induced colitis in mice.

Quercetin-3-rutinoside protected male mice against radiation-induced hematopoietic toxicity, suggesting cancer patients may also benefit from supplementation (Dutta et al. 2021). Rutin exhibits antioxidant and anti-inflammatory activity and may protect against male infertility. A mini review by Rotimi et al. (2023) found that it mitigated induced oxidative stress, apoptosis, inflammation, and related physiological processes that cause testicular dysfunction.

The root and the frond accumulate selenium, suggesting benefits for phytoremediation (Srivastava et al. 2005). Ten ferns were tested, and ray fern was determined to be the best overall for phytoremediation. Rabbit's foot fern (*Davallia griffithiana*) was the best accumulator of selenate, while ladder brake fern (*Pteris vittata*) showed the highest accumulation when treated with selenite.

The fern has been screened for anti-stress and anti-allergic response in asthma, using in vivo animal models. An ethanol extract showed significant inhibition of leukocytosis (Vadnere et al. 2013) and liver protection (Manubolu et al. 2014). A methanol extract has been found to exhibit antidiabetic activity (Chand Basha et al. 2013). Both water and ethanol extracts show analgesic activity, and the fern wax inhibits growth of *Salmonella typhi*, *Staphylococcus aureus*, and *Escherichia coli* (Manubolu et al. 2013; Naik and Jadge 2010). The frond extract exhibits larvicidal activity against malaria and dengue-infested mosquitoes, with insignificant toxicity to non-target aquatic organisms (Kamaraj et al. 2018). Earlier work by Deharo et al. (1992) identified n-hentriacontanol to possess antimalarial activity.

ADIANTUM

California Fern Five-Fingered Jack Maidenhair Ferns

Geographic Range: Alaska, Belgium, British Columbia (Canada), Canary Islands, Ecuador, Ethiopia, France, India, Iran, Iraq, Ivory Coast, Jamaica, Latin America, Malaya, Nepal, Newfoundland (Canada), Pakistan, Pennsylvania, Perak (Malaysia), Philippines, Quebec, South Africa, Spain, Turkey, United States

Habitat: temperate zones, hot springs, acidic soil conditions, epiphytic (growing on trees), lithophytic (growing on rocks)

Practical Uses: alcoholic beverages, basket decoration, fish food, hair blackness and shininess (ashes), hair rinse, opening and enlarging earlobes, staple food

Medicinal Applications: Alzheimer's disease, abdominal cramps, analgesic, antianxiety, anti-biofilm, anti-hair loss, anti-inflammatory, anti-lithiatic, anti-obesity, anti-ulcer, antiasthma, antiurolithiatic, antibacterial, antidiarrheal, antidysenteric, antifungal, antioxidant, anticonvulsant, antidepressant, antihistaminic, anuria, aphrodisiac, asthma, bee stings, blisters, blood, brain, bronchitis, cancer, centipede bites, chest, cholesterol, colds, colic, colitis, contraceptive, cough, cystitis, demulcent, debility, diabetes, diarrhea, dysentery, dog bites, diuretic, diabetes, earlobes, edema, emetic, emmenagogue, epilepsy, expel placenta, expectorant, childbirth, fainting, fever, flu, gonorrhea, gastric issues, hair loss, hayfever, heartburn, heart, hoarseness, headaches, heartbeat, menstruation, infertility in women, endurance, intestinal distress, jaundice, kidneys, liver, lung infections, menstruation, mental health, mouth ulcers, nasal congestion, pneumonia, postpartum, pulmonary catarrh, urination, pleurisy, rabies, rheumatism, reduce blood sugar, respiratory, scorpion stings, scrofula, leprosy, snake bites, sore back of infants, spleen, stimulant, stomach cramps, stomach conditions, swollen glands, spermicidal, tonic, urinary

Warning: Caution is advised regarding reproductive health and fertility, as certain species are known to have contraceptive and/or abortifacient effects.

The genus name derives from the Greek adiantos, meaning "unwetted" or "unmoistened," referring to the ability of fronds to repel water. The Greek *dianinein* means, "to wet." There are about 150 *Adiantum* species worldwide, mostly to be found in tropical regions.

The species name *capillus-veneris* (Venus maidenhair fern) derives from the Latin and means "hair of Venus," alluding to the Roman goddess Venus, whose hair was dry and perfectly arranged when she arose from the waters near Cyprus. The Catholic Church later renamed the fern virgin's hair (Dowling 1900). Pedatum derives from the Latin "footed," referring to the pinnae that radiate outward from the horseshoe-shaped rachis.

The genus is popularly known as *hansraj* in ayurvedic medicine, and is used for treating colds, tumors of the spleen, liver, and other viscera, skin diseases, bronchitis, and inflammatory diseases.

The common maidenhair fern (*Adiantum aethiopicum*) is used in Ethiopia for respiratory and liver conditions. The Basotho people of South Africa dry the frond and smoke it for head colds. In parts of Europe, demulcent tea is consumed for asthma and other mucus-congested bronchial conditions (Watt and Breyer-Brandwijk 1962).

MAIDENHAIR FERN ESSENCE

This essence of *Adiantum aethiopicum* imparts the ability to see the deeper meaning behind one's choices, decisions, patterns, and events in one's life, and to appreciate the soul's purpose. It introduces a heightened sensitivity that alters one's vibration, lifting resonance and allowing for changes in the life path. This essence facilitates hearing and listening to the inner voice for guidance, encouraging reliance on internal rather than external support. Find at the South African Flower and Gem Essences company.

Venus maidenhair fern (*Adiantum capillus-veneris*) is a well-known medicinal herb used both traditionally and in modern times; in North America, it is known as southern maidenhair or black maidenhair fern. Southern maidenhair fern is common to temperate zones worldwide, with a few ferns found growing around hot springs in the Black Hills of South Dakota and Fairmont Hot Springs in British Columbia (Canada), over one thousand kilometers from its usual range.

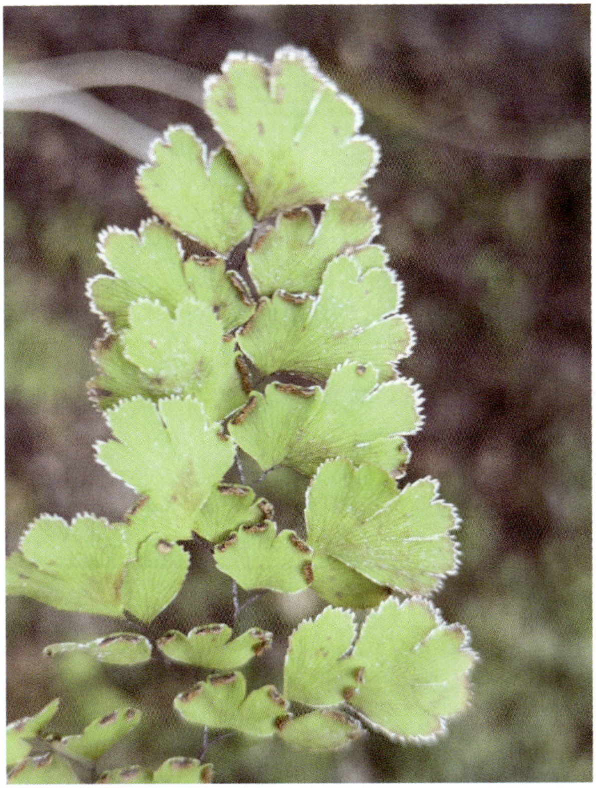

Adiantum capillus-veneris
(Venus Maidenhair Fern)
Photo by Alan Rockefeller

The Roman naturalist Pliny wrote "In vain, do you plunge the Adiantum into water, it always remains dry." He noted that, when soaked in wine, the fern was believed to break urinary stones (now known as bladder or kidney stones). The frond was crushed and applied to centipede bites. The fern was also known as *terrae capillus* and used to treat intestinal distress and reduce menstrual flow and remove afterbirth.

The frond has been utilized since the times of Dioscorides, mainly for respiratory conditions. He mentions in his five volumes *de Materia Médica* that the root is useless but the fronds are beneficial for asthma, jaundice, spleen, and pain with urination.

Aelius or Claudius Galenus (130–210 CE) was a Greek physician, whose writings influenced European medicine for nearly 1400 years. He suggested the fern "maketh things thin that are thick." Short and to the point.

To this day, the Venus maidenhair fern is prepared in a honey syrup and flavored with orange flowers in France. This is known as *sirop de capillaire* and used to treat pulmonary catarrh. Several fresh fronds are immersed in hot water for half an hour, strained, and about one cup of sweetener and 30 ml of neroli or orange flower hydrosol are added. Prepared this way, the syrup will keep fresh in the fridge for several weeks.

The fern has a lily-like fragrance. It symbolizes fascination, magic, discretion, secrecy, and the bond of love.

Maud Grieve (1858–1941), herbalist and horticulturist, (1931) notes "It also enters into the composition of *Elixir de Garus*. It is employed on the Continent as an emmenagogue under the names of polytrichid, polytrichon or kalliphyllon administered as a sweetened infusion of 1 oz. to a pint of boiling water." Grieve's *A Modern Herbal* was a standard resource for many herbal students in the 1960s.

My distant relative, the renowned English botanist and astrologer Nicholas Culpeper (1616–1654) (1652) wrote in his book, *The English Physician* (1652), "This and all other Maiden hairs is a good remedy for coughs, asthmas, pleurisy, etc., and on account of it being a gentle diuretic also in jaundice, gravel and other impurities of the kidneys. All the Maidenhairs should be used green and in conjunction with other ingredients because their virtues are weak." He further noted "Maidenhair distilled in May, the water cleanses both liver and lungs, clarifies the blood and breaks the stone." This book, written in English instead of Latin, brought herbal medicine to everyone and was used by the medical establishment.

The distillation and production of hydrosols were popular in parts of Europe, helping preserve plant constituents that would be lost in dry plant material.

Hieronymus Brunschwig, German surgeon, alchemist, and botanist (1450–1512) suggested that a water distillation of the whole maidenhair fern be applied to alopecia of the scalp to promote hair retention. He also claimed it could break stones, clear yellow jaundice, and alleviate colic in the stomach and intestine. His book *Liber de arte de distillandi de simplicibus* (1500), describes the distillation of plants and the use of hydrosols for various health conditions.

John Gerard, English botanist and surgeon, wrote in (1597), "It consumeth and wasteth away the King's Evil and other hard swellings, and it maketh the hair of the head or beard to grow that is fallen and pulled off." King's Evil was an old term for tuberculous cervical lymphadenitis (scrofula).

In the Hebrew Talmud, the fern called *yo'ezer* was recommended for liver complaints. Towards the end of the 17th century Dr. Joseph Garrus, living in Paris, developed an elixir that contained maidenhair fern, which became a popular panacea during the following century. However, after his death, he was accused of improving a formula by Paracelsus called élixir de propriété. It is still considered one of the finest aperitif liquors for stimulating digestion (Labrude 2010).

The Irish herbalist John K'Eogh (1735) wrote "It helps cure asthma, coughs and shortness of breath. It is good against jaundice, diarrhea, spitting of blood and the bites of mad dogs. It also provokes urination and menstruation, and breaks up the stone in bladder, spleen and kidneys."

Today, frond infusions are used in Spain, Belgium, and the Canary Islands for bronchitis and whooping cough as well as for painful menstruation. Meanwhile, the rhizomes have been used as expectorant in Iran and Iraq, highlighting the plant's similar medicinal applications across different cultures (Quisumbing 1951). In Turkey, the fronds are fed to Mohair goats to produce a high-quality milk product (de Baïracli Levy 1973).

The fronds contain eight carotenoids, four pheophytins, and two chlorophylls. Lutein (806 μg/g), chlorophyll b' (410 μg/g), chlorophyll a (162 μg/g), 9'-Z-neoxanthin (142.8 μg/g) and *E*-violaxanthin (82.2 μg/g) are present in high amounts. Lutein is well-known for its benefits in eye health, preventing retinal and macular degeneration.

Hexane fractions of the alcohol extract reveal isoadiantone, isoadiantol-B, 3-methoxy-4-hydroxyfilicane, 3,4-dihydroxyfilicane, and quercetin flavonoids.

Various phenolics include 4-hydroxybenzoic acid, chlorogenic acid, caftaric acid, kaempferol glycosides, p-coumaric acid, rosmarinic acid, 5-caffeoylquinic acid, and quercetin glycosides. Kaempferol-3-sophorotrioside is present in significant amounts with 58.7 mg/g (Zeb and Ullah 2017). Quinic acids and shikimic acids are also present. Caftaric acid is the ester of caffeic acid. Work by Tanyeli et al. (2019) found the compound to possess antioxidant and anti-inflammatory activity in indomethacin-induced gastric ulcers in rats.

Frond infusions were traditionally used in Iran to treat jaundice (Tewari et al. 2017). In early medical and pharmaceutical textbooks of traditional Iranian medicine, it was named *pare-siavashan*. A review of the literature by Dehdari and Hajimehdipoor (2018) found maidenhair fern to possess a number of medicinal benefits, including antidiabetic, anticonvulsant, analgesic, hypocholesterolemic, goitergenic, antibacterial, antifungal, wound healing, anti-obesity, anti-hair loss, antiasthma, anti-inflammatory, antidiarrheal, antispasmodic, diuretic, and anti-urolithiatic properties.

Follicular density and the anagen/telogen ratio suggest that maidenhair fern possesses significant activity against testosterone-induced alopecia (Noubarani et al. 2014).

An excellent recent review by Kashkooe et al. (2021) provides a comprehensive synopsis of its properties and toxicology. The benefits include remodeling of lung alveolar epithelial cells in hypoxic environments (or during high-intensity exercise), wound healing, protection from free radical damage to fibroblast cells, effectiveness against testosterone-induced alopecia (male pattern baldness). Additionally, it possesses anticonvulsant, antidepressant, analgesic, diuretic, anti-inflammatory, antimicrobial, anti-lithiatic (stone reduction and removal), hypothyroid balancing, antidiarrheal, antispasmodic, antiasthmatic, antihistaminic, and anticancer properties, and inhibition enzyme beneficial in Alzheimer's disease, diabetes, and skin conditions.

In the Amazon regions of Brazil and Peru, the fern is traditionally used as an expectorant, for rheumatism, heartburn, gallstones, hair loss, and urinary issues. In Nepal the fronds are pounded into a paste and applied to the forehead for headaches.

The genus is popularly known as *hansraj* in ayurvedic medicine, and is used for treating colds, tumors of the spleen, liver, and other viscera, skin diseases, bronchitis, and inflammatory diseases. Hansraj is an Indian cough medicine widely available, containing the fern. Fresh frond tea has been traditionally used for irregular menses, and to facilitate childbirth and aid the

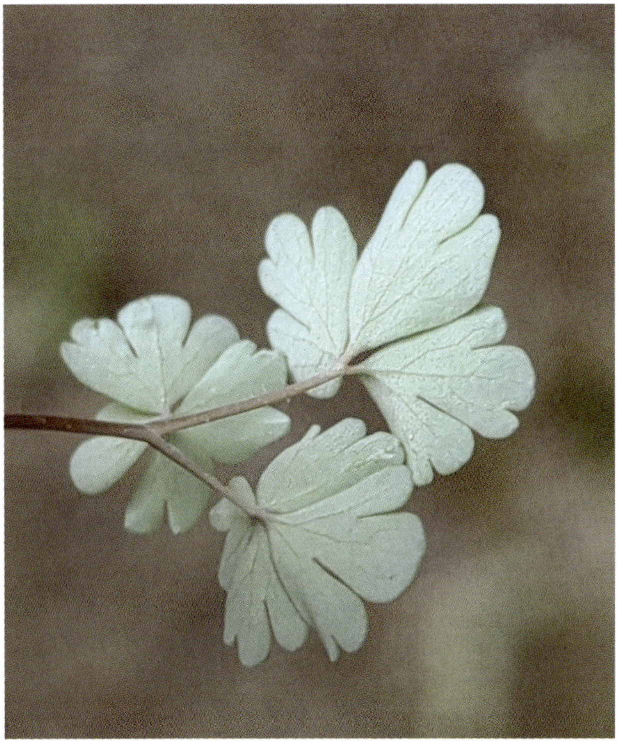

Underside Close-Up of
Adiantum capillus-veneris
(Black Maidenhair Fern)
Photo by Alan Rockefeller

expulsion of the placenta from the uterus after childbirth. The frond decoction was given to infertile women, and the whole fern was used as an aphrodisiac to arouse sexual desire or increase pleasure (Singh and Singh 2012).

In India, the fronds are mixed with honey to treat seasonal fevers (Singh et al. 1989). The juice has been traditionally used to treat cough and to reduce blood sugar levels, the fronds chewed for mouth ulcers and a tea used as a diuretic.

The ethyl acetate fraction exhibits superior analgesic and anti-inflammatory benefits compared to ibuprofen and indomethacin, respectively (Haider et al. 2011).

Isolated compounds in alcohol extracts show in vivo anti-inflammatory and significant hypoglycemic activity (Ibraheim et al. 2011). Water extracts applied to late-radiation-induced injury, bedsores, and burns exhibit skin tissue repair (Nilforoushzadeh et al. 2014). Both crude and gold nanoparticles of the fern possess antiproliferative and apoptosis-inducing properties against MCF-7 and BT47 breast cancer cell lines (Rautray et al. 2018). In rats, water and hydroalcoholic extracts reduce acetic acid-induced colitis, significantly lowering levels of myeloperoxidase compared to the control drugs prednisolone and mesalazine

(Khoramian et al. 2020). An extract given to mice exposed to hypoxia and then strenuous exercise, reduced P53 and TNF-α expression and increased the surface area of lung tissue (Yadegari et al. 2019). An in vivo rat study found that the fern reduced the serum levels of calcium, phosphorus, and blood urea, validating its traditional use by Unani physicians for urolithiasis. However, creatinine levels remained unchanged (Ahmed et al. 2013).

Like acarbose, the fern extracts are potent in vitro dual inhibitors of alpha-amylase and alpha-glycosidase. Unlike guar gum, the fern does not hinder glucose diffusion.

The fern extract is equivalent to orlistat in inhibiting pancreatic triacylglycerol lipase. However, it does not exhibit antihyperglycemic activity comparable to metformin and glipizide in a rat study. However, the extract is superior to atorvastatin, showing significant anti-obesity effects in rats fed a high cholesterol diet for ten weeks (Kasabri et al. 2017). The fern also exhibits in vivo glucose tolerance (Neef et al. 1995). The methanol extract has a very low MIC value of 0.48 micrograms/ml against *Escherichia coli* (Singh et al. 2008).

The fronds, stems, and rhizomes of the maidenhair fern were extracted with various solvents and tested against ten Multi-Drug Resistant bacterial strains and five fungal strains. Significant activity against most of the studied MDR bacteria was noted (Ishaq et al. 2014).

ESKAPE drug-resistant bacteria are a group of pathogens found in both community and hospital-acquired infections known for their high levels of antibiotic resistance and their ability to "escape" the effects of antibacterial drugs. The acronym "ESKAPE" stands for the following bacteria: *Enterococcus faecium*, *Staphylococcus aureus*, *Klebsiella pneumoniae*, *Acinetobacter baumanii*, *Pseudomonas aeruginosa*, and the *Enterobacter* species. Ethanol extracts of the maidenhair fern inhibited growth of all six MDR ESKAPE pathogens (Khan et al. 2018).

In 2019 the CDC published a list of eighteen antibiotic-resistant microbes that threaten the lives of Americans. In addition to the six mentioned above, they are *Clostridium difficile*, *Neisseria gonorrhoeae*, *Campylobacter*, *Enterococcus* ssp., *Salmonella* and *Salmonella enterica* serotype, *Typhi*, *Shigella*, *Streptococcus pneumoniae*, *Candida albicans*, and *Mycobacterium tuberculosis*.

In 2019, an estimated 1.7 million people died from drug-resistant bacteria worldwide. It is unfortunate that three quarters of people believe that it is the person taking the drug who becomes resistant, not the microbes. And about two-thirds of people ingest unnecessary antibiotics for viral infections.

The fern may offer benefits for commercial freshwater fish farming growth and health; Research by Hoseinifar et al. (2020) found that adding leaf powder to fish food increases carp growth, enhances resistance to various bacteria, and boosts the overall immune health of carp. Notably, it improves resistance to *Yersinia ruckeri*, a gram-negative bacterium that causes enteric red mouth disease in some fish species.

An endophytic fungus, *Chaetomium globosum*, was discovered on healthy leaves of the fern in Egypt. An ethyl acetate extract of this fungus exhibited strong antioxidant activity and potent cytotoxicity against HepG2 (liver) and FGC4 (rat hepatoma) cancer cell lines. This extract is moderately antibacterial, inhibits butyrylcholinesterase, one of the neurohydrolase enzymes that may play a role in Alzheimer's disease, and prevents the herpes simplex virus 2 from attaching to VERO cells (Selim et al. 2014).

Further research by Selim et al. (2016) replicated the findings and revealed significant inhibition of butyrylcholinesterase and strong cytotoxicity against HepG2 (liver) as well as UACC62 (melanoma) cell lines. A rat study using an ethanol extract suggests significant antidepressant and antianxiety effects due to reduced malondialdehyde levels as well as increased antioxidant levels (Rabiei and Setorki 2019).

Secondary metabolites of the endophytic fungus exhibit significant anti-inflammatory effects, specifically in reducing inflammation associated with rheumatoid arthritis. This was demonstrated in an adjuvant-induced arthritis rat model (Abdel-Azeem et al. 2016).

Carbendazim (CBZ) is a toxic fungicide widely used in agriculture and veterinary practice, known for its persistence and residues in food products. Fern extracts have been shown to reduce liver toxicity in CBZ-treated rats by reducing inflammation and enhancing antioxidant activity (Seif et al. 2023). Previous research found that the fern protects the female reproductive system (Madboli and Seif 2021).

Bisphenol A is a plastic pollutant that causes liver and xeno-toxicity. Fern extracts appear to ameliorate the toxicity due to antioxidant activity (Kanwal et al. 2018).

The main volatile compound in the fern is (E)-2-decenal, which exhibits a scent that is plastic-like, but described by some as a stink bug odor. The tincture of this fern is used in hair tonics and some alcoholic beverages.

Give me the strong, rank scent of fern in the spring for vigour.

HENRY DAVID THOREAU

Historically, this fern has been an official drug in several countries, including France, Austria, Belgium, Croatia-Slavonia, Denmark, Portugal, Romania, Russia, Serbia, Spain, Sweden, and Switzerland.

In France and India, trailing or walking maidenhair fern (*Adiantum caudatum*) fronds have been used for cough and fever. In the Philippines, the fronds are applied externally for various skin conditions, in India they are applied as a paste to blisters and wounds and the rhizome prepared as a tea for elevated blood sugar, and in Malaya and Perak, decocted fronds and rhizomes are used to treat chest complaints (Burkill 1966).

Isaac Henry Burkill (1870–1965) was an English economic botanist and author working in India and what is now known as Singapore. He was honored with the Linnean Medal in 1952, recognizing his significant contributions to the field of botany.

The triterpenoid- and phenolic-rich fraction of *Adiantum caudatum* exhibits alpha-amylase and alpha-glucosidase inhibition comparable to that of acarbose (Telegari and Hullatti 2015). Water extracts of the fronds show potent activity against *Escherichia coli*, *Bacillus subtilis*, and *Pseudomonas aeruginosa*, with the latter bacteria being more susceptible to the aqueous extract than to amoxicillin (Ahmed et al. 2015).

Amoxicillin is the most common antibiotic prescribed to children, and in the pork industry it is used to control systemic infections such as *Streptococcus suis*. Its overuse in treating human *Helicobacter pylori* has led to antibiotic resistance and increasing antimicrobial resistance in patients with endodontic infections (Ardila et al. 2023).

Delta maidenhair fern (*Adiantum cuneatum* syn. *A. raddianum*) is used in traditional Jamaican medicine. Its common name is derived from the dark, shiny stipes, which look like human hair.

It is native to South America and grown indoors all around the world. Despite its popularity as an indoor plant, its introduction to Hawaii has led to it becoming invasive. There are several cultivars, varying in shapes and sizes, including 'Fragrans,' 'Fritz Lüthi,' 'Ocean Spray,' 'Pacific Maid,' 'Brilliantelse,' and 'Kensington Gem.' The latter two cultivars won the Royal Horticultural Society's Award of Garden Merit.

Delta maidenhair fern (*Adiantum cuneatum*) was investigated for its phytochemical composition. Hexane fractions revealed filicene and filicenal extracts, which, when injected intraperitoneally, exhibited potent analgesic activity in two mice models of pain. Filicene was seven times more potent than reference drugs such as ASA (aspirin) and acetaminophen and inhibited both neurogenic and inflammatory phases of the formalin test (Bresciani et al. 2003).

Filicene, when tested against acetic acid-induced abdominal constrictions, was more potent than acetaminophen, diclofenac, and ASA at equivalent doses. Filicene produced dose-related inhibition of pain caused by capsaicin and glutamate. The antinociceptive action was significantly reversed by atropine, haloperidol, various GABA(A) and GABA(B) antagonists (bicuculline and phaclofen, respectively). It was not affected by L arginine nitric oxide, serotonin, adrenergic, or opioid systems. This suggests that, although not completely understood, the mechanism of action involves interaction with the cholinergic, dopaminergic, glutamatergic, GABAergic, and/or tachykinergic systems (de Souza et al. 2009).

Hepatonic acid, an unsaturated fatty acid with a cyclopropane moiety, isolated from fan-leaved maidenhair fern (*Adiantum flabellulatum*) possesses anti-protein tyrosine phosphatase activity (Chen et al. 2022c). This fern thrives in acidic soil conditions.

Protein tyrosine phosphatases (PTPs) are involved in various conditions, including diabetes, Alzheimer's and Parkinson's diseases, allergies, and inflammation. These enzymes, along with protein tyrosine kinases, regulate phosphorylation within cells, and their alteration and mutation are associated with cancer, diabetes/obesity, autoimmune, and infectious diseases. Although numerous studies suggest PTPs are "undruggable," the potential benefits of natural fatty acids, such as hepatonic acid, warrant further research.

The fragile maidenhair fern (*Adiantum fragile* syn. *Dennstaedtia anthriscifolia*) is used medicinally in Jamaica.

The rough maidenhair fern (*Adiantum hispidulum*), known for its beautiful red-pink new foliage, is also called rosy maidenhair or five-fingered jack. It is native to tropical and temperate regions and has been naturalized in the Southeastern United States. This fern is sometimes grown indoors as it cannot tolerate cold winters. The species name *hispidulum* derives from the Latin hispis meaning "hair," "minutely hairy," or "bristly."

Tailed maidenhair fern (*Adiantum incisum*), harvested in Pakistan, contains significant levels of alkaloids, possesses antioxidant activity, and shows moderate to significant antifungal activity against *Aspergillus niger* (Kazmi et al. 2019). The dried leaf dust of the fern is consumed with butter to alleviate the feeling of burning in the body. The fronds are used to relieve cough, lower blood sugar levels, and treat skin disorders (Singh and Upadhyay 2012).

A water/ethanol extract of the whole fern has been shown to effectively treat STZ-induced type 2 diabetes in rats, owing to both antioxidant and alpha-amylase inhibition. The fern contains compounds such as cardiac glycosides, flavonoids, phenolics, saponins, and fixed oils (Bilal et al. 2022).

California maidenhair (*Adiantum jordanii*) was harvested by the Mendocino people of California for its thin black midrib, which was used to open and enlarge earlobes (Lloyd 1964).

The Costanoan living around the San Francisco Bay Area decocted the fern to purify blood, treat stomach troubles, expel afterbirth, and address various postpartum issues. Other groups have used the decocted fern to treat pain below the shoulders (Moerman 1986).

Broadleaf maidenhair fern *Adiantum latifolium* is used in Latin American traditional medicine for anxiety, and as an analgesic and anti-inflammatory. A methanol extract was tested on mice and demonstrated pain reduction and anti-inflammatory benefits through the inhibition of IL-1β production (Nonato et al. 2011).

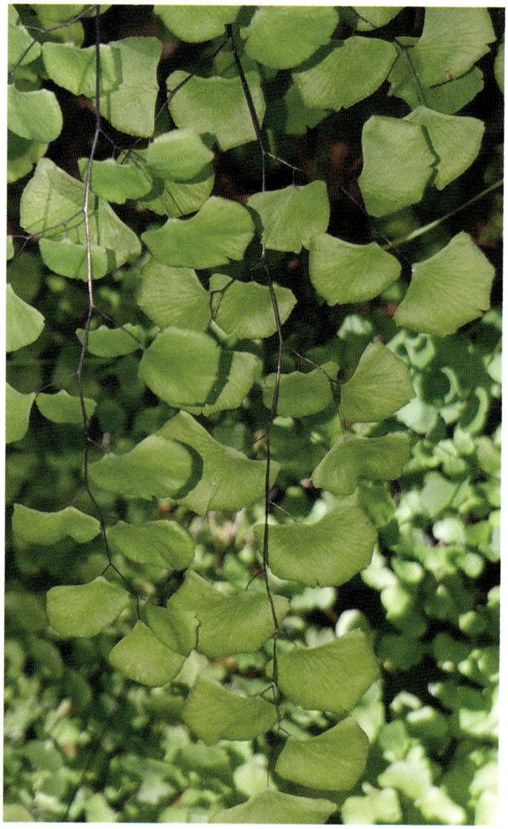

Adiantum jordanii
(California Maidenhair)
Photo by Alan Rockefeller

The SARS-CoV-2 virus pandemic resulted in millions of people losing their lives, and hundreds of millions more suffering short and long-term health consequences. A compound, 22-hydroxyhopane (diplopterol), derived from the fronds of *Adiantum latifolium*, binds to six enzymes essential for viral replication, as well as to RNA binding protein, spike protein, membrane protein, and ACE2 receptors (Kumar and Siddique 2022).

Whole fern extracts from *Adiantum lunulatum*, which grows in India, reveal the presence of various triterpenes including mollugogenol A, an antifungal saponin. In India, powdered dried rhizome is used for snakebites (Singh et al. 1989), and bites are treated with a paste made from both fronds and rhizomes. Traditionally, the fern has been used to treat rabies, epilepsy, fever associated with elephantiasis, abdominal cramps, flu, and Hansen's disease (leprosy) caused by *Mycobacterium leprae.*

The compound has potential spermicidal activity, causing significant damage to the sperm membrane in both head and tail regions and affecting sperm motility and viability (Rajasekaran et al. 1993). Strangely, a decoction of the fresh ferns is given to cure irregular menstrual cycles, and a paste made from the fronds is given to help women conceive (Rout et al. 2009).

Ethanol extracts of the fern possess hepatoprotective and antioxidant characteristics (Kakadia et al. 2020). In India, ten grams of the whole fern is mixed with black pepper and prepared into a paste or into pills, with two pills taken twice daily for a month to cure bronchitis or asthma (Singh et al. 1989).

Malaria accounts for over 3% of total disease burden worldwide. A natural ozonide, 1,2,4-trioxolane, derived from monosorus maidenhair fern (*Adiantum monochlamys*) was first isolated in 1976. More research may result in new applications of various ozonide derivatives for this major infectious disease (Tiwari et al. 2019).

Artemisinin, derived from sweet wormwood (*Artemisia annua*) contains 1,2,4-trioxolane derivatives. Tu Youyou was honored with the 2015 Nobel Prize for her work on artemisinin and its derivates, which have saved millions of lives.

The fern exhibits two-stage carcinogenesis in mouse skin papilloma models (Konoshima et al. 1996).

Northern maidenhair (*Adiantum pedatum* syn. *A. aleuticum*) has been used by the Lenni Lenape and Iroquois of the Delaware River valley region for heart problems, rheumatism, asthma (smoked), and skin wounds. The name *pedatum* derives from the Greek "foot" and refers to the fronds' bird's foot shape.

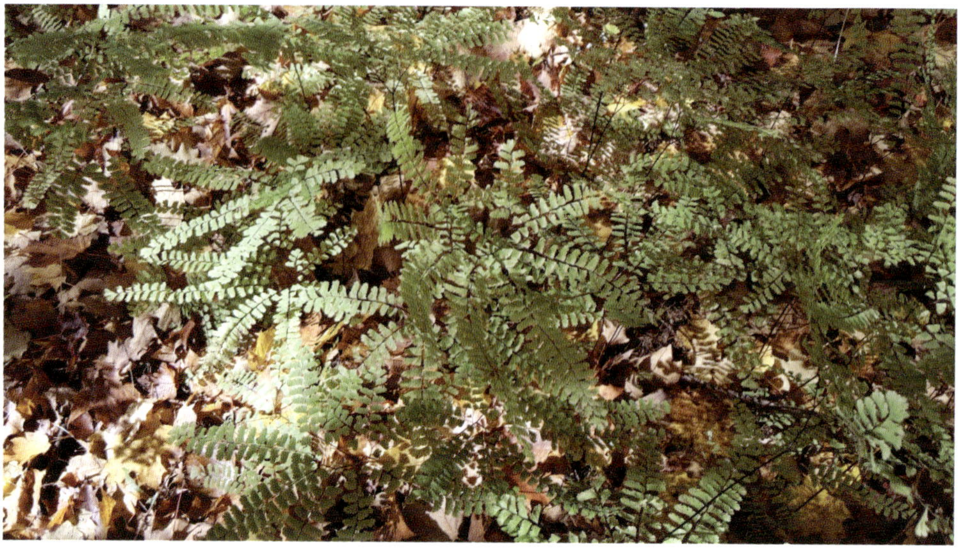

Adiantum pedatum (Northern Maidenhair)
Photo by Alan Rockefeller

The Iroquois used decoctions of the roots to promote menstruation and possibly abortifacient. It was ingested or used as an external wash for gonorrhea. It was also given to children to relieve stomach cramps or rubbed externally on the sore backs of infants. Decoctions of the rhizome were taken for anuria and fresh rhizomes were prepared as a foot bath for rheumatism. The fern infusions were used ceremonially as an emetic remedy for love medicine (Moerman 1986).

The Forest Potawatomi, a Native American tribe originally from the Great Lakes region in the Northeastern and Midwestern United States, infused northern maidenhair fern roots and drank the tea to cure breast engorgement, or mastitis. The fern is known as black leg or *memakate'wiga'teuk*.

The Meskwaki, also known as the Fox people, used the whole fern to cure children who "turn black" (Moerman 1986). The condition remains unknown.

Before being relocated westward, the Cherokee used fern poultices to treat rheumatic muscle pain. The doctrine of signatures involved the young fronds uncurling and straightening, relating to standing tall without pain. The fern, known as *kâ'gaskû'ntagî*, meaning "crow shin," was combined with hawthorn berry and *Aralia racemosa* rhizome as a powerful medicine for women with irregular heartbeats. They also dried and powdered the fronds as a smoke for heart trouble or asthma. A slow decoction of roots was taken to stop excessive menstruation, and rhizomes were taken for respiratory conditions (Smith 1924).

The Cherokee infused or decocted the fern for ague and fevers. It was also used for "sudden attacks such as bad pneumonia in children." (Moerman 1986).

The fern is an expectorant, stimulant, demulcent, and a mild astringent tonic.

The Menominee of the Wisconsin/Michigan region used the rhizome in combination medicines for dysentery and the whole fern for "female maladies" (Moerman 1986). The Menominee, or O-Maeq-No-Min-Ni-Wuk, meaning "People of the Wild Rice," relied on wild rice as staple food. The Mi'kmaq drank fern decoctions to treat fits, possibly epilepsy (Moerman 1986).

Herbalists have traditionally used this fern for fever, coughs, hoarseness, asthma, pleurisy, and *Streptococcus* infections of the lungs.

Formerly known as one species, *Adiantum pedatum* is now considered the Northeastern species, and western maidenhair (*Adiantum aleuticum*) is found west of the Rocky Mountains. The two species are difficult to distinguish, with the latter fern also found in Newfoundland, Quebec, and south to Pennsylvania. Where the two species grow together, a fertile hybrid, green mountain maidenhair (*Adiantum viridi-montanum*), has developed.

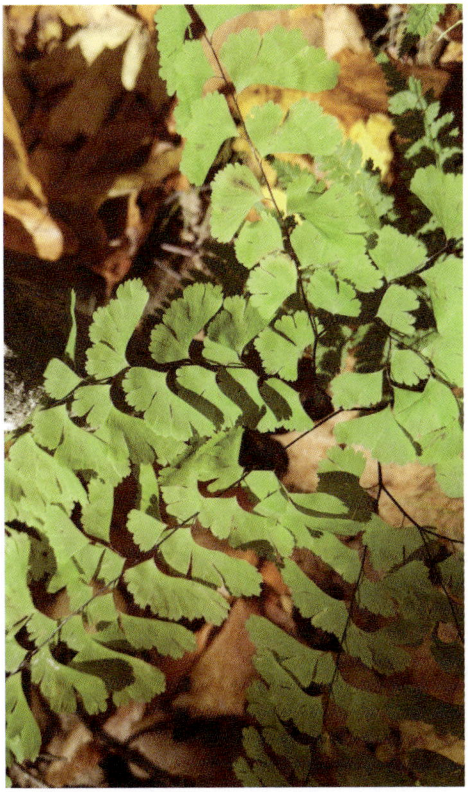

Adiantum pedatum
(Northern Maidenhair)
Photo by Alan Rockefeller

The Haida of Alaska and Skidegate refer to western maidenhair as *ts'aagwaal* and *ts'aagul*. The beautiful, black, and shiny stems have been used to decorate baskets (Turner 2004). (This may also refer to lady fern Athyrium filix-femina, which you can see in a photo on page 66.) The fern was used by various tribes of Western Washington (Gunther 1945).

The Lummi know it as *tungwëltcin* meaning "hair medicine." They shared with the Makah and Skokomish the use of this fern for hair care. The Skokomish and Twana name *aiya'o'lgad* translates as "hair bigger." The Gitxsan call this and other ferns *demtx* or *damtx*. The Haisla call this fern, or ferns in general, *saʔit'*, meaning "finger plant."

The Makah chewed the leaves of the *tlotlotc'sa'dit* (dry fern) for sore chests and stomach trouble, and internal hemorrhage. An alternate name is *yuyuuxlts-bitsaal*, meaning "the leaves work even when there is no wind."

Infused frond water was used as hair rinse by Makah, Skokomish, and Lummi of the Pacific Northwest. The Nuu-chah-nulth refer to this fern as "the real one," or *yuxsmapt*.

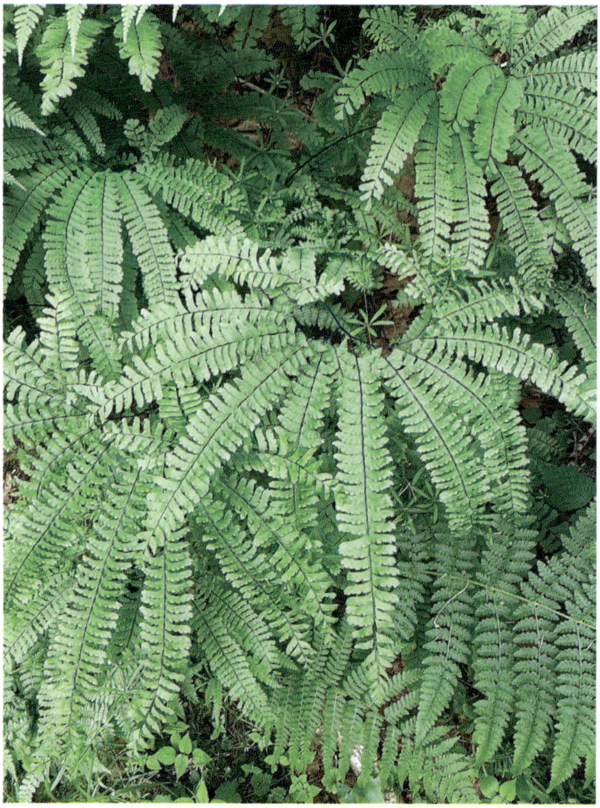

Adiantum aleuticum var. *aleuticum*
(Western Maidenhair Fern)
Photo by Drew T. Henderson

The Kwakwaka'wakw name for this fern and ferns in general is *salʔidana*. The Quinault burned the leaves to ash and rubbed them into the scalp to make hair blacker and shinier (Gunther 1945). They call the fern *pilápila*, *pal-pulth* or *hah-polk-pulth*. The Twana also refer to the fern as "hair bigger," *aiyaʔólgad*.

The Ditidaht refer to the fern as "resembling whale baleen," or *tl' iitl' iidqw aqsibak' kw*. The Lushootseed name is *pepech*, and the Southern Lushootseed call it *tsábtsub*. The plant was dried and powdered as a snuff or smoked to relieve asthma. The Hesquiat chewed the fronds for shortness of breath. Infusions were used by dancers in the winter to keep them "light on their feet" and increase endurance.

The Mahuna of Southern California applied the fern externally for rheumatic pain, and the Navajo used infusions as part of a combination for bee and centipede stings. They dried the fern and smoked it or consumed a tea for mental problems (Wyman and Harris 1951). The Nlaka'pamux of British Columbia call it "creek's little black fringe" or "grizzly bear's friend."

The famous Eclectic physician Dr. John King (1898) noted the leaves are slightly bitter, with a faintly sweetish, aromatic, feebly astringent taste. He suggested it is a useful tonic, expectorant and refrigerant, with sub-astringent activity.

In China, the fronds and rhizome are used to treat impetigo and as a bronchial expectorant. Michael Moore (2003) notes northern maidenhair fern is useful for upper respiratory issues and disrupted menstruation. For a cough syrup, prepare an infusion with one tablespoon of the frond in hot water, or use the roots with two parts honey, one part water, and two parts finely chopped fronds by volume. The fern exerts similar action on the mucous membranes of the bladder and uterus and is used for cystitis with mucus and burning urination. To stimulate delayed menstruation, simmer 30 grams of finely chopped frond, fifteen grams of chopped, dried rhizome, and one-half liter of water for twenty minutes. The tea does not stimulate cramping.

The fern contains the bitter naringin, which is about one-fifth as bitter as quinine. This bioflavonoid reduces inflammation in people with type 2 diabetes (Al-Aubaidy et al. 2021). Extracts of the fern exhibit potential protection from induced colon cancer in male albino rats through antioxidant and apoptosis mechanisms (Khamis et al. 2023).

Walking maidenhair or black maidenhair fern (*Adiantum philippense*) is commonly known in India as *goyali lota* or *kalijhant* in Bengali, and *hamsapadi* in Hindi. Two to three teaspoons of the dried powdered rhizome is stirred in water and swallowed once daily for three to five days during the menstrual period to enhance fertility (Parihar and Parihar 2006). Conversely, it is also used by tribal women in India as a contraceptive with one gram of the powdered rhizome mixed with water, taken once every three to five days during menstruation. Decoctions of the rhizomes are used for dysentery and as an antidote for snake and dog bites. The fresh fronds are decocted and used for abnormal or irregular menses (Singh and Singh 2012).

Other traditional uses include treatments for chronic nasal congestion, bronchitis, and swollen glands. For gastric issues, the fresh frond paste is given in one-gram doses twice daily on an empty stomach for two weeks. The widely available Hansraj an Indian cough medicine most commonly contains this fern as well.

Diabetes is a growing global epidemic. Work by Paul et al. (2017) found that ethanol extracts actively utilize glucose in an isolated pancreatic cell uptake assay. The fern extracts inhibit differentiation of pro-adipocyte to adipocyte in the 3T3-L1 cell lines, suggesting possible use of the fern in managing diabetes associated with obesity. Earlier work by Paul et al. (2012) demonstrated the hypoglycemic effect of the fern extract on alloxan-induced diabetic rats.

Phomalactone, derived from the endophytic fungus *Nigrospora sphaerica*, exhibits activity against human and phytopathogenic bacteria and fungi (Ramesha et al. 2020). The compound inhibits the growth of *Phytophthora infestans*, a serious mold also known as late potato blight, which was responsible for the potato famines in Ireland and Scotland in the mid-1800s and is considered a re-emerging pathogen today.

Nigronaphthaphenyl, derived from the endophyte *Nigrospora sphaerica*, exhibits activity against *Bacillus subtilis* and *B. cereus*, shows *cytotoxicity* against the HCT 116 (human colon) cancer cell line, inhibits alpha-glucosidase, and has anti-inflammatory properties (Ukwatta et al. 2019). Six out of twenty-one metabolites show binding energy higher than acarbose, indicating potential as alpha-glucosidase inhibitors and suggesting antidiabetic activity (Kantari et al. 2023). Earlier work by Metwaly et al. (2014) isolated nigrosphaerin A and identified previously known compounds cytotoxic to HL60 (leukemia) and K562 (myelogenous leukemia) cancer cell lines, exhibiting moderate activity against leishmania, and antifungal activity against *Cryptococcus neoformans*.

The fern extracts inhibit bacterial biofilm formation and show synergistic activity with chloramphenicol against *Escherichia coli*, *Staphylococcus aureus*, and *Pseudomonas aeruginosa*. An additive effect is noted against *Shigella flexneri* (Adnan et al. 2020).

Brittle maidenhair fern (*Adiantum tenerum*) has bright green foliage that reminds one of miniature *Ginkgo biloba* leaves. The tree, also known as maidenhair tree, is considered one of the oldest "living fossil" trees on the planet. It is widely cultivated for its flavonoid-rich leaves, which benefit brain health and increase blood flow to the extremities. One cultivar grown indoors is 'Farleyense,' named for a Barbados sugar plantation where first discovered.

I lived in Peru and studied plant medicine in the early 1980s and became familiar with the mental health condition called *susto*, also known as "fright" or "soul loss," characterized by a range of symptoms such as anxiety, depression, insomnia, and fatigue. Susto is believed to be caused by a traumatic event that caused the soul to leave the body. Traditional healing practices often involve rituals and herbal remedies, using various plants either solo or in combination, to bring the soul back to the body.

Four leaf maidenhair fern (*Adiantum tetraphyllum*) was commonly used by curanderos, brujos, and other traditional healers as revealed through interviews conducted by Bourbonnais-Spear et al. (2007). It is uncertain which species of the genus *Adiantum* was used by The Q'eqchi' (Quechua) Maya for susto and epilepsy, but it may be the same one.

Ethanol extracts were tested for their ability to inhibit GABA-transminase (GABA-T) and bind to GABA-A benzodiazepine (BZD) receptors. Both are sites targeted for anxiety and epilepsy. Work by Awad et al. (2009) examined thirty-two plants and found ten of those plants showed greater than 50% GABA-T inhibition at 1mg/ml, and twenty-three plants showed greater than 50% binding to GABA-A-BZD receptors at 250 micrograms/ml. A strong correlation was found between GABA-A binding and the frequency of use for susto, suggesting validation of its traditional use.

Giant or diamond maidenhair fern (*Adiantum trapeziforme*), found in Mexico, is more aromatic but less valuable as a medicinal plant (Grieve 1931).

Methanol extracts of the Himalayan maidenhair fern (*Adiantum venustum*) show activity against the fungus *Aspergillus terreus*, and the multidrug-resistant bacterium *Staphylococcus aureus* (Singh et al. 2008). Incidentally, the fungus *Aspergillus terreus* is used today in the production of lovastatin, a lipid-lowering drug. Oyster mushrooms and other medicinal fungi contain the natural lovastatin, which can help lower cholesterol without the side effects associated with statin drugs. Traditionally, this fern has been used for headaches, scorpion stings, and skin wounds.

An anticancer screening of an ethanol extract demonstrated significant activity against Ehrlich Ascites carcinoma in an animal model. It also reduced levels of lipid peroxidation, likely due to its terpenoid and flavonoid content (Viral et al. 2011).

The Himalayan maidenhair fern is hardy to -34°C/29.2°F and is a popular choice for fern gardeners in northern climates.

On the Ivory Coast, Vogelii maidenhair fern (*Adiantum vogelii* syn. *A. tetraphyllum*) was used to treat fainting, debility, edema, and skin lesions of leprosy (Bouquet 1974). The species is named in honor of the German botanist and plant collector Johann Reinhold Theodor Vogel (1812–1841).

An excellent review of *Adiantum* species and their uses and benefits was published by Rastogi et al. (2018). The genus possesses antidysenteric, antiulcer, antimicrobial, antitumor, and antiviral activity. Traditional uses include treating respiratory problems such as coughs, colds, fevers, and pneumonia, as well as providing expectorant activity.

New species are continually being identified and named. For instance, in 2015, the fern *Adiantum shastense*, which is endemic to Shasta County, California, was officially classified and named as a new species.

PLUMED MAIDENHAIR FERN ESSENCE

This essence of *Adiantum formosum* facilitates healing, peace, and stillness at the soul level, particularly after experiences of spiritual trauma or deep sorrow that have impacted the soul and are locked into cellular memory. It helps those who have issues surrounding religion or spirituality, those who have strict religious or spiritual views and those with a restrictive morality. It is also deemed useful for those who have a fear of losing spiritual control or who feel scarred by their religious or spiritual experiences. Find as First Light Flower Essence of New Zealand's No. 43 Plumed Maidenhair Fern.

AGLAOMORPHA

Basket Ferns   Bear Paw Fern

The genus name may derive from the Greek agláos meaning "shining," and *morpha* "having a form." Worldwide, there are about fifty species, often referred to as basket ferns.

Bear paw fern (*Aglaomorpha coronans*) is native to tropical Asia and cannot tolerate the least amount of frost. It is either epiphytic (growing on trees) or lithophytic (growing on rocks). In the wild, it can grow up to two meters, and it is often prized as an indoor plant.

In East Timor, various parts of oakleaf fern (*Aglaomorpha quercifolia* syn. *Drynaria quercifolia*) are used for food and medicine. The name *quercifolia* refers to the oak leaf-like appearance of the fronds. The rhizomes are made into a broth and used to increase breast milk production, while the young fronds are added to rice dishes.

The fern is used in several areas of the world for its antioxidant, antibacterial, analgesic, and anti-inflammatory properties (Costa et al. 2021).

ALEURITOPTERIS

Attractive Fern   Silverback Fern
Flattering Fern   Silver Cloak Fern

The genus contains about 40 species, especially after folding in the genus *Allosorus* in 2020.

For *Aleuritopteris albomarginata* see *Cheilanthes albomarginata* on page 86.

Extracts of silver cloak fern (*Aleuritopteris anceps*) inhibit the growth of *Staphylococcus aureus* and *Pseudomonas aeruginosa* bacteria (Joshi et al. 2020).

Silverback fern (*Aleuritopteris argentea* syn. *Cheilanthes argentea*) contains alepterolic acid. Fifteen amide derivatives were synthesized and tested against four different cancer cell lines. One compound inhibited HeLa (epithelial/cervical) cancer cells and is nearly nontoxic to noncancerous cells. The compound induced apoptosis by decreasing the mitochondrial membrane potential (Zhang et al. 2020).

A piperazine-tethered derivative of alepterolic acid exhibits cytotoxicity to HepG2 (hepatoma) and MDA-MB-231 (triple negative breast) cancer cell lines. In the latter case, the compound inhibited growth, prevented colony formation, and induced apoptosis (Liu et al. 2023).

Extracts from *Aleuritopteris bicolor* syn. *Hemionitis bicolor* exhibit significant inhibition of alpha-amylase, suggesting potential benefits for blood sugar regulation (Pandey and Sharma 2022).

ALSOPHILA

Fuzzy Spleenwort Maquique Fern Tree Ferns

The binomial name of these tree ferns has also been assigned to a genus of moths. It derives from the Greek alsos, meaning "grove" or "glade," and phila meaning "loving."

In Mexico, maquique fern (*Alsophila firma* syn. *Cyathea mexicana*) has been used in traditional medicine for the symptoms of type 2 diabetes. A tea of the rhizome was drunk throughout the day while fasting. The tree fern is known in Spanish as helecho maquique, and in Nahuatl as peshma.

The rhizome contains flavanones and dihydroflavonoids. When given to induced hyperglycemic rats in vitro the extract significantly reduced blood sugar levels and inhibited glucose-6-phosphatase and fructose1,6-bisphosphatase.

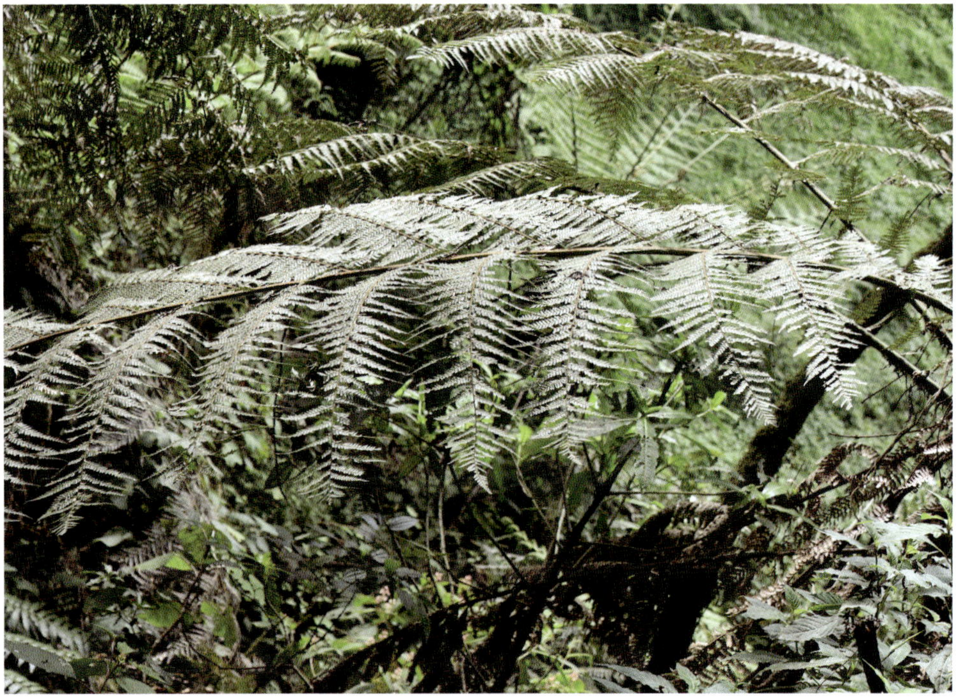

Alsophila firma (Maquique Fern)
Photo by Alan Rockefeller

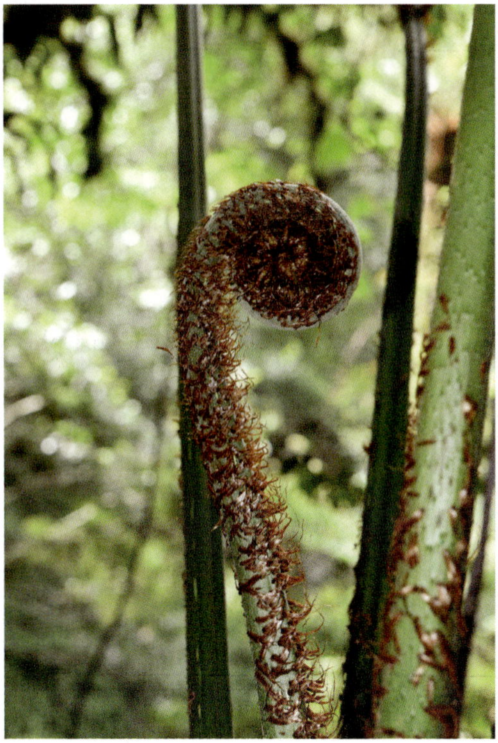

Young Frond of *Alsophila firma*
Photo by Alan Rockefeller

This inhibition may help decrease glucose production, thereby regulating blood sugar levels. Another potential mechanism is the inhibition of hepatic glucose output, which plays a role in controlling glucose levels during fasting (Andrade-Cetto et al. 2021).

In India, ten grams of giant tree fern (*Alsophila gigantea* syn. *Gymnosphaera gigantea*) rhizome is gathered fresh, crushed, and then mixed with one gram of black pepper powder and some cow's milk. This combination is taken twice daily for a week on an empty stomach to cure leucorrhea (white vaginal discharge) (Panda et al. 2011).

An extract of shiny tree fern or sheshino (*Alsophila mannianna*) shows significant antifungal activity against *Candida albicans* (Bisso et al. 2022).

An extract from setosa fern, or fuzzy spleenwort, (*Alsophila setosa*) shows 82.21% inhibition of monoamine oxidase-A (MAO-A) (Andrade et al. 2014). MAO-inhibitor drugs were first approved for depression in the late 1950s and recent studies suggest that MAO-A mediates the growth of several cancers, exhibiting cancer-nerve cell crosstalk, and is effective in disrupting perineural invasion (Wu and Shih 2023).

The flying spider-monkey tree fern (*Alsophila spinoulosa*) is a rare fern that can grow up to five meters tall or more with fronds one to three meters in length. It is found in shaded forests of Asia including China, Nepal, India, Burma, Myanmar, and Japan.

The fronds have been traditionally used for hepatitis, gout, rheumatism, and tumors. The stems are edible and rich in starch. They are chipped, dried and used as a substrate for orchid cultivation. The leaf is composed of various sugars, including galactose, arabinose, glucose, rhamnose, mannose, fucose, and galacturonic acid, a type of uranic acid derived from galactose. An ethanol extract of this fern revealed diploptene, β-sitosterol, caffeic acid, astragalin, and various glucopyranose compounds.

Astragalin (kaempferol-3-glucoside) has been shown to have anti-inflammatory, antioxidant, neuroprotective, cardioprotective, anti-obesity, anti-osteoporotic, anticancer, anti-ulcer, and antidiabetic properties (Riaz et al. 2018). According to PubMed, there are 468 studies on the benefits of astragalin.

Various compounds were tested for inhibition of xanthine oxidase, a measure of benefit in gout. Among them, caffeic acid was the most potent inhibitor of the enzyme (Chiang et al. 1994). A water extract of the dried stem augments both humoral and cellular immune response, in an animal model (Kao et al. 1994).

Research by Pei et al. (2022) suggests that the leaf should be considered a functional food ingredient due to its effects on prolonging lifespan increasing anti-oxidative enzymes (SOD and CAT) and decreasing the level of radical oxygen species (ROS) and malondialdehyde (MDA) in the roundworm *Caenorhabditis elegans*.

AMPELOPTERIS

Scrambling Ferns

Riverine scrambler fern (*Ampelopteris prolifera* syn. *A. elegans* syn. *Thelypteris prolifera*) fronds are used in traditional Indian medicine as a laxative. In Tanzania, the frond sap is added to mixtures and taken as a tea for meningitis and encephalitis. In India, the fronds are eaten raw or cooked but considered less tasty than *Diplazium esculentum* (see page 120). Frond extracts exhibit activity against the cucumber mosaic virus, a commercial crop pathogen. It grows under full sun in freshwater swamps of West Africa, the tropical mainland of Asia and Northeastern Australia.

ANEMIA

The genus name derives from the Greek *aneimon* "without clothing," in reference to the absence of blade tissue in sporangia. Around 120 species are native to the United States, Mexico, Brazil, Africa, and India. They are sometimes referred to as flowering ferns, more commonly applied to *Osmunda* genus.

Anemia phyllitidis spores and prothallia contain a protein with properties similar to calmodulin, a protein found in the human placenta. Calmodulin regulates metabolism, muscle contraction, apoptosis, memory, inflammation, and the immune response (Tidow and Nissen 2013). Downregulated calmodulin expression is responsible for endothelium dysfunction and angiogenesis damage in diabetes. Many of the phytochemicals proposed to treat Alzheimer's disease (AD) work through calmodulin-mediated mechanisms. Some directly bind and inhibit calmodulin directly, while others modulate calmodulin-binding proteins, including amyloid-β and BACE-1 (β-site amyloid-precursor-protein-cleaving enzyme 1) (O'Day 2023).

Over the past twenty years, over 300 drug trials have been conducted to treat this devastating disease, but with only minimal success. These efforts primarily focused on dissolving beta-amyloid clumping or tau tangles.

Researchers may be addressing the symptoms rather than the root cause of AD. Over 120 publications have implicated herpes simplex virus type 1 (HSV-1) in the progression of AD (Itzhaki et al. 2017).

One study found that in 70% of cases, HSV-1 was present within amyloid-beta plaques, suggesting that a leaky gut and a faulty blood-brain barrier may allow the virus to enter brain microglia. The brain's defense is to encapsulate the virus and thereby preventing it from causing further damage.

In his brilliant book *Psychobiotic Revolution*, Scott Anderson (2017) writes "[the plagues and tangles] are, it seems, the firemen—not the arsonists."

Rogers (2019) notes that over 60% of North Americans carry the herpes simplex virus, which can proliferate during high stress period and with excessive arginine intake, among other factors. Furthermore, the spore extracts have been shown to damage K562 (human premyeloid leukemia) cells (Simán et al. 2000).

ANGIOPTERIS

Cochinchina Fern
Dragon Scales Fern
Elephant Fern
King Fern
Mule's Foot Fern
Narrow-Leaved Fern
Turnip Fern
Vessel Fern

Geographic Range: tropical and subtropical Asia, South Sea islands, Northeastern India, China
Habitat: deep soil, shady environments
Practical Uses: food, stems used for starch, income source at local markets, alcoholic beverages, perfume
Medicinal Applications: analgesic, anti-adipogenic, antibacterial, antifungal, antihyperglycemic, anti-inflammatory, cancer, cytotoxic, HIV-1 reverse transcriptase inhibition, tuberculosis

The genera name derives from the Greek *aggeion* meaning, "vessel," and *pteris*, meaning "fern" or "wing." These ferns are noted for their spores, which are dispersed explosively.

When extracted, the narrow-leaved fern (*Angiopteris angustifolia* syn. *A. evecta*) exhibits cytotoxicity against MCF-7 (human breast) cancer cell lines (Komala et al. 2022).

Angiopteris caudatiformis is a tropical Asian fern. In China, the rhizome is known as *ji ma*, or *pi zhen lian zuo jue* and is used in Dai folk medicine to treat infections such as enteritis, dysentery, and tuberculosis. The rhizome and fibrous roots are a commonly used ingredient in herbal formulas, such as cough with lung heat, venomous snakebites, furuncle, and bleeding wounds.

Angiopterlactones A and B, osmundalactone, osmundalin and 3,4-dihydroxy-γ-capralactone have been isolated from the rhizome. Angiopterlactone A is slightly cytotoxic against HeLa (epithelial/cervical) cancer cell lines, whereas osmundalactone and osmundalin show moderate antifeedant activity against the diamondback or cabbage moth (*Plutella xylostella*) and the tobacco budworm (*Heliothis virescens*) (Yu et al. 2009). The former pest damages members of the cabbage family, and the latter, despite its misleading common name, attacks alfalfa, clover, flax, soybean, okra, and tobacco.

A global patent to produce synthetic angiopterlactone B has been filed (WO20170775491).

Cochinchina fern (*Angiopteris cochinchinensis*) extracts have been shown to reduce the nitric oxide production in murine macrophages stimulated by lipopolysaccharide (LPS), and to decrease edema and injury in lung tissue. The primary target in alleviating inflammation was Src protein kinase. The fern extract binds directly to this kinase, significantly mitigating lung injury (Jang et al. 2022b).

The edible fern *Angiopteris esculenta* is widely collected in various parts of China, where it serves both as food, and as a source of income at the local market. The stems are particularly valued for their edible starch.

Elephant, or mule's foot, fern (*Angiopteris evecta*) has the longest fronds of any fern in the world. The name evectus derives from the Latin, meaning "to carry out," "raise," or "elevate." Another common name is turnip fern.

In Northeastern India, the massive stems of this fern are cooked and eaten, and a traditional alcoholic beverage called ruchshi is also made from them. In the South Sea islands, an aromatic oil is produced to perfume coconut oil for cosmetic purposes.

All extracts from the leaves, stem bark, stem heartwood, roots, and tubers, using five different solvents, revealed significant antibacterial activity. The dichloromethane and ethyl acetate fractions of leaves and stem bark were the most effective and were the only fractions to also exhibit antifungal activity (Khan and Omoloso 2008).

The leaf extract exhibits significant antituberculosis activity (Mohamad et al. 2011).

Oral ingestion of ethanol extracts of this fern by lab mice significantly reduced blood glucose levels and prevented increases after a glucose challenge (Hoa et al. 2009). Additionally, an in vivo study on Swiss albino mice by Sultana et al. (2014) found that the fern exhibits both antihyperglycemic and analgesic activity.

The large rhizome contains angiopteroside, succinic acid, β-sitosterol, and stigmasterol. Angiopteroside ethanol extracts exhibit activity against HIV-1 reverse transcriptase and ChaGo (human lung) cancer cell lines. The level of cytotoxicity was very similar to the control chemotherapy drug doxorubicin (Taveepanich et al. 2000). Angiopteroside, extracted from the leaves, inhibits the growth of the bacterium *Bacillus subtilis* (Anggia et al. 2015).

Angiopteris helferiana is a huge, expansive fern growing in subtropical Asia, with fleshy rhizomes containing (–)*epi*-osmundalactone and angiopteroside. These compounds were tested for their anti-adipogenic and anti-inflammatory activities by Lamichhane et al. (2020). Adipogenesis is the process whereby fat-laden cells (adipocytes) develop and accumulate as adipose tissue in various parts of the body. Both compounds inhibited lipid production by 35% and 25% using 3t3-L1 cells. The former compound, in tests on RAW264.7 cells, inhibited nitrite production by 82%, suggesting anti-inflammatory benefits. Both compounds suggest possible application in treating obesity and related health concerns.

The rhizome of turnip, vessel or dragon scales fern (*Angiopteris lygodiifolia*) also contains angiopteroside. A common Chinese term for the fern is Ljuwbintai.

Angiopteris palmiformis leaves were extracted with methyl alcohol. Chen et al. (2010) isolated and identified two new fernane triterpenoids, 7α-hydroxyfern-8-en-11-one and 11β-hydroxyfern-8-en-7-one, two new filicane triterpenoids, 3-β-hydroxyfilic-4(23)-ene and filicenol; as well as the previously identified 3alpha-hydroxyfilic-4-(23)-ene. Like other tropical and subtropical plants, this fern emits methyl chloride (Yokouchi et al. 2007). *Osmunda banksiifolia* syn. *Plenasium banksiifolium* is also a strong emitter of this volatile compound.

ARACHNIODES

Climbing Shield Fern
East Indian Holly Fern
Floral Fern
Iron Fern
Leather Fern
Leatherleaf Fern
Seven Weeks Fern

Geographic Range: China, Germany, India, Japan, United States
Habitat: shady environments, cultivated indoors
Practical Uses: used in the floral industry
Medicinal Applications: antibacterial, anti-inflammatory, analgesic, antioxidant, antipyretic, bone healing, cancer, hepatoprotective, sedative

The genus is widely misspelled as *Arachinodes*, *Arachnioides*, or *Arachnoides*. The genus name derives from the Greek *arachnion* meaning "spider's web," referring to the intricate, miniature pinnae in the frond.

Leatherleaf (*Arachniodes adiantiformis* syn. *Rumohra adiantiformis* syn. *Polypodium adiantiforme*) has a variety of names including leather fern, leathery shield fern, iron fern, seven weeks fern, and climbing shield fern. The species name *adiantiformis* derives from the Greek *adianton*, meaning "unwettable," alluding to the fronds' ability to shed moisture.

The leatherleaf fern or floral fern is a tropical fern which is the source of income for thousands of people in Brazil who harvest and sell the wild fern for the floral industry. It has also been imported from the United States to Germany since 1996 and cultivated in Germany shortly thereafter.

The fungi *Dematophora bunodes* (Rosellinia bunodes) is a well-known plant pathogen, which causes root rot in both leatherleaf and taro (*Colocasia esculenta*), a major food staple.

Leatherleaf fern or *knysna* fern has been traditionally used as a treatment for syphilis, with some evidence suggesting its efficacy.

Arachniodes exilis is a traditional medicine used in China for its antibacterial, anti-inflammatory, and sedative properties.

The fern contains phenolic compounds including aspidin BB, 4-methyl-2-butyl-3,5-dihydroxyphenol, eriodictyol, epicatechin, miscathoside, eriodictyol-7-O-β-D-glucopyranuronide, and luteolin-4'-O-β-D-glyco-pyranuronide; polyphenols include araspidin BB, arachniodesin A and B, as well as epicatechin and procyanidin B2.

Aspidin BB induces cell cycle arrest and apoptosis in HO-8910 (human ovarian) cancer cell lines (Sun et al. 2013). The compound is also active against *Propionbacterium acnes*, a bacterium responsible for acne and related skin eruptions (Gao et al. 2016).

Eriodictyol plays a role in brain, cardiovascular, liver, and pancreatic health, in skin protection and in treating obesity. It is analgesic, antioxidant, antipyretic, and anti-inflammatory and helps to prevent various diseases via multiple cellular signaling pathways (Deng et al. 2020). In a mouse study, the compound ameliorated cognitive deficits and suppressed aggregation of amyloid-beta and tau phosphorylation in the brain (Li et al. 2022a).

Retinoblastoma is an intraocular malignancy in children that often causes vision loss. Eriodictyol inhibits proliferation, migration, and invasion of retinoblastoma cell lines, and induces apoptosis, possibly by blocking the Pl3K/Akt signaling pathway (Wen et al. 2021).

Ethanol extracts of eriodictyol show potent antioxidant activity, evidenced by reducing power, lipid peroxide, DPPH, ABTS, superoxide anions, and hydroxyl radical, and hydrogen peroxide. Improved levels of glutamate oxaloacetate, transaminase, glutamate pyruvate transaminase, malondialdehyde, and superoxide dismutase in a mice liver assay suggest hepatoprotective activity (Zhou et al. 2010).

Total flavonoids derived from the fern inhibit the tumor growth of HepG2 (hepatoma) carcinoma in nude mice, through apoptosis and inhibition of angiogenesis in tumor tissue (Li et al. 2017a). Many ferns are traditionally used to promote fractured bone healing and bone diseases such as osteoporosis. Total flavonoids extracted from the fern also resulted in a significant downregulation of osteogenic markers (Col1a1, OPN, Runx2, and Osx), compared to the control. The extract promotes odonto/osteogenic differentiation of human umbilical cord mesenchymal stem cells via activation of the estrogen receptor ER (Yu et al. 2020). Previously, the fern was shown to promote differentiation of rat bone marrow mesenchymal stem cells through bone morphogenetic protein signaling.

Arachniodes rhomboidea contains kaempferol, kaempferol-3-O-α-L-rhamnoside, kaempferol-3-O-β-D-glucoside, kaempferol-3,7-O-α-L-dirhamnoside, quercetin-3-O-β-glucoside and kaempferol-3-O-β-D-rutinoside.

The latter flavonoid exhibits high cytotoxic effects against MCF-7 (breast) and HepG2 (hepatoma) cancer cell lines. It also exerts synergistic cytotoxicity with doxorubicin, the well-known chemotherapy drug. The flavonoid inhibits aldose reductase, suggesting the cardiotoxic effect from the drug may be reduced. Thus, it increases sensitivity to cancer cells and protects against the side effects of chemotherapy (Osman et al. 2020).

The East Indian holly fern (*Arachniodes simplicior*) is so named for the stiff, waxy, evergreen fronds that resemble holly leaves. The fern is native to Japan and China. It is grown indoors and, when purchased from a garden center, is often listed as *Arachniodes aristata* 'Variegata.' The leathery frond has a yellow-green stripe down the center.

ASPIDOTIS

Golden Serpentine Fern   Dense Lace Fern   Indian's Dream Fern

Golden serpentine, dense lace, or Indian's dream fern (*Aspidotis densa*) is native to the West Coast of North America, growing mainly on serpentine soils, hence its common name. Serpentine soil is formed by weathered ultramafic rock containing antigorite, lizardite, and chrysolite (white asbestos). Ultramafic rocks are igneous or metamorphic rocks contains more than 70% iron or magnesium.

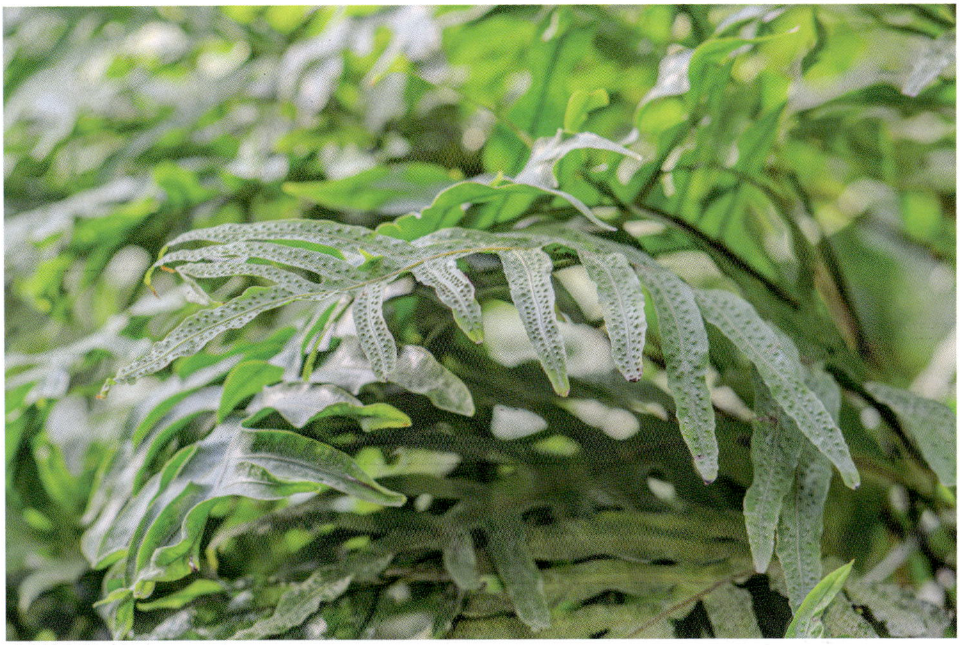

Aspidotis densa (Golden Serpentine Fern)

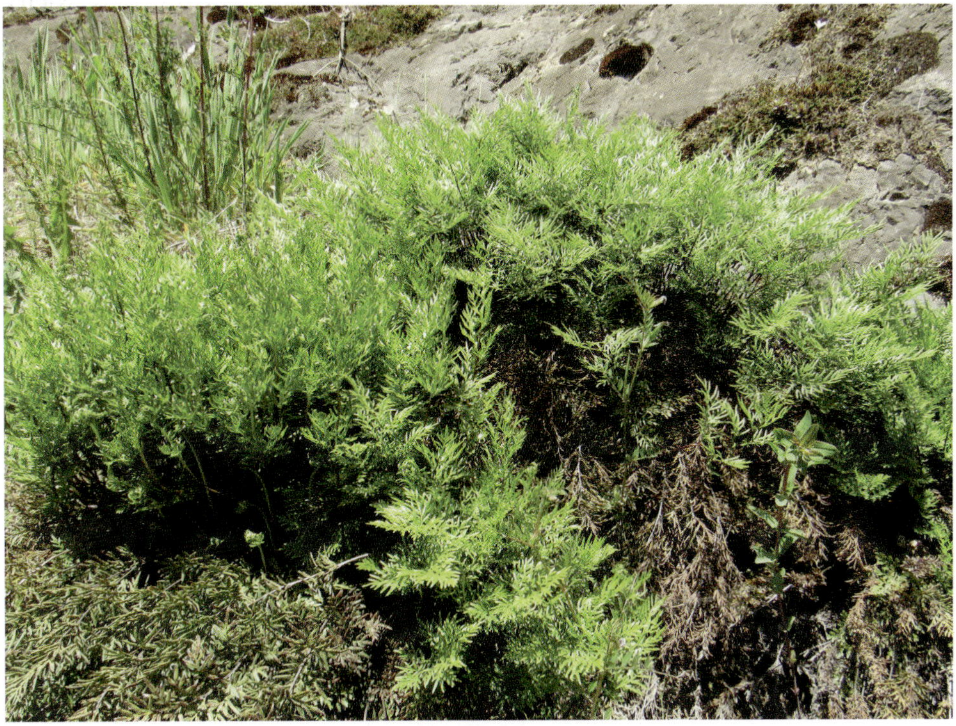

Aspidotis densa (Serpentine Fern)
Photo by Drew T. Henderson

ASPLENIUM

Bird's Nest Ferns
Black Spleenworts
Brownstem Spleenwort
Buttonhole Fern
Countess Dalhousie's Spleenwort
Cow's Tongue
Creeping Spleenwort
Dragon Tail Fern
Ebony Spleenwort
God's Hair
Green Spleenwort
Hart's Tongue Fern
Hen and Chicken(s) Fern
Hind's Tongue
Horse Tongue
Long-tail Spleenwort
Mare's Tail Fern
Mole Ladder Fern
Mother Spleenwort
Norfolk Island Spleenwort
Rock Spleenwort
Rustyback Fern
Scaly Fern
Scott's Spleenwort
Sickle Spleenwort
Single-sorus Spleenwort
Smooth Rock
Subarctic Lady Fern
Verdon Spleenwort
Walking Ferns
Wall Rue Fern

Geographic Range: Africa, Asia, Australia, Canada (British Columbia), Europe, India, Iran, Ireland, Japan, Lesotho, Malaysia, New Zealand, North America (Eastern U.S.), Peru, South Africa, Vanuatu

Habitat: calcareous rocks, humid tropical environments, limestone boulders, moss-covered rocks, shaded woods, temperate zones, tropical and subtropical regions, warm and shady areas

Practical Uses: food, hair wash, houseplant, ornamental baskets, rachis used as toothpicks, used in perfumery for fougère scent

Medicinal Applications: anthelmintic, anti-inflammatory, antioxidant, antibacterial, cancer, demulcent, diuretic, emmenagogue, expectorant, hepatoprotective, laxative, menstruation, mucilaginous, nephroprotective, promotes bone healing, skin

Warning: Some species may have abortifacient properties and can cause antifertility effects.

The genus name derives from the Greek *splen* meaning spleen, hence spleenwort or miltwort (*milt* from the German *milz* for spleen).

Black spleenwort (*Asplenium adiantum-nigrum* syn. *A. andrewsii*) is a common evergreen fern in Africa, Europe, and Asia. However, it is quite rare

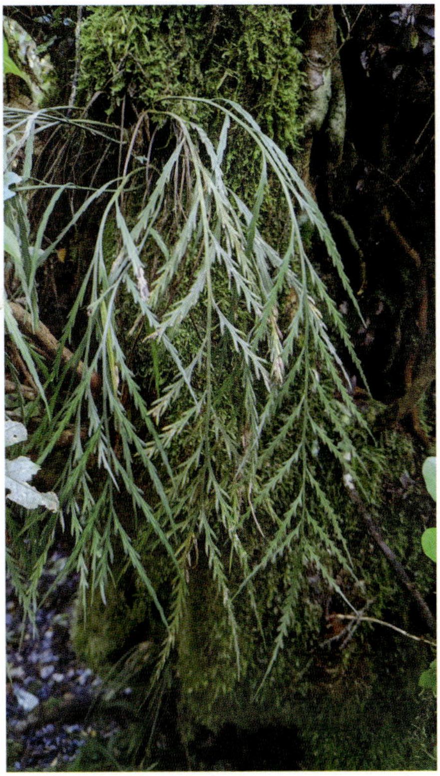

Asplenium flaccidum
(Drooping Spleenwort)
Photo by Alan Rockefeller

in Southwestern North America, where it has been introduced but has not become widespread.

The Greek physician and botanist Dioscorides noted,

> *Asplenon* has many leaves (similar to the creatures called centipedes and millipedes) growing round about out of one root . . . The leaves (boiled in vinegar and taken as a drink for forty days) are able to reduce the spleen, but you must also rub the spleen with the leaves pounded into small pieces with wine. It helps slow painful urination, hiccups and jaundice and breaks stones in the bladder. . . . They say that to cause barrenness it must be dug up when the night is moonless. It is also called scolopendrium, splenium, hemionion, pteryx . . . while the Magi call it the blood of a weasel.

John Gerard wrote that it is called *Asplenium* because "it is special good against the infirmities of the spleen or milt and Scolopendria of the likeness that it hath with the bear-worm."

Nicholas Culpeper (1652) noted that the distilled water of spleenwort

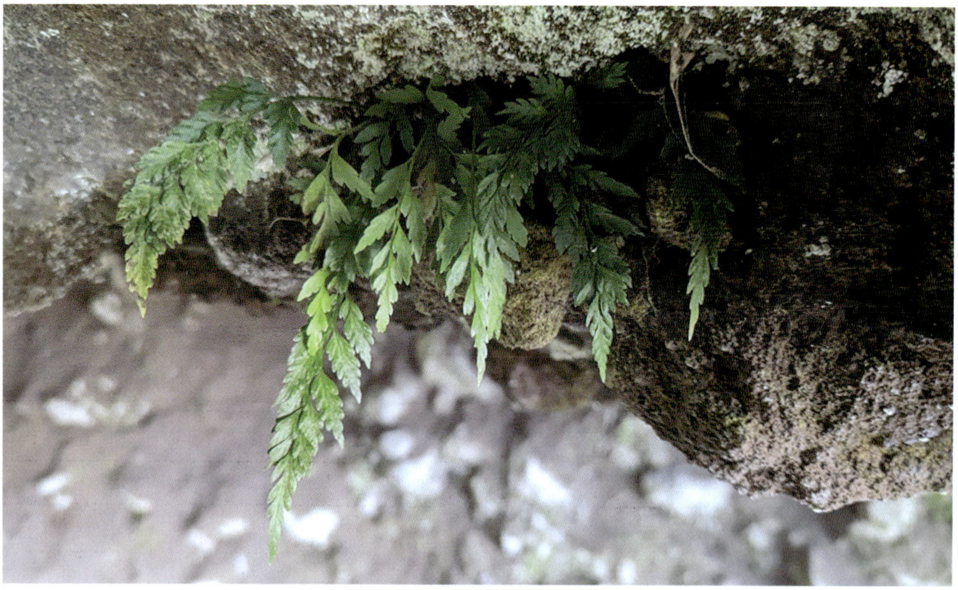

Asplenium appendiculatum (Spleenwort)
Photo by Alan Rockefeller

thereof being drank, it is very effectual against the stone in the reins and bladder. John K'Eogh noted that *Asplenium* has a temperate nature, and he repeated some of the writing of Dioscorides. He noted that "it has a hot dry nature. Either internally or externally applied, it is very good for obstruction or swelling of the spleen. It is also beneficial for wounds, as it protects them from inflammation" (K'Eogh 1735).

Grieve (1931) called it black maidenhair (*Asplenium nigrum*) and described similar uses as other maidenhair ferns: "A decoction of it relieving a troublesome cough and proving also a good hair wash."

Medicinal uses include diuretic, contraceptive, emmenagogue, expectorant, pectoral, and laxative properties. A tea was prepared for issues involving the spleen, liver jaundice, and ophthalmia. A syrup has been traditionally prepared for coughs, and a decoction for rinsing hair. It was once believed to cause sterility in women.

In the Western Himalayas, the fronds are used to treat jaundice (Khoja et al. 2022). In South Africa, the rhizome was used as anthelmintic and ceremonial emetic. In Iran, the fern rhizome has been traditionally decocted and used for kidney disease and inflammation (Bahadori et al. 2015). The rhizomes exhibit significant activity against *Staphylococcus aureus* and *Escherichia coli*.

Egyptian spleenwort (*Asplenium aethiopicum* syn. *Asplenium furcatum*) methanol extracts exhibit antioxidant activity, while crude acetone extracts induce high mosquito larvae mortality (Antonysamy et al. 2014).

Also known as *'iwa 'iwa a kane* by the Māori, the rhizome has been traditionally used as an anthelmintic by Indigenous people of Lesotho (Chopra et al. 1956).

Japanese bird's nest fern (*Asplenium antiquum*) looks very much like bird's nest fern (*Asplenium nidus*). It is smaller and more compact, making it an attractive house plant.

The fronds of the bird's nest fern (*Asplenium australasicum*) contain a considerable amount of fucose-rich mucilage and p-coumaric acid, showing an enhanced effect on collagen production and the growth of fibroblast (NIH-3T3) cells. A randomized controlled clinical trial showed an emulsion with 1% extract exhibited good moisturizing effect and improved elasticity of human skin. The extract also exhibits suppression of B16-F10 melanoma viability, suggesting a natural hypopigmenting agent (Zeng and Lai 2019a; 2019b).

Consumption of the fern extract reduced damage to the exposed skin of hairless mice by UVA radiation. A study by Masuda et al. (2022) found that the extract enhanced superoxide dismutase 2 expression and downregulated apoptosis in the mice epidermis.

Kim et al. (2022) conducted a randomized, double-blind, placebo-controlled comparative study involving women aged forty to sixty years. The edible bird's nest extract was consumed for twelve weeks and significantly improved skin wrinkles compared to control group.

The Māori of New Zealand use *pikopiko*,* the young fiddleheads of mother spleenwort or hen and chicken(s) fern (*Asplenium bulbiferum*) for food. The young, uncurled frond is harvested, washed, then steamed, or chopped up and added to bread dough. It is also known as hen fern, chick fern, or mother fern. This fern is native to New Zealand, Australia, Malaysia, and India. It propagates with small bulbils on the upper side of the lacy fronds that develop into small plants that drop off and grow as clones. The fronds contain antioxidant flavonoids such as kaempferol glucosides. Traditionally, the fronds were applied externally to hemorrhoids, and a tea taken for liver problems (Baskaran et al. 2018).

---

*The term *pikopiko* may also apply to the common shield fern (*Polystichum richardii*).

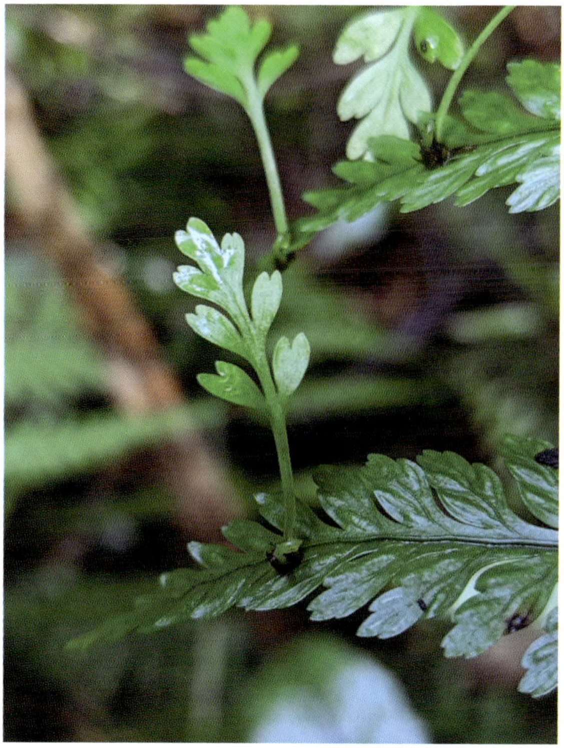

Asplenium bulbiferum
(Hen and Chicken(s) Fern)
Photo by Alan Rockefeller

Weinstein (2020) notes in his highly recommended *The Complete Book of Ferns* that DNA testing has revealed many ferns sold as this species are actually misidentified.

One sterile hybrid, the false hen and chicken(s) fern (*Asplenium* × *lucrosum*) is produced by crossing this species with Norfolk Island spleenwort (*Asplenium dimorphum*). This hybrid will not produce fertile spores, but bulbils.

Rustyback fern, scaly fern, or finger fern (*Asplenium ceterach* syn. *Ceterach officinarum*) is widespread throughout Europe and used in Italy for its diuretic effect. The species name suggests its use in monasteries and apothecaries. The term *officinarum* is often associated with plants that have medicinal properties and were used in officinas, the workshops, or pharmacies of monasteries and apothecaries.

Its range extends from Southern Europe to North Africa, and Western Asia to the Himalayas, tolerating very alkaline soil. It is a hardy fern surviving down to -25°C/-13°F. In the Western Himalayas, the fronds are used to treat kidney stones (Khoja et al. 2022). In the mountains of Central-Southern Italy, the fern has been traditionally used to regulate menstruation (Guarrera et al. 2008).

Other medical uses include expectorant, pectoral (combined with mucilaginous herbs), aperient, and diuretic activity, including treatment for kidney and bladder stones. Gerard (1545–1612) notes the spleenwort, also called *asplenum* or *ceterach*, was said to be used by Dioscorides for infirmities of the spleen, strangury, and yellow jaundice.

Nicholas Culpeper (1616–1654) notes that the fern is owned by Saturn. He cites Matthiolus, who claimed that a mixture of a drachm of the dust (spores) from the backside of the fronds is mixed with half a drachm of powdered amber, taken with the juice of purslane or plantain, would help cure gonorrhea. He also notes that boiling the frond and root can help those suffering from melancholy, especially when associated with sexually transmitted infections (Culpeper, 1652).

The distilled water was noted for treating kidney and bladder stones some five hundred years ago.

Maud Grieve (1931) noted the early name *miltwaste*, recognizing its ability to cure disorders of the milt or spleen, especially enlargement. In the doctrine of signatures the lobular milt-shaped fronds resembled the shape of the spleen. The doctrine of signatures was a means by which early people (who could not read) used the color, shape, or other distinguishing features to relate medicinal plants to their use for various ailments.

Grieve wrote, "It was also used as a pectoral and as an aperient in obstructions or the viscera, and an infusion of the leaves was prescribed for gravel. . . . Pliny considered that it caused barrenness."

In vitro, the water extracts induce calcium oxalate crystallization, showing their critical role in kidney stone formation and/or elimination. Increasing doses inhibit calcium oxalate monohydrate growth and effectively increase the number and reduce the size of the crystals, which became progressively thinner, rounded, and concave. These crystals are less adherent and more easily excreted through the urinary tract. The water extract promotes the formation of calcium oxalate dihydrate, rather than monohydrate so that a significant number of crystals are reduced in size (de Bellis et al. 2019).

An extract from the fern displayed strong inhibitory activity against HeLa (human cervical) cancer cell lines and possessed antibacterial activity against *Bacillus cereus* and *Pseudomonas aeruginosa* (Petkov et al. 2021a).

The volatiles in this fern are composed mainly of fatty acid derivatives: isomeric heptadienals (>25%), and decadienals (>20%) Živković et al. (2021).

Ceterach officinarum extract contains hyperoside and chlorogenic acid. It did not demonstrate cytotoxic or phototoxic activity in this study, but its cytoprotective properties against hydrogen peroxide-induced oxidative stress in NIH-3T3 (mouse embryonic fibroblast) and HaCaT (human keratinocyte) cell lines bode well for future skin health conditions (Farràs et al. 2022).

Hyperoside is cited in over one thousand studies on PubMed. It is widely recognized by many herbalists as a compound in Saint John's wort and is often erroneously promoted as the active component of the medicinal herb. Hyperoside has a broad spectrum of activity, including anticancer, anti-inflammatory, antibacterial, antiviral, anti-sepsis, anti-arthritis, anti-colitis, and protective effects against diabetic nephropathy, myocardial ischemia-reperfusion, and pulmonary fibrosis (Wang et al. 2022b).

Constituents of an extract from this fern and Hart's-tongue fern (*Asplenium scolopendrium*) act as agonists of 5-HT2 receptors and cause muscle contraction by activating the serotonergic signaling system (Petkov et al. 2021b).

Wedgeleaf spleenwort (*Asplenium cuneatum*) was used as an emetic in South Africa (Watt and Breyer-Brandwijk 1962) and as an anthelmintic enema in Ghana.

Subarctic lady fern (*Asplenium cyclosorum* syn. *Athyrium filix-femina* ssp. *cyclosorum*) was used by Bella Coola, a community in British Columbia, Canada, as a simple or compound decoction of the root for washing sore eyes. The Indigenous people Tlingit infused the fern for chest inflammation associated with catarrh (Moerman 1986).

Countess Dalhousie's spleenwort (*Asplenium dalhousiae*) is a traditional medicine in Pakistan and elsewhere. This perennial evergreen and diminutive fern is named in honor of the Earl of Dalhousie. The specific Dalhousie is uncertain, as the lineage and title have been held by the Chief of Clan Ramsay in Scotland and have been passed down since 1617. Several members of the Ramsay family served in the Bengal army in the late 1700s and onward.

A study on male rats was conducted on the effects of methanol extracts from the frond on antifertility. The results suggest that the extract might induce antifertility effects via oxidative stress and interference with testicular architecture, thus lowering sperm motility, viability, and sperm production rates (David et al. 2019). Extracts of the fern are antioxidant and exhibit antiproliferative effects on MDA-MB-231 (breast cancer) cells (Al-Assar et al. 2021).

Rock spleenwort (*Asplenium delavayi*) is an easily grown fern and a useful model for studying mutual bacteria/fern relationships. Both bacterial and fungal endophytes have long been an area of personal interest, and further study may reveal that these organisms are responsible for the health benefits of many plants.

Dragon's tail fern (*Asplenium ebenoides*) is native to the Eastern United States, growing on or near calcareous rocks. It has been hybridized from American walking fern (*Asplenium rhizophyllum*) and ebony spleenwort (*Asplenium platyneuron*) to become syn. *Asplenosorus* × *ebenoides* in order to induce sterility (not producing spores) for the commercial market. It is also known as Scott's spleenwort, named after R. Robinson Scott, who identified the fern as a new species in 1861. It is probably the result of happenstance hybridization between *Asplenium platyneuron* and the American walking fern (*Asplenium rhizophyllum*), formerly *Camptosorus rhizophyllus*. It is hardy down to -30°C/-22°F.

Falcate spleenwort (*Asplenium falcatum* syn. *A. lunulatum*) has been used in traditional Indian medicine for treating malaria, enlarged spleen, calculi, jaundice, and urinary incontinence (Chopra et al. 1956). In North Africa the rhizome is used for jaundice and prolonged malaria symptoms (Hare et al. 1916).

Sheen-ghass, also known as fountain spleenwort or smooth rock spleenwort, (*Asplenium fontanum* ssp. *pseudofontanum*) fronds, found in rock crevices in the Western Himalayas, are used to treat respiratory conditions (Khoja et al. 2022).

Gaston's spleenwort (*Asplenium gastonis*) contains the flavanone hesperidin. The compound has been widely studied with over 3,200 PubMed citations. Hesperidin is commonly found in citrus fruits, and its bioavailability and benefits to humans may depend upon gut microbiota composition (Mas-Capdevila et al. 2020).

Long-tail spleenwort (*Asplenium incisum*) extracts significantly inhibit the proliferation of *Porphyromonas gingivalis*, with the activity lasting for three days. The extract also exhibited anti-inflammatory and anti-osteoclastogenic activity, suggesting therapeutic potential for treating periodontal disease (Moon et al. 2021).

Five grams of *Asplenium indicum* rhizomes were made into a paste, mixed with 10 ml of cow milk, and taken twice daily for a week in an attempt to cure gonorrhea (Singh and Upadhyay 2012).

A paste of the rhizome with cow's urine was used in India for the treatment of leucorrhea (Rout et al. 2009). A survey of traditional medicinal plants in Ethiopia led to reports of single-sorus spleenwort (*Asplenium monanthes*) being used to treat coughs (Bogale et al. 2023). The dried leaves were smoked

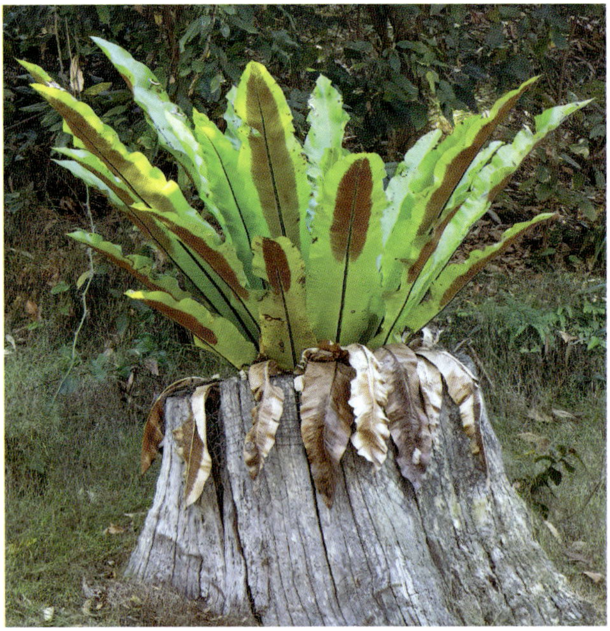

Asplenium nidus
(Bird's Nest Fern)

for head colds in South Africa (Watt and Breyer-Brandwijk 1962) and used as a diaphoretic in Peru (Tryon 1959).

Bird's nest fern (*Asplenium nidus*) is a popular vegetable in Asian cuisine and a well-known houseplant. The stems are sometimes plaited for ornamental baskets.

An actinobacteria named *Gordonia asplenii* was isolated from humic soil on the fern. The cell wall peptidoglycan contains meso-diaminopimelic acid, sugars (ribose, arabinose, galactose) and the menaquinone MK-9 (H2). Suriyachadkun et al. (2019). The latter compound is a vitamin K_2 homolog that acts as a prothrombogenic agent and a functional electron transfer compound in nitrate reductase. Meso-diaminopimelic acid biosynthetic enzymes are unique to bacteria and absent in mammals. Work by Usha et al. (2012) suggests that the structure and function may be useful for *Mycobacterium tuberculosis* chemotherapy.

Work by Chen et al. (2019) found that water extracts of this fern show significant antifungal activity and highest total activity against *Candida krusei* (syn. *Issatchenkia orientalis*), without toxicity to African monkey kidney epithelial (Vero) cells.

The fern has been traditionally used in the South Pacific island of Vanuatu to induce female sterility. This effect is said to be reversed by taking *Hemigraphis reptans* as the antidote (Bourdy and Walter 1992).

In the Philippines, the fern is used as a depurative and sedative (Quisumbing 1951).

The fronds of ebony or brownstem spleenwort (*Asplenium platyneuron*) are a popular diurnal resting spot for mosquitoes. While nothing can be done about it, one researcher in Florida suggests that physically removing the vegetation could help control the insects (Samson et al. 2013). Good luck with that!

Mare's tail fern or sickle spleenwort (*Asplenium polyodon*) is used in traditional Indian medicine for cancer (Singh 1999).

Extracts of *Asplenium polypodioides* syn. *Diplazium polypodioides* show antioxidant and antiproliferative effects on MDA-MB-231 (breast cancer) cells (Al-Assar et al. 2021).

Asplenium species are rich in volatile compounds, highly prized for their fougère fragrance in perfumes. The main odorous lipidic derivates are (E)-2-decanal (fatty and waxy odor), nonanal (aldehydic and waxy odor with a fresh green nuance), (E)-2-heptenal (green odor with a fatty note), and 1-octen-3-ol (mushroom odor). Various species exhibit different variations. For example, Verdon spleenwort (*Asplenium jahandiezii*) is rich in 9-oxononanoic acid, Irish or western black spleenwort (*Asplenium onopteris*) is rich in hydroxyacetophenone, with its sweet and floral note, and rock spleenwort (*Asplenium foreziense*) is rich in 4-hydroxybenzoic acid.

Asplenium repandum syn. *A. variabile* fronds were decocted in Malaya to treat gonorrhea (Burkill 1966). It is commonly found in Africa.

Walking fern (*Asplenium rhizophyllum* syn. *Camptosorus rhizophyllus*) is found on moss-covered limestone boulders in shaded woods. The species name derives from *rhizal*, meaning "root" and *phyllon*, meaning "leaf" due to its habit of rooting leaves. The name "walking fern" refers to the frond tips poking into their mossy neighbors and taking root to produce new plants.

Walking fern has been traditionally used by Indigenous people of Eastern North America and the Southeastern United States, such as the Cherokee, for treating coughs, irregular menstruation, and for topical applications for swollen breast disease, potentially mastitis. A combination of horse balm or stoneroot (*Collinsonia canadensis*), walking fern, wild ginger (*Asarum canadense*), and sharp-lobed hepatica (*Hepatica acutiloba*) was infused and used four times before noon for four days as a ceremonial emetic (causing vomiting). The fern is astringent, mucilaginous, and tonic.

Asian walking fern (*Asplenium ruprechtii* syn. *Camptosorus sibiricus*) is used in Chinese, Korean, and Japanese traditional medicines to treat Buerger's disease, or Winiwarter-Buerger's disease, thromboangiitis obliterans. The common name *walking fern* comes from a new fern developing when a leaf tip touches the ground. Buerger's disease is a progressive inflammation and clotting (thrombosis) of small and medium arteries and veins in the hands and feet. It may be exacerbated by tobacco use, worsens with walking and increases sensitivity to cold weather. Ulceration and gangrene can result in amputation. This condition is often mistaken for Raynaud's syndrome.

Cycloartane glycosides from the whole fern were tested for cytotoxicity against A375-S2 (human melanoma) and HeLa (cervical) cancer cell lines (Zhang et al. 2008).

Two compounds, disaccharose and disaccharoside, derived from an ethanol extract were tested against two human tumor cell lines by Li et al. (2008b).

The fern contains aspleniumsides A through E (cycloartane glycosides). Research by Wang et al. (2020) found cytotoxicity against HL-60 (acute leukemia) and HepG2 (liver) cancer cells lines.

Wall rue fern (*Asplenium ruta-muraria*) grows on limestone and calcareous rocks in Europe, East Asia, and Eastern North America. It is a rather small fern, only a few centimeters tall. Older common names include white maidenhair, tentwort, or *Salvis vitæ*. Tentwort refers to its use in treating rickets, previously known as the "taint." In Kashmir, the leaves were used for exactly this purpose (Chopra et al. 1956). The rhizomes were traditionally used in North Carolina as an astringent and anthelmintic, and the fronds as a pectoral and diuretic (Jacobs and Burlage 1954).

Grieve (1931) noted its use for coughs and ruptures in children, and to prevent hair loss.

Culpeper (1652) wrote,

> This is used in pectoral decoction . . . being drunk helps those that are troubled with coughs, shortness of breath, yellow jaundice, diseases of the spleen, stoppings of the urine, and helps to break the stone in the kidneys. . . . It cleanses the lungs, and rectifying the blood causes a good colour to the whole body. The herb boiled in oil of camomile dissolves knots, allays swellings and dry up moist ulcers.

A distilled water of the fronds was used for various eye conditions. The fern was applied to scrofula, also known as the king's evil. Today it is termed mycobacterial cervical lymphadenitis (tuberculosis) in the neck.

In Ireland, the fern was known as a "herb of the seven gifts," valued in the county Tipperary to cure seven diseases. It was boiled in milk and taken for epilepsy and decocted for kidney troubles.

Asplenium ruta-muraria contains caffeic glycosides and glucopyranosides, as well as 1-O-caffeoyl glycoside, sucrose, diploptene, and β-sitosterol. Work by Fan et al. (2012) showed aromatase inhibitory potential of the extracts. Aromatase inhibitors are widely used to treat hormone-sensitive cancers. Several medicinal plants, such as the stinging nettle (*Urtica dioica*) root, also exhibit this benefit.

Hart's tongue fern (*Asplenium scolopendrium* syn. *Phyllitis scolopendrium*) is native to North America (var. *americanum*, but very rare), and parts of Europe and Asia. The species' name derives from the resemblance of sori, the clusters of sporangia, to the tropical centipede *Scolopendra*. Ontario has the densest occurrence of this fern in North America, with over one hundred sites reported.

The common name originates from Europe, where mature red male deer were known as harts in medieval times. The name refers to the long, strap-like fronds that unfurl and look like extra-long tongues. Other common names are hind's tongue, fox tongue, cow's tongue (Ireland), buttonhole, horse tongue, god's hair, and *lingua cervina* (deer's tongue), a name found in older apothecaries.

The fern contains thiaminase, tannins, flavonoids such as kaempferol, mucilage, and the invert sugar saccharose.

The unfurled fiddleheads of this fern were copied as a pattern for the necks of violins.

The Greek physician and pharmacologist Pedanius Dioscorides recommended drinking the fern in wine for snakebite and as an infusion for diarrhea and dysentery (De Materia Medica III.121). The 15th century *Herbarius Latinus* suggested decoctions be taken for forty days to dissolve spleen blockages.

Fuchs's (1543) (see Dobat and Dressendorfer 2001) woodcut articulates the small, serrated indents along the edge of the frond. The name *spleenwort* is so named because when the body retains too much dampness (according to Traditional Chinese Medicine) the tongue swells and becomes serrated from imprints of the teeth. Fuchs noted "Therefore those who have a spleen disease should use this herb often and industriously." The sori on the underside of the frond are also considered a representation of the doctrine of signatures for the spleen.

William Coles (1657), the famed English herbalist, also recommended spleenwort for enlarged or hardened spleen in humans and animals. In Wales and the Highlands of Scotland, a frond ointment is used for burns, scalds, and hemorrhoids. John Pechet (1694) noted "the powder of it is of excellent use for the Palpitation of the heart, for Mother Fits, and Convulsions, being taken in small beer and Posset-drinks."

The fern decoction was considered useful for Bright's disease (nephritis) and given in combination with goldenseal for diabetes. Grieve (1931) noted its use to remove obstructions of the liver and spleen, and to remove urinary gravel. She also mentioned that "an ointment is made of its fronds for burns and scalds and for piles." Other uses included treating gout, clearing eyes, reducing fever, and removing warts and pustules. Decoctions were used as a hair wash and to astringe oily skin or a facial poultice was prepared for delicate skin. The fern was used in Devon and Hebrides for colds and lung congestion, in Wiltshire for warts, and on the Isle of Wight to cool erysipeloid skin eruptions on the legs. In Ireland, an ointment was used for burns and scalds, ringworm, dog and insect bites. In Meath, it was the main ingredient to treat jaundice, and in Wexford in a combination for treating asthma (Allen and Hatfield 2004).

Roy Vickery (1995) reported a Devonshire myth about the fern. The Son of Man used it as a pillow when he needed to lay his head and, in return, left two hairs, which the fern is said to treasure in the stipe. Children search for and find these two auburn hairs.

An extract of the fern reveals itself to be a potent inducer of necrotic cancer cell death (Petkov et al. 2021a).

Hildegard von Bingen, abbess and mystic, wrote,

> Hart's Tongue fern (hirtzunge) is hot, and it is very effective for the liver, lungs, and painful intestines. Therefore, take Hart's-Tongue fern and boil it in wine. Add pure honey and bring it to a boil once again. Then pulverize pepper and twice as much cinnamon, and bring it, with the above-mentioned wine, to a boil once again. . . . It benefits the liver, purges the lungs, heals aching intestines, and carries away internal decay and mucus (Throop 1998).

Culpeper (1652) suggested, "It is a good remedy for the liver, both to strengthen it when weak and ease it when afflicted. . . . It is commended for hardness and stoppings of the spleen and liver, and the heat of the stomach. The distilled water is very good against the passion of the heart, to stay hiccough, to help the falling of the palate, and to stay bleeding of the gums by gargling with it."

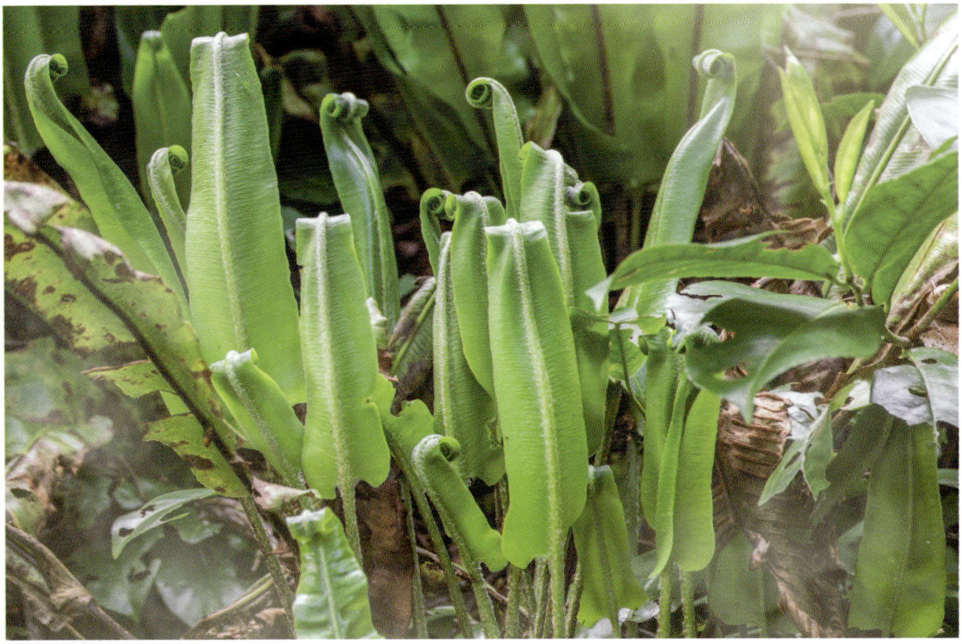

Asplenium scolopendrium (Hart's Tongue Fern)

Over four hundred varieties of Hart's tongue fern were documented and classified during the Victorian era in England.

In the Northern Albanian mountains, the fern is used to treat various respiratory conditions (Pieroni et al. 2005). In Iran, the fern rhizome has been traditionally infused for spleen enlargement, fever, and bronchitis (Bahadori et al. 2015). The rhizomes exhibit significant activity against *Staphylococcus aureus* and *Escherichia coli*.

A screening of vulnerary plants against major oral pathogenic bacteria was conducted by Ferrazzano et al. (2013). The activity against *Streptococcus mutans*, *S. sobrinus*, *Lactobacillus casei*, and *Actinomyces viscosus* was evaluated. The fern was identified as one of five plants showing activity against cultured gingival fibroblasts. Both *Streptococcus mutans* and *S. sobrinus* bacteria are implicated in dental caries. The latter bacteria use a novel protein, enolase, to suppress the antibody response and help them survive and colonize. Pre-treatment of mice with enolase suppressed a primary immune response against T-cell dependent antigen. Enolase stimulated early production of IL-10, an anti-inflammatory cytokine, but not IFN-γ, a pro-inflammatory cytokine (Veiga-Malta et al. 2004). This suggests enolase is an immune suppressive protein. The enzyme inhibits cholesteryl ester hydrolases and is regulated by liver X receptors (de Boussac et al. 2015).

Actinomyces viscosus is part of the normal flora of the human oropharynx. In rare cases, however, it can develop biofilm, cause endophthalmitis after cataract surgery, endocarditis in organ transplant patients, and resemble lung cancer.

The homeopathic preparation is used for sinus complaints, as well as cancer of the mouth and hard palate.

Creeping spleenwort (*Asplenium serra*) extract contains the xanthone mangiferin. The fern exhibits high antichemotactic (94.06%) and antioxidant activity (Andrade et al. 2014).

Mangiferin possesses antioxidant, antimicrobial, antidiabetic, anti-allergic, anticancer, hypocholesterolemic, and immune-modulating activities. It protects against various human cancers, including lung, colon, breast, and neural cancers, by suppression of TNF-α expression and apoptosis. Specifically, it protects against neural and breast cancers by suppressing MMP-9 and MMP-7 and activating the β-catenin pathway (Imran et al. 2017).

Mole ladder fern (*Asplenium sibiricum* syn. *Diplazium sibiricum*) should not be confused with the American walking fern (*Asplenium rhizophyllum* syn. *Camptosorus rhizophyllus*). Mole ladder fern is used in herbal medicine for vasculitis and cancerous tumors. Water extracts of the fern prevent lung tumorigenesis by reducing reactive oxygen species (ROS) and DNA damage, suggesting benefits in lung carcinoma (He et al. 2018).

Asplenium singaporianum fronds were decocted and used to stop hemorrhaging after childbirth in Malaya (Burkill 1966; May 1978).

Maidenhair spleenwort (*Asplenium trichomanes*) was traditionally used for coughs and is found in temperate zones on all continents except Antarctica.

The Cherokee prepared the fern for irregular menstruation and liver complaints. An infusion was taken for coughs, "breast disease," and "acrid humors" (Moerman 1986). The Haida (Skidegate) name *sil tl' xida* means "leaf that shakes its hands." The ethnobotanist Newcombe recorded *snaaljang* or *snaaljaang* as other names for *Asplenium* ferns (Newcombe 1897). Fern Woman, *snanjang jaad*, is mentioned by Swanton (1905) as a mythical superpower. When the roots are used for medicine, they are called snanjang k'ul by elders. The fern was also called *sgaana jaad xad.dalaa*, meaning "little killer-whale women" or "little spirit women."

Grieve (1931) noted that the fern is demulcent, sweet, mucilaginous, and expectorant. "In Arran, the fronds have been dried and used as a substitute for tea; it acts as a laxative." The Isle of Arran, found off the West Coast of

Scotland, is known for this use. In Ireland, a cough remedy known as "maidenhair" was very popular in Londonderry. It was boiled with honeysuckle and oatmeal and taken for dysentery in Cavan (Allen and Hatfield 2004).

In the mountains of Central-Southern Italy, the fern has been traditionally used to regulate menstruation (Guarrera et al. 2008). A decoction of the frond (two to three teaspoons) is used for abscesses of the uterus, while a teaspoon of the dried fronds is taken orally for a week to promote menstruation.

A medieval skeleton dating back to the 9th or 10th century was found on the Spanish Balearic Islands with residue of this fern in dental calculus. Herbal texts suggest possible uses for skin conditions, urinary tract issues (kidney stones), or as a respiratory decongestant (Fiorin et al. 2018).

The fronds of *Asplenium trichomanes*, locally referred to as guewtheer, from the Western Himalayas are used to treat jaundice (Khoja et al. 2022). The rachis is used as a toothpick and employed after ear piercing for a week before the earrings are permanently placed. In parts of India, the fern is known locally as *do patiya chhoti*.

In Europe, the fern has traditional ethnopharmacological usage as an expectorant, cough suppression, laxative, emmenagogue, and for irregular menses and as an abortifacient. Frond infusions, decoctions, and methanol extracts were tested for in vitro estrogenic activity by Dall'Acqua et al. (2009). Both infusions and methanol extracts exhibit activity against MCF-7 (breast cancer) model. Various compounds were identified and exhibited selective activation of the estrogen receptor β.

Polyphenols extracted from the fern through cold methanol maceration revealed the presence of the flavanol hyperoside and phenolic chlorogenic acid. The extract is neither cytotoxic nor phototoxic but may be useful for health applications associated with skin health (Farràs et al. 2022). However, work by Petkov et al. (2021a) found that an extract from the fern appears to be a potent inducer of necrotic cell death.

Further research found that the fern extract's production of contractions in rat gastric smooth muscle tissue was significantly reduced by atropine, an antagonist of muscarinic receptors, and turned into relaxation by galantamine. After combined pre-treatment with galantamine and L-arginine, the relaxation was more pronounced. The dominant contraction is initiated by inhibition of acetylcholinesterase, and relaxation develops with pre-inhibited acetylcholinesterase and is significantly potentiated by L-arginine. This is associated with the nitrergic signaling pathway (Petkov et al. 2021b).

The fern contains the tyrosinase inhibitor 4-ethenylphenyl 6-O-(6-deoxy-a-L-mannopyranosyl)-β-d-glucopyranoside. The whole fern contains volatile compounds with an oily or waxy odor. The fougère scent in perfumery is based on the green odor.

Green spleenwort (*Asplenium viride*) from the Western Himalayas is locally referred to as *lakitguewtheer* and its fronds are used to treat sunburn (Khoja et al. 2022).

Asplenium yoshinagae var. *planicaule* is also known in India as *do patiya badi*. The fresh rhizome paste is mixed with milk and given orally to females affected with gonorrhea three times daily for a week (Panda et al. 2011).

ATHYRIUM

Japanese Painted Fern   Lady Ferns

Geographic Range: China, Eastern Asia, Sino-Himalayan regions, Western Pacific islands, Europe, Japan, Northeastern China, Pacific Northwest (U.S.), South Korea, Tlingit regions, Vancouver Island (Canada), Yukon/Alaska

Habitat: cedar and alder trees, Pacific Northwest rainforests, skunk cabbage wetlands

Practical Uses: compost degradation, cosmetics, food, tea, wine preservation

Medicinal Applications: anti-HIV potential, anti-inflammatory, antibacterial, antifungal, antihyperglycemic, antimicrobial, antioxidant, antiparasitic, asthma, cholera, coughs, expectorant, fever, frequent urination, immune system, kidney, pain, breast milk, mastitis, pain, pneumonia prevention, rheumatic fever, scorpion stings, sores, tuberculosis, ulcers, UV protection, vomiting of blood, wounds

Warning: Induction of female infertility or premature delivery by some species.

The *Athyrium* genus is composed of more than 230 fern species, mainly endemic to Sino-Himalayan regions and western Pacific Islands. The genus name derives from the Greek *athyros*, meaning “doorless,” referring to the late opening of the indusium (the membrane covering the sori of the frond).

The ferns have long been traditionally used for a variety of ailments, including cough, rheumatic fever, scorpion stings, sores, burns and scalds, intestinal fever, pain (specifically breast pain), low breast milk production, parasites, and as digestive carminatives.

An excellent review of the fern properties by Salehi et al. (2018) is worth reading. Although *Athyrium multidentatum* (see page 68) is the most studied, many species demonstrate antimicrobial, anti-inflammatory, antioxidant, antiproliferative, and anti-HIV potential.

Extracts of southern lady fern (*Athyrium asplenioides*) exhibit radical scavenging potential (antioxidant), antifungal activity against four *Candida* species, and induces antihyperglycemic activity (Wadaan et al. 2023).

Northern lady fern or lady in red (*Athyrium filix-femina* var. *angustum*) was a traditional remedy used by Indigenous healers of Eastern North America for intestinal fevers, vomiting of blood, and to prevent water breaking too early during pregnancy.

The Chippewa (Anishinaabe) call the fern *a'sawan* and used a tea combination for anuria or stoppage of urine flow (Densmore 1928). Four root lobes of stinging nettle were added to decoctions as a vermifuge. Some Indigenous tribes use root tea to stimulate breast milk production during mastitis. The Ojibwa (Anishinaabe) infused the rhizome as a tea to induce milk flow in women with caked breast (Moerman 1986).

The Potawatomi call the fern *nonagon-a-wusk*, meaning "milkweed," in reference to this usage. They also used rhizome infusions for the same purpose. The Ojibwa grated the dry rhizomes and used the powder on skin sores and the Iroquois combined the fern rhizomes of *ies-ka-ron-ioka* with New England aster (*Athyrium novae-angliae*) for intestinal fever, and *Rhus typhina* for frequent urination.

Tea made from the stalk was given to ease back pain associated with labor, and root powder was dusted on skin ulcers. The Fox (Meskwaki) decocted the rhizome to cure pain in women's breasts due to childbirth.

Western lady fern (*Athyrium filix-femina* var. *cyclosorum*) grows up to two meters tall in parts of the rainforests of the Pacific Northwest. The Yupik (Chugach) of Yukon/Alaska call it *kun'aq* or *kun'aqutaq* and prize it for its edible roots. Similarly, the Tlingit name is *kw'álx*, meaning "fern with edible root" (Turner 2014). The Lime Village Tanaina of Alaska boiled lady fern for kidney trouble and asthma. The Haida refer to it as *ts'aagul* and *saagwaal* or perhaps *jáadaa sáagwaal* (woman's fern) (Turner 2004). The Wsánec of the Saanich Peninsula on Vancouver Island know it as *leklekā*. It grows among

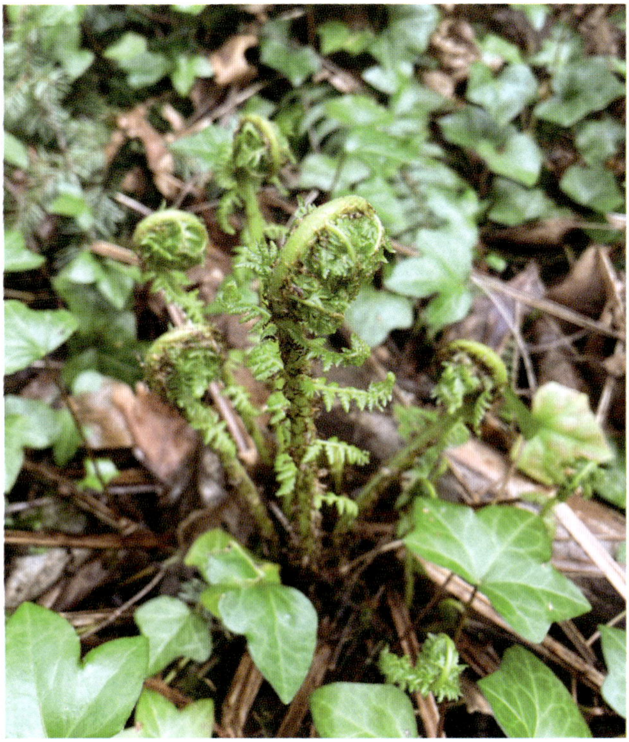

Athyrium filix-femina
(Lady Fern)
Photo by Drew T. Henderson

skunk cabbage under western red cedar and red alder trees. An alternate name is *leq'leq'éy*. The fiddlehead tea was used to treat tuberculosis (Turner and Hebda 2012).

The Coast Salish ate the new shoots and rhizomes (Moerman 2010). The Dena'ina (Tanaina) call the rhizome *ux*, and the fronds *ux t'una' ux* (Turner 2014). The Quileute of Washington State steam pit roast and peel the yellow-centered rhizome, *tseqwë*, for food. The Makah ate the "bulbs" (on top of the rhizome), and the Klallam ate the new shoots. The Quinault traditionally dug the rhizomes and served them cooked with dried salmon eggs. They called the fern *kuwáalsa* or *tsamxaih*. The Cowlitz decocted the stems and drank the tea to reduce inflammation (Moerman 1986). The upper Cowlitz call it *qálqali*.

The appearance of the lady fern resembling a cedar branch led to the Nlaka'pamux name *kwatkwlp-éke?*. The Stl'atl'imx (Pemberton) called this fern, and possibly others, *xan'q*.

The Makah pounded four stipes of fern, boiled them, and gave the tea to women to ease labor pains (Gunther 1945). "In preparing this medicine the fronds of the fern were stripped from the stalk with a downward motion toward the roots and a prayer was offered that the child would 'slip' as easily as the fronds of the fern were removed." (Densmore 1939).

Indigenous groups of Washington State boiled the stems to halt postpartum hemorrhage, while the Nlaka'pamux in British Columbia used fern infusions to stop vomiting blood. The Klallam believed if the fern was used to cover berries, you will end up with less. They called it *q'enq' an ts' isilch*.

The European lady fern (*Athyrium filix-femina* var. *filix-femina* was widely used on the continent medicinally in former times. Dioscorides noted that the fern could induce female barrenness or cause women to deliver prematurely. He suggested that dried frond powder be applied to old ulcers and used to heal galled necks of oxen and other cattle.

Hildegard von Bingen observed that "Female fern (polypodium) is hot and dry. If a lean person, who is not very sick, ails in his intestines, he should pulverize female fern and a third as much sage. Eating this powder diminishes his humors" (Throop 1998).

Culpeper (1652) wrote "the fern is under the dominion of Mercury. "The roots . . . being bruised and boiled in mead or honeyed water, and drank, killeth both the broad and long worms in the body, and abateth the swelling and hardness of the spleen. . . . The roots bruised and boiled in oil, or hog's grease, make a very profitable ointment to heal wounds or pricks gotten in the flesh."

K'Eogh (1735) repeated Culpeper's treatise but added that around midsummer, the fronds are burned to produce ash for washing linens.

Grieve (1931) notes the medicinal uses are similar to those of male fern but less strong. William Cole, the English herbalist, wrote that "if the Asse be oppressed with melancholy, he eats of the herbe Asplenium [lady fern]."

The rhizome was reported to keep wine in a hogshead from turning sour. During the fern frenzy of the late 1800s, over 300 varieties were cultivated.

Akkarghoda lady fern (*Athyrium hohenackerianum*) contains trans-linalool oxide (furanoid), loliode, phytol, 4,8,12,16-tetramethylheptadecan-4-olide, γ-sitosterol, polypodosaponin, oslandin, glucocaffeic acid, methyl salicylate, triterpenes, ecydysterones (polypodine A and 5-β-hydroxy-ecdysterone), p-aspidin, albaspidin, margaspidin, polystichalbin, methylene-bisapidinol, desaspidin and catechin tannins, including 7-L-arabinofuranoside.

The fern, found in Sri Lanka and India, is most potent before sporulation, showing activity against both gram-positive and gram-negative bacteria (Stetsenko et al. 1984). Ecdysterones are most concentrated when the fern first emerges. Work by Bahadori and colleagues (2015) reported the decocted rhizome being traditionally used for intestinal parasites. The rhizomes were found to exhibit moderate activity against *Staphylococcus aureus*.

Loliode has strong antioxidant and anti-inflammatory activity both in vitro and in vivo, and its photoprotective activity may be useful in cosmeceutical products, which combine cosmetic and pharmaceutical benefits. The compound has been isolated from *Sargassum horneri* (brown seaweed).

Ethanol extracts of this fern are cytotoxic and induce apoptosis in breast, lung, and colon cancer cell lines (Elasbali et al. 2022). Gamma sitosterol inhibits MCF-7 (human breast) and A549 (human lung) cancer cell lines through growth inhibition, cell cycle arrest, and apoptosis (Sundarraj et al. 2012).

The fronds are used as an expectorant and possess choleric activity. The main volatile compounds in the fern are 2-phenylethananl (lilac and hyacinth-like) and 1-octen-3-ol (mushroom-like). Traditional recipes suggest ten to twenty drops of frond tincture as needed for digestive benefits.

Athyrium mesosorum syn. *Rhachidosorus mesosorus* contains compounds that inhibit xanthine oxidase, suggesting possible benefits in treating gout (Noro et al. 1984). Its native range include China, where it is known as *zhou guo jue*, as well as South Korea and Japan.

Multi-toothed lady fern (*Athyrium multidentatum*) has fronds that are widely used as an edible vegetable in Northeastern China.

Extracts of this fern possess strong antioxidant activity and show cytotoxic activity against HepG2 (liver) cancer cell lines (Qi et al. 2015; 2017). Not only do the extracts significantly suppress tumor growth, but they also evoke oxidative stress and apoptosis. Aerial parts of the fern, extracted with ethanol, are anti-inflammatory and reduce LPS-induced acute lung injury by inhibiting nitric oxide and PGE2. By suppressing TLR4 signaling, this fern may help prevent pneumonia caused by microbial infection. The effects of a 10 mg/kg extract are similar to the positive control, dexamethasone (Han et al. 2018).

The compound striatisporolide (a butanolide metabolite) damages the cell wall and membrane of *Escherichia coli* (Sheng et al. 2019). Stratisporolide A exhibits significant cytoproliferative and minor cytoprotective effects on human umbilical vein endothelial cells (HUVECs). The authors suggest the mechanisms involve interference with reactive oxygen species (ROS) generation and cell apoptosis (Liu et al. 2016).

Polysaccharides derived from the fern rhizome attenuate D-galactose-induced oxidative stress and cell apoptosis by activating the PI3K/AKT pathway in an aging mouse model (Jing et al. 2019). Aging in humans is associated with several factors such as oxidative stress, telomere erosion, DNA damage, and oncogenic activation. Excessive D-galactose may induce the formation of reactive oxygen species (ROS) via oxidative metabolism and advanced glycation end products. Chronic administration for six to ten weeks can cause deterioration of cognitive and motor function in mice and is considered a good model of accelerated aging.

Polysaccharide fractions enhance macrophage phagocytosis and promote macrophage proliferation. Increased production of NO, IFN-γ, IL-1β, IL-2, IL-6, and IL-10 suggest immune enhancement (Wang et al. 2022c).

The Japanese painted fern (*Athyrium niponicum*) is popular among gardeners and was named the Perennial Plant Association's 2004 Perennial Plant of the Year. The fern exhibits antiviral activity in vitro (Mizushina et al. 1998).

Eared lady fern (*Athyrium oblitescens*), previously known as *Athyrium otophorum*, is native to Eastern Asia. It has beautiful burgundy to raspberry-colored stems, with lime green fronds that mature into a blue-tinged, ashy medium green (Weinstein 2020).

The decaying fern (*Athyrium wallichianum* syn. *A. brunonianum*) contains a novel *Sphingobacterium* gram-negative bacterium, proposed as *Sphingobacterium athyrii* sp. nov., which degrades both cellulose and xylan, the predominant polysaccharides found in land plants cell walls (Cheng et al. 2019). This suggests potential applications to enhance compost degradation.

Bisphenol A (BPA), a toxic endocrine disruptor, was investigated for its effects on A549 (lung) carcinoma cells. At higher doses, it exhibits cytotoxicity, but an extract from the alpine lady fern (*Athyrium yokoscense*) protected against bisphenol A cytotoxicity. Both oxidative stress and inflammation were downregulated via ERK1/2 and NF-κB pathways (Lee et al. 2022b). The fern hyperaccumulates cadmium, lead, and arsenic. In Japan, the fern is known as *hebino-negoza*.

The Finnish name for the alpine lady fern *Athyrium distentifolium*, *tunturihiirenporras*, means "field mouse's stair."

AZOLLA

Mosquito Ferns Water Fern

Geographic Range: Asia, Central America, North America (Southern Ontario), South America

Habitat: aquatic environments, freshwater, rice paddies, tropical and subtropical regions

Practical Uses: aquaculture feed (catfish, tilapia), bio-adsorbent for wastewater, bioremediation (phenanthrenes, petroleum hydrocarbons), nitrogen source in rice paddies, potential as nutraceutical products, organic cultivation, potential as functional food, pollution removal, water filter

Medicinal Applications: anti-inflammatory, antimicrobial, antioxidant, cancer, cardioprotective, cytotoxic, hepatoprotective, neuroprotective, osteoblast differentiation, radiation-protective

Warning: There are potential negative liver effects at high doses in broiler chickens.

Water or mosquito ferns (*Azolla species*) are aquatic ferns that possess a symbiotic relationship with cyanobacteria such as *Anabaena azollae*, living in frond cavities.

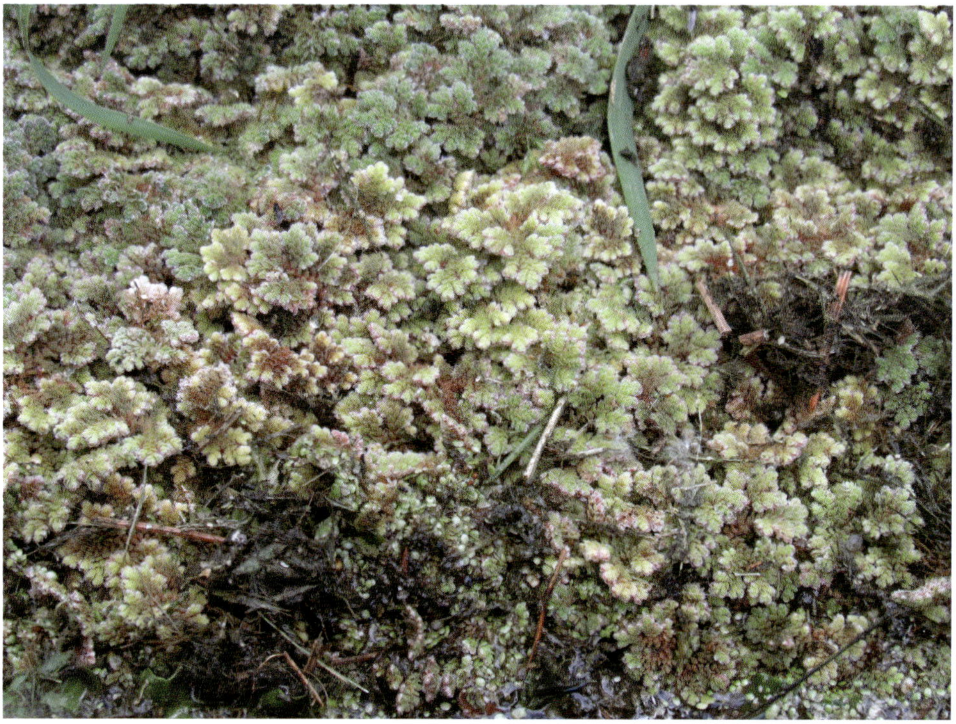

Close-up of *Azolla microphylla* (Mexican Mosquito Fern)
Photo by Drew T. Henderson

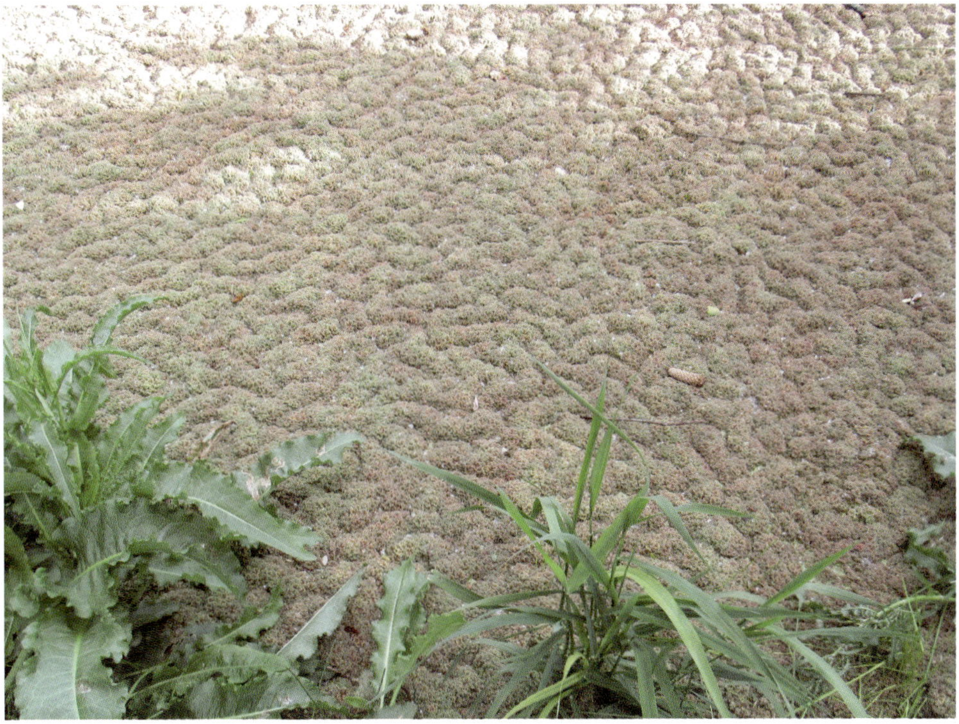

Azolla microphylla (Mexican Mosquito Fern)
in the Background
Photo by Drew T. Henderson

This relationship allows for rapid growth and the production of nitrogen, enabling the ferns to cover water surfaces quickly by doubling in mass every few days.

There are seven species worldwide, including the large mosquito fern (*Azolla filiculoides*) and the Mexican mosquito fern (*Azolla cristata*), both of which are widely used in Asia for rice cultivation because the ferns release nutrients into the water that enhance the growth of rice plants.

The fern extract contains peonidin-3-O-glucoside, vitexin, rutin, thiamine, choline, tamarixetin, hyperoside, astragalin, and quercetin. Peonidin-3-O-glucoside inhibits cancer growth, improves liver health, suppresses inflammation, and increases osteoblast differentiation. Numerous citations in PubMed highlight its various benefits.

Vitexin exhibits antioxidant, anticancer, anti-inflammatory, antihyperalgesic, and neuroprotective properties. In the latter case, it appears to exert antioxidant activity and antagonism to protein misfolding and aggregation in Parkinson's disease. Vitexin also acts as an inhibitor of monoamine oxidase B

(MAO-B), an enzyme that increases striatal dopamine levels (Mustapha and Taib 2023).

Tamarixetin (a quercetin metabolite) has been well researched, showing benefits in preventing allergic inflammatory diseases, antibacterial activity including the prevention of sepsis, protection against cardiac hypertrophy, anti-cancer effects (e.g. liver, and leukemia), and enhancement of antiplatelet effects. Research by Stainer and colleagues (2019) found that tamarixetin exhibits anti-thrombotic activity and that, in combination with aspirin, may be a good strategy for stroke prevention.

There are over 450 citations in PubMed on the health benefits of astragalin. A paper by Riaz et al. (2018) notes its various pharmacological benefits, including anti-inflammatory, antioxidant, neuroprotective, cardioprotective, anti-obesity, anti-osteoporotic, anticancer, anti-ulcer, and antidiabetic potential.

All this combined evidence suggests enormous potential to cultivate the fern organically for functional food and nutraceutical products. Asian rice farming makes use of this nitrogen-rich fern by inoculating paddies with *Azolla*, releasing nitrogen to the crops as the fern decomposes. Catfish and tilapia can also be fed the ferns in an aquaculture system.

It is speculated that around fifty million years ago, the Arctic Ocean was a large warm lake, perfect for *Azolla* growth. As the thick bundles died and sank to the bottom over a million years, they took the carbon from the atmosphere, cutting carbon dioxide levels in half and creating an oxygen-rich atmosphere. The reduction in CO_2 may have contributed to cooler climates, ice ages, and today's atmospheric conditions. Maybe.

It appears that increased carbon dioxide levels from fossil fuels are influencing today's climate change crisis. The ferns also filter gray water, are edible, and can be used as immune protectors in raising tilapia.

Azolla caroliniana is the smallest fern on the planet (Patel and Reddy 2018). It is a freshwater aquatic fern found in Southern Ontario and southward into Central and South America. It is suggested that it may be a type specimen of *Azollla filiculoides*.

Methanol extracts of these two ferns exhibit moderate antimicrobial activity against *Geotrichum candidum*, *Enterococcus faecalis*, and *Klebsiella pneumonia*, as well as antioxidant and anti-inflammatory activities. *Azolla caroliniana* exhibits higher cytotoxicity against HepG2 (hepatoma) cells compared to *Azolla filiculoides* (Rahman et al. 2023).

Geotrichum candidum is a common yeast that colonizes human skin, the respiratory tract, and the gastrointestinal tract. It is also used as a culture in cheese making, brewing, and various fermented milk products. The yeast has been the subject of over 6,500 scientific papers from 2017–2022. Despite its uses, it can cause geotrichosis, especially in individuals with neoplasms, leukosis, HIV infection, diabetes mellitus, or following kidney transplants, and is rarely involved in urinary tract infections (Bilman and Yetik 2017).

The mosquito fern (*Azollla filiculoides*) removes pollutants from dairy wastewater, making it an efficient, inexpensive, and affordable bio-adsorbent (Hosseini et al. 2021).

Phenanthrenes, found in members of the orchid family, are used synthetically in dyes, plastics, pesticides, drugs, and explosives. The freshwater fern is highly effective in remediating phenanthrene pollution (Kösesakal and Seyhan 2023). Earlier work by Kösesakal et al. (2016) found that the fern phytoremediates petroleum hydrocarbons (crude oil) in contaminated fresh water sources.

Mosquito fern (*Azolla imbricata*) is used in Traditional Chinese Medicine, though little was known of its compounds until recent work by Qian et al. (2020). The research team identified ninety-three compounds including derivatives of chlorogenic acid, flavonoids, cinnamoyl tyrosine, cinnamic acid derivatives, fatty acids, coumarins, and lignans. Sixty-four of these compounds, including the newly discovered brainin D, exhibit antioxidant activity.

Ethanol extracts of the fern protect against lead-induced hepatotoxicity in rats (Elrasoul et al. 2020). The compound 3,4,5-O-tricaffeoylquinic acid relieves inflammation and exhibits radiation-protective benefits, potentially aiding clinical radiotherapy (Liu et al. 2022a).

Azolla leaf meal (ALM) (5%) improved broiler chicken growth performance. A 10% addition created negative liver effects, but up to 45% inclusion showed no adverse reactions and reduced production costs by over 30% (Abdelatty et al., 2021; Al-Shwilly 2022).

The fern can replace sunflower meal protein in dairy goats, rabbits, and potentially humans as a functional food, containing significant protein, vitamin B12, and growth promoters (El-Fadel et al. 2020).

BLECHNUM

Alpine Water Fern
Brazilian Blechnum
Centipede Fern
Deer Fern
Hammock Fern
Hard Fern
Little Hard Fern
Mountain Hard Fern
Palm Leaf Fern
Star Fern
Swamp Fern
Toothed Midsorus Fern
Wedge Water Fern

Geographic Range: Brazil, Central and South America, Chile, China, Europe, Fiji, India, Malaysia, New Zealand, Pacific Northwest, Papua New Guinea, United States

Habitat: aquatic environments, forests, freshwater regions, temperate and tropical climates, wetlands

Practical Uses: bio-remediation (PAHs), fish slime removal, nutraceutical products, perfume, skin care, survival food

Medicinal Applications: anti-inflammatory, anti-cancer, anticonvulsant, antidepressant, antidiabetic, antimicrobial, antioxidant, antiparasitic, antithrombotic, anxiolytic, cardioprotective, cytotoxic, flu, hepatoprotective, MAO-A inhibition, nematocidal, neuroprotective, sedative, typhoid treatment, urinary infections

Warning: The fern genus is a bio-absorbent of harmful chemicals such as PAHs, so caution is advised for food use. It may also induce sterility.

The genus *Blechnum* is composed of approximately 236 species, widespread in tropical regions of the world, with a few found in all parts of Europe and in the Pacific Northwest of North America.

Various *Blechnum* species are used in Traditional Chinese Medicine (TCM), ayurvedic medicine, and Mapuche medicine, the traditional medicine in Chile. Globally, various species have been used for typhoid, urinary infections, influenza, wounds, pulmonary complaints, blisters, boils, and anthelmintic infections. Over ninety compounds have been identified in *Blechnum* species to date, including chlorogenic and blechnic acid, anthocyanidins, steroids, flavonols, flavones, lignans, fatty acids, phytosterols, sesquiterpenes, aldehydes, and carotenoids.

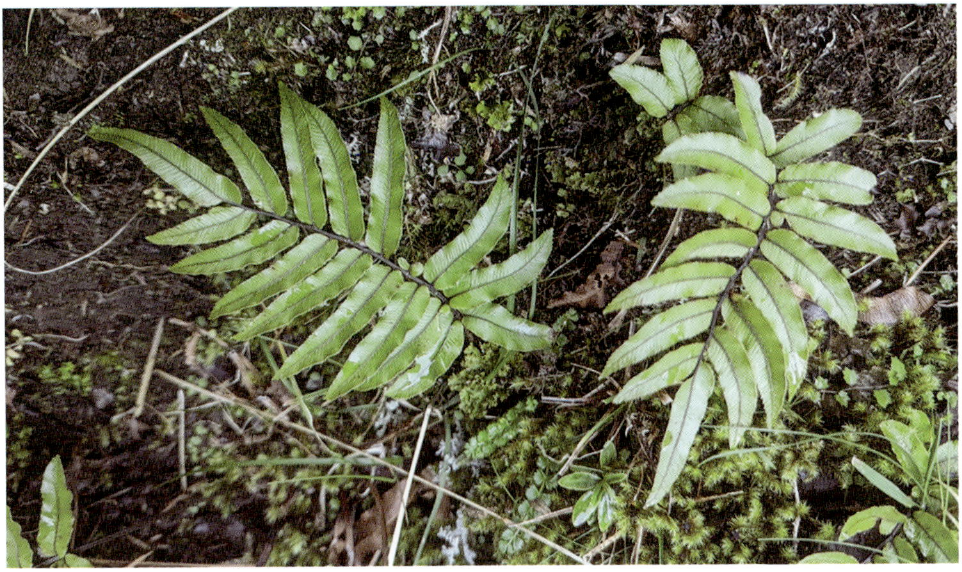

Blechnum montanum (Mountain Kiokio)
Photo by Alan Rockefeller

Blechnum binervatum contains neophytadiene, a compound with anti-anxiety, antidepressant, anticonvulsant, and sedative properties, possibly acting through the GABAergic system (Gonzalez-Rivera et al. 2023). Neophytadiene is also found in algae and the seaweed *Sargassum polycystum*. Neophytadiene exhibits activity against *Bacillus cereus* (Ngobeni et al. 2020) and is also present in alder (*Alnus nitida*) leaves and fruit, as well as in anise, pennyroyal, and dill essential oils.

This compound may inhibit biofilm formation associated with multidrug-resistant pathogens involved in difficult foot ulcer infections (Mashamba et al. 2022). The fern has been shown to exhibit MAO-A inhibition.

Brazilian blechnum (*Blechnum brasiliense*) exhibits antioxidant activity and MAO-A inhibition (de Mello Andrade et al. 2017) and contains chlorogenic and rosmarinic acids. Rosmarinic acid inhibits neuroinflammation in neurodegenerative diseases, based on a study with zebrafish brain tissue (Fasolo et al. 2021). Combining rosmarinic acid and its derivates with antibiotics could enhance their efficacy against drug-resistant microbes (Kernou et al. 2023).

Star fern (*Blechnum fluviatile*) contains the pungent tasting compound polygodial with antifungal, antibacterial, anti-inflammatory, anticancer (human prostate cells), antiparasitic, and anti-allergenic properties.

STAR FERN ESSENCE

This essence of *Blechnum fluviatile* facilitates healing, peace, and stillness at the soul level, after experiences of trauma or deep sorrow that have impacted the soul and are locked into cellular memory. Use in everyday situations where one's 'reality is influenced by external opinions or media such as television advertising. This essence is beneficial for those who have been brainwashed or programmed to accept a reality contrary to their own experience. Find as First Light Flower Essence of New Zealand No. 42 Star Fern.

Palm leaf fern or *kiokio* (*Blechnum novae-zelandiae* syn. *Parablechnum novae-zelandiae*) contains laminaribioside, a marker compound against which antibodies are found in Crohn's disease patients (Dotan et al. 2006). Its fronds start pink when young and turn dark green with age.

The hammock fern (*Blechnum occidentale*), found from the Southern United States to South America, has been traditionally used in Brazil for various pulmonary ailments, inflammation, and infections of the urinary tract and liver. The fronds contain rosmarinic acid and neophytadiene, both mentioned on the previous page, and are known for their MAO-A inhibitory properties. Its traditional uses for reducing pain and inflammation were confirmed in a mouse study by Nonato et al. (2009).

The centipede fern (*Blechnum orientale* syn. *Blechnopsis orientalis*) is known in TCM as *paku lipan*. Its fronds are traditionally used for intestinal wounds, pulmonary issues, stomach pains, skin disorders (wounds, boils, abscesses), urinary tract infections, and as a contraceptive.

The young shoots are pounded and applied to boils, blisters, sores, and carbuncles while the fronds are ground and mixed into cow's milk for asthma, bacterial infections, intestinal parasites, and to enhance female fertility (Baskaran et al. 2018). In Papua New Guinea, the fern is known as *hastajori*. The new frond leaves are eaten by women twice for three days with a break of two weeks, to induce sterility (Holdsworth 1980; Kumar et al. 2015). The fern's condensed tannins help treat diabetic ulcer wounds. Lai et al. (2016) found fern hydrogels were able to close diabetic wounds by day twelve, on average. Re-epithelization, higher fibroblast proliferation, collagen synthesis, and angiogenesis were all observed.

Various lignans have been found in the fronds including blechnic acid,

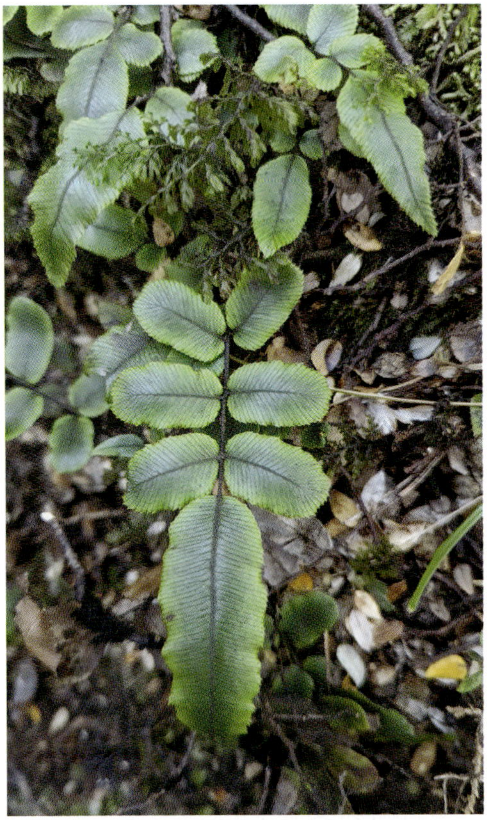

Blechnum procerum (Small Kiokio)
Photo by Alan Rockefeller

7-epiblechnic acid, 8-epiblechnic acid, brainic acid, and flavonols such as quercetin-3,7-digalactoside, quercetin-7-4'digalactoside, querceitin-3,4'diglucoside, and various flavones including lucenin-2.

In India, the fronds are used for urinary bladder issues, the extracted juice is used for intestinal wounds, and the rhizomes for typhoid fever. In China, the rhizomes are used to treat intestinal parasites.

Work by Kalpana et al. (2020) found that the fern extract produced moderate termiticidal activity against the sheep nematode *Gastrothylax crumenifer.*

A U.S. patent has been filed for its use in the treatment of influenza.

In Fiji, the fern is known as *vula walu*. Methanol extracts have higher total phenolic content than vanillic acid and significant α-amylase inhibition, suggesting possible benefits for type 2 diabetes (Mala et al. 2022).

Fatty acids derived from extracts exhibit antimicrobial, anti-inflammatory, antioxidant, anti-ulcer, and nematocidal properties (Devi et al. 2016). The root, leaves, and stems show cytotoxicity to MCF-7 (human breast) cancer cell lines (Aini et al. 2008) and butanol, ethyl acetate, and water extracts show cytotoxicity against colon adenocarcinoma (HT-29), human colon carcinoma (HCT-116), breast carcinoma (MCF-7) and human leukemia (K562) cell lines (Lai et al. 2010).

In the same study, three extracts showed efficacy against *Bacillus cereus*, *Micrococcus luteus*, methicillin-resistant *Staphylococcus aureus* (MRSA) and *Staphylococcus epidermidis*.

A follow-up study by Lai et al. (2017) found that water extracts are active against five gram-positive bacteria and possess selective cytotoxicity against HT-29, and HepG2 (hepatic) cancer cell lines. Activity of four extracts against *Escherichia coli*, *Pseudomonas aeruginosa*, and *Candida albicans* was noted in work by Deepa et al. (2013). The fern also exhibits α-glucosidase inhibition, suggesting possible benefits in treating diabetes (Chai et al. 2015a).

This fern has the ability to absorb harmful chemicals known as polycyclic aromatic hydrocarbons (PAHs) from its surroundings. While this means we should be cautious when using the fern for food medicine, it also opens up possibilities for using the plant to clean up polluted environments (Zhu et al. 2013a). The fern may also be a useful feeding additive to help treat sheep infected with trematode worms.

Alpine water fern or little hard fern (*Blechnum penna-marina*) is a delicate fern found in parts of Chile, New Zealand, Australia, and Pacific Ocean islands. In temperate climates, fern gardeners will use this fern to fill crevices in rock walls or plant between paving stones with little foot traffic. It is easy to cultivate, helping fill in areas near ponds and wet areas.

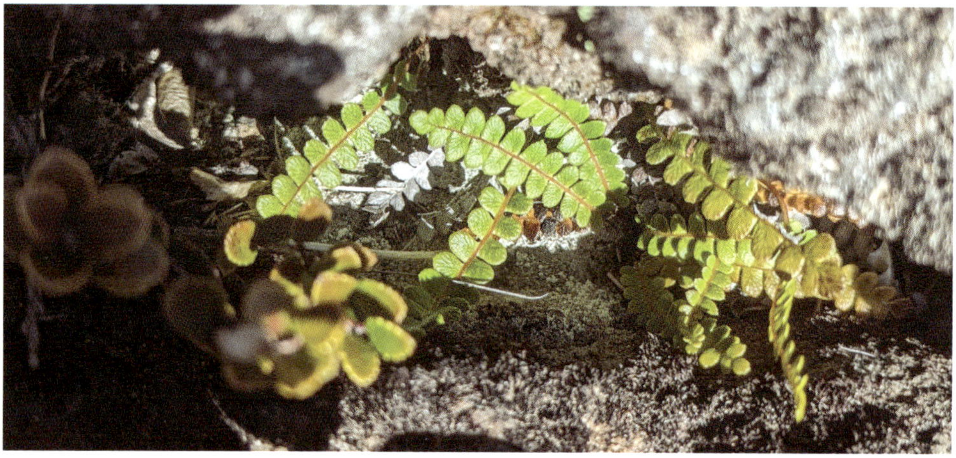

Blechnum penna-marina ssp. *alpina* (Alpine Water Fern)
Photo by Alan Rockefeller

Research by Torres-Benítez et al. (2023) examined four *Blechnum species*, and found this one exhibited the highest levels of phenolics, flavonoids, antioxidant activity, and cholinesterase inhibition.

Swamp or toothed midsorus fern (*Blechnum serrulatum*) rhizome is prepared as an infusion for intestinal worms in French Guiana, and the fronds are applied to skin abscesses (DeFilipps et al. 2004).

In Malaysia, the frond leaflets of hard fern or deer fern (*Blechnum spicantum* syn. *B. spicant* syn. *Struthiopteris spicant*) are chewed to treat internal cancer, lung and stomach complaints, and used externally for skin sores (May 1978). The roots are decocted for diarrhea. Midwives in the Faeroe Islands during the 18th century used the fronds to staunch bleeding during childbirth.

The Indigenous people of Haida Gwaii call the edible rootstock *snaal jaad* (Turner 2004). The Coastal Salish used the rhizome and fronds as emergency food (Turner and Bell 1971) and the Central Salish know the root as *palaʔ*. The Squamish name is similar, *pálapála*. The Quileute know the fern as *kêstola'put*. They boiled the fronds and drank the tea for general ill health and applied a poultice of the fresh fronds to affected parts of the body suffering paralysis (Moerman 1986). Another name, *lak^{w} aʔáa*, means "to wipe," referring to its use for wiping slime from fish. A legend from the tribe involves telling a child when it is lost to look for this fern as food. The Hesquiat peeled the stems and ate the center portion when hungry and nothing else to eat (Moerman 2010). The Nitinaht also considered it a survival food. The Nuu-chah-nulth call the fern *kaatskuuxsmapt*, meaning "standing up plant." The Quinault chewed the raw fronds of *ska'ê êtskl'o* for colic. The neighboring Makah ate the green fronds for respiratory and stomach complaints (Gunther 1945). The Makah call this fern *iʔits'bak'kuk* and placed the ferns under food being cooked to add flavor.

The Kwakiutl made a compound decoction with the rhizome or simply held the fresh or dried rhizome in the mouth for diarrhea (Moerman 1986). The Kwak'wala (Kwakwaka'wakw) call it *k'ak'osam'a*.

Like many ferns, Indigenous groups used these ferns to remove the slime from harvested fish. The Ditidaht call this fern *bibeʔtak'kw apt*, meaning "sockeye-like plant."

The aerial parts contain ethyl vanillate, and (E)-nerolidol sesquiterpene which exhibits anticancer, antioxidant and antimicrobial activity. Various blechnic acids, trans-blechnic acids and brainic acids are also present. Ethyl vanillate cream (20%) was used in a double-blind, placebo-controlled clinical trial on thirty cases of vitiligo patients receiving phototherapy. One group applied the cream or placebo on assigned lesion twice daily for three months. There was a significant change in pigmentation after applying ethyl vanillate compared to the placebo (Namazi and Shotorbani 2015).

The main volatile compounds in this fern are 2-phenylethananl (lilac and hyacinth-like) and 1-octen-3-ol (mushroom-like) and are valued as absolutes in fougère perfume blends.

The fronds of wedge water fern or mountain hard fern (*Blechnum vulcanicum*) contain phytoecdysteroids, including ecdysone, ponasterone, and shidasterone. Ecdysterones and ecdysteroids are naturally occurring anabolic steroids used to enhance physical performance without predictable side effects.

A ten-week clinical trial by Isenmann et al. (2019) of young men involved in strength training found significant increases in muscle mass when consuming these compounds. In contrast, illegal anabolic steroids such as clenbuterol, stanozolol, and metandienone, can cause severe health issues including supraventricular tachycardia, atrial fibrillation, hypotension, chest pain, myocardial injury, myocarditis, myocardial infarction, cardiomyopathy, hepatomegaly, hyperglycemia, and death (Kumari et al. 2023).

BOTRYCHIUM

Grape Ferns   Moonwort   Rattlesnake Fern

Geographic Range: China, North America, Newfoundland, New England, Nova Scotia, West Mabou Beach

Habitat: areas with mycorrhizal fungi for symbiosis, environments with sunlight and shade

Practical Uses: food

Medicinal Applications: abscesses, asthma, labor pain, tongue, boils, bronchial asthma, chronic cough, diuretic, dysentery, ears, eyes, expectorant, febrile convulsive twitch disease, headaches, immune modulation, kidney health, lunacy, memory, promoting labor, snakebites, soothing the central nervous system, stomach issues, tuberculosis, vomiting induction, whooping cough, wounds

Warning: Potential for moonwort poisoning associated with organ dysfunction and rhabdomyolysis, caution with ingestion due to toxicity of certain species of grape ferns.

The genus name *Botrychium* derives from the Greek *botrus*, meaning "cluster of grapes," referring to the fruiting structure. Thus, these are commonly known as grape ferns.

Grape ferns are intriguing due to their prolific progeny despite their small size, with almost half the fern being small, buoyant spores. The spores are light and germinate when they sense a month or more of darkness in their new environment. The gametophyte has only a few days or weeks to attach to a symbiotic fungus for nutrition, making the fern a mycoparasite. When the first fronds finally emerge to photosynthesize, the relationship with the fungus does not end. In fact, in times of stress the fern may go underground for years, subsisting on the mycorrhizal fungi. There are about thirty species of grape ferns in North America. In China, various species are used for asthma and chronic coughs (Li et al. 2020).

Upswept or triangle-lobed moonwort (*Botrychium ascendens*) is generally found in Western North America, with a few extant species in Newfoundland, New England, and on West Mabou Beach in Nova Scotia. Its rarity in these regions may contribute to conservation efforts, such as preventing the construction of golf courses.

There have been four documented cases of moonwort poisoning associated with organ dysfunction and rhabdomyolysis, a condition where damaged muscle tissue releases toxins into the bloodstream, potentially leading to kidney failure. All patients recovered after treatment (Li et al. 2020).

Woolly grape fern (*Botrychium lanuginosum*) contains compounds including sucrose, luteolin-7-O-glucoside, β-sitosterol, apigenin, daucosterol, thunberginol A, luteolin, and various glucosides. Daucosterol inhibits cell proliferation and induces cell cycle arrest and apoptosis in prostate cancer cells (Gao et al. 2019). This effect is mediated through the activation of JNK signaling. Daucosterol also suppresses dextrate sulphate sodium-induced colitis in mice by increasing natural killer cell activity and inhibiting excessive IgA levels (Jang et al. 2019).

Thunberginol A may be effective against type 1 and type IV allergies (Yamahara et al. 1995) and exhibits antimicrobial activity against oral bacteria. It suppresses B and T lymphocyte activation, contributing to its effectiveness against type IV allergies. Type I allergies are mediated by IgE antibodies and include asthma, rhinitis, and dermatitis. Type IV allergies involve a delayed cellular response and include food sensitivities, poison ivy, contact dermatitis, and reactions to drugs like allopurinol.

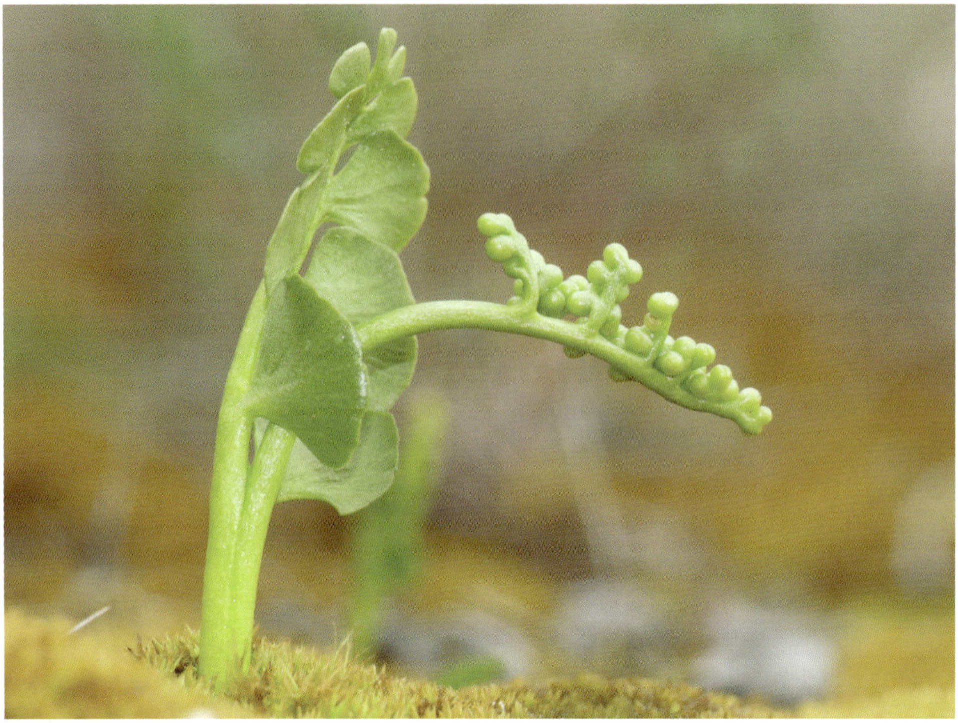

Botrychium lunaria (Moonwort)

I titled my first book *Sundew Moonwort . . . and More Medicinal Plants of Alberta* (1992). I had been recently introduced to moonwort (*Botrychium lunaria*) in a local forest and liked the juxtaposition of Sun and Moon. The large sporangia, resembling a cluster of grapes, made a distinct impression on this young botanist. Lunaria derives from the Latin *luna*, meaning "moon."

In Europe, moonwort was one of many ingredients in witches' salves. "In the Middle Ages moonwort was used as a remedy for abscesses and wounds. A common name for the plant, which grows in mountain meadows, is Walpurgis herb. It is said to assist in finding hidden treasure" (Müller-Ebeling et al. 1998). Other sources suggest it turned quicksilver to pure silver or unlocked any door. Swiss folklore held that carrying the rhizome in the right pocket protected from daggers and bullets.

Moonwort looks similar to the French tea cake *obletje* (*oublie*), meaning "forgetfulness." It is said that a French count, taken prisoner and left unransomed for too long, painted a branch of moonwort and sent it to his estate to reproach them for not securing his freedom (Powell 1979).

Hildegard von Bingen suggested moonwort for issues related to the eyes, ears, and tongue. The ancient Greeks used anointing oil from rue juice and nine drops of dew collected from moonwort for protection.

Nicholas Culpeper (1652) noted, "the Moon owns the herb. Moonwort is cold and drying . . . the leaves boiled in red wine, and drank, stay the immoderate flux of women's courses, and the whites. It also stays bleeding, vomiting and other fluxes. . . . It is good for ruptures, but is chiefly used, by most with other herbs, to make oils or balsams to heal fresh or green wounds."

In Nepal, the fronds are crushed into a paste and applied to ripen boils. In Wales, the fern has been traditionally made into oils, ointments, and balsams for skin wounds, and rubbed onto the kidney region to cure dysentery.

Moonwort is known to the Algonquin as *kanodan*, a magical plant gathered by moonlight. It was used in sorcerer incantations; and by alchemists who gave it credit for converting quicksilver (mercury) to pure silver. The fern was gathered on the full moon for curing lunacy; and is said to wax and wane with the moon. Folklore has it that the leaves always face the Moon, and that moonwort caused the loss of calves in herds. It was believed to have the power to open locks or cause horses to throw shoes.

The doctrine of signatures suggests that the fronds are shaped like a crescent moon (Rogers 2014b).

The Canadian author and historian Barnard Assiniwi (1988) writes that moonwort is considered a panacea among the Algonquin, similar to ginseng in TCM, and suggests it improves memory. Other sources suggest its benefits in soothing the central nervous system.

MOONWORT FERN ESSENCE

This essence of *Botrychium lunaria* is associated with childbirth and supports first-time mothers. Fears projected from the unconscious or even from well-meaning friends can create stress and anxiety about the birthing process.

Moonwort essence helps both mother and fetus trust in the natural rhythms of labor and have faith in the timing of the birth experience. On the physical level, it can alleviate back pain associated with labor and ensure the placenta is fully expelled. This essence is of course prepared under the full moon. This fern is part of my Prairie Deva Essences research line.

Leather grape fern (*Botrychium multifidum* syn. *Sceptridium multifidum*) is noted for its evergreen, leathery, shiny green leaves. The species' name *multifidum* refers to the various segments of the leaf. This fern is known as *bayakhra* in Nepal. A paste of the root was applied to the forehead for headache, as well as blemishes on the tongue. Fresh frond juice was given for stomach trouble.

Botrychium schaffneri has been used in TCM for whooping cough, bronchial asthma, and febrile convulsive twitch disease in young children, a transient fever-induced condition. A fern rhizome ethanol extract reduces the viability of non-small cell lung carcinoma (NCI-H1299) by inducing apoptosis and slowing tumor growth in a nude (hairless) mice study by Liu et al. (2021b).

The related glabrous-ternate grapefern (*Botrychium ternatum*) has been used in TCM for thousands of years, with over thirty compounds, including seventeen flavonoid glycosides.

A water-soluble polysaccharide named BTp1 extracted from this fern was shown to significantly enhance cell viability and promote the release of nitric oxide in RAW264.7 cells, suggesting potential immune modulation (Zhao et al. 2017b).

Rattlesnake fern (*Botrychium virginianum*) is named for its rattlesnake appearance of the gathered sporangia. In Appalachia, the presence of the fern suggests the right conditions for growing ginseng, bloodroot, black cohosh, and other sang* sign root picking.

The fern was a traditional remedy by Indigenous healers of Eastern North America, including the Lenni Lenapes and Iroquois, for tuberculosis-related coughs. The species name *virginianum* means "of Virginia." The Iroquois consumed a cold infusion of the rhizome for (tuberculosis) cough, as did the Ojibwa. The Chippewa (Ojibwa, Anishinaabe) used the fern for snakebites (Densmore 1928). It was also used in a formula for dreaming of snakes, helping one trust their intuition to resolve issues.

A decoction of rattlesnake fern and bark of tulip poplar (*Liriodendron tulipifera*) was applied both externally, to the place where a person dreamt they were bitten, and internally as a tea, which induced ceremonial emesis.

The Cherokee decocted the rhizome to induce vomiting and boiled it down to a syrup that was rubbed on the snakebite (Moerman 1986).

**Sang* is a local term for ginseng used by the regional population.

The Chickasaw originally lived in Northern Mississippi and Alabama, before withdrawing to Oklahoma. They decocted the root as emetic, expectorant, and diaphoretic. They also applied the mashed fresh rhizome to snakebites (Moerman 1986).

"Warm infusions of the fronds induce a gentle and warm perspiration, while at the same time soothing the nervous system, and are mildly diuretic.... The root was decocted by the Fox [tribe] to treat tuberculosis (Rogers 2014b).

BRAOMEA

Braomea insignis exhibits strong antioxidant activity (Ding et al. 2008).

CERATOPTERIS

Floating Antler-fern Water Ferns

Ceratopteris is a genus of aquatic ferns, commonly referred to as water ferns. The genus name *Ceratopteris* may derive from the Greek *kerat*, meaning "horn" and *pteris* meaning "fern" or "wing." The word "cerate" comes from the Latin word *ceratum*, which means "waxed." This water fern effectively sheds water, so I lean toward the latter explanation.

The fern possesses four genes related to MKN6, the gene responsible for controlling the production of sporophytes in mosses. According to Beerling (2019), it acts as a gene silencer, blocking gametophyte development to allow for sporophyte maturation.

In Liberia, water ferns are "cultivated" for food (Hartley 1962).

Floating antler-fern (*Ceratopteris pteridoides*) is a semi-aquatic fern, traditionally used in Northern Columbia as a diuretic and for treating gallstones. Alviz et al. (2013) conducted a rat lab study with ethanol and decocted water extractions, and found significant diuretic, natriuretic, and kaliuretic effects compared to the control. The fern has been shown to tolerate high cadmium levels.

Water sprite or Indian water fern (*Ceratopteris thalictroides*) frond and rhizome are edible, cooked as potherb or eaten raw in sub-Saharan Africa (Maroyi 2014).

The fern contains pterosin A and its derivatives, which help regulate blood sugar homeostasis, protect pancreatic β cells, prevent their death, and reduce reactive oxygen species (Chen et al. 2015).

When fed to diabetic mouse models for four weeks, pterosin A improved hyperglycemia and glucose intolerance, significantly reversing increased serum insulin and insulin resistance. In cultured human muscle cells, the compound enhanced glucose uptake and AMPK phosphorylation (Hsu et al. 2013).

CHEILANTHES

Floury Cloak Fern	Rock Fern
Lip Ferns	Silver Fern
Poison Rock Fern	Wooton's Lace Fern

Geographic Range: Bhutan, Ethiopia, India, Mexico, Nepal, Nigeria, Pakistan, Southwestern United States

Habitat: desert-like environments, dry and sunny areas, higher altitudes, rock crevices

Practical Uses: nasal and ear ornaments, peptic ulcers, pyrexia, stimulant, stomach pain, typhoid fever, wound treatment

Medicinal Applications: anti-adipogenic, anti-inflammatory, anti-proliferative, antioxidant, cytotoxic, immune system, menstruation, pain, stimulant

Warning: Genus toxic to sheep and cattle; contains carcinogenic compounds.

The genus name derives from the Greek *cheilos*, meaning "lip," and *anthos*, meaning "flower." Of course, there are no flowers. About 180 species are presently known worldwide.

The lip ferns (*Cheilanthes* sp.) have evolved to thrive in dry, sunny, desert-like environments. They protect themselves from full sun with woolly hairs, scales, or a waxy cuticle (farina), giving the underside of the frond a whitish-gray appearance.

White-margined lip fern (*Cheilanthes albomarginata* syn. *Aleuritopteris albomarginata*) is found at higher altitudes in India, Nepal, Pakistan, and Bhutan, growing in rock crevices. The juice from the rhizome was traditionally used to treat peptic ulcers.

In Southern Nigeria, the dried, powdered fronds were mixed with ginger rhizome powder to treat infertility in women (Nwosu 2002). Frond extracts have been investigated, and ethyl acetate fractions exhibit the highest in vitro anti-inflammatory and anti-adipogenic activity. An in vivo study on high-fat-diet-induced obese rats found a crude methanol extract lowered plasma triglyceride levels and reduced the weight of adipose tissue (Lamichhane et al. 2014).

Silver lip fern (*Cheilanthes bicolor* syn. *Aleuritopteris bicolor*) leaves and rhizomes are used in India as a stimulant and remedy for preventing fear among children. Young girls use the stems as nasal and ear ornaments (Singh and Upadhyay 2012).

Floury cloak fern (*Cheilanthes farinosa*) is valued by the Gaddis tribe of India. It was traditionally used to treat liver and menstrual issues. Fronds were decocted and taken orally for one week to treat menstrual irregularities. The decoction was also taken for colds and pyrexia, and the rhizome paste applied to wounds and atopic dermatitis. Rhizome tea was consumed internally for stomach pain (Singh et al. 2005). In parts of India, the fern was given for mental disorders. An extract of the washed rhizome, with scales removed, was given to those suffering from epileptic seizures.

A decoction of the fronds was taken orally for a week to treat irregular menstrual cycles (Jain 1991). In Ethiopia, the fronds are used to treat inflammatory disorders and pain.

The methanol extract potentiates the anti-inflammatory activity of acetylsalicylic acid, and in animal studies, it relieved pain better than the drug both early on and later. The content of chlorogenic acid is believed responsible for complete or partial reduction of inflammation and thus provides pain relief (Yonathan et al. 2006).

Chlorogenic acid has been widely researched and is found in numerous edible and medicinal herbs. It primarily relieves pain by increasing antioxidant activity against inflammatory conditions.

Water extracts of this fern exert significant cytotoxicity, anti-proliferative effects, and induce apoptosis in Hep3B (hepatoma) cancer cell lines without causing substantial damage to non-cancerous cells (Radhika et al. 2010).

Cheilanthes fragrans syn. *C. pteridioides* is an evergreen fern traditionally used as tea. It is known in French as *cheilanthes de madere*, in Italian as *felcetta du madera* and *felcetta odorosa*.

Poison rock fern (*Cheilanthes sieberi*) rhizomes were traditionally used in parts of Asia for treating typhoid fever and colds. The fern is toxic to sheep and cattle and contains carcinogenic compounds.

Rock fern (*Cheilanthes tenuifolia*) frond paste was applied to exude pus from skin abscesses. In India, the root and rhizome tea was consumed to improve immune health (Dixit 1989).

Wooton's lace fern (*Cheilanthes wootoni* syn. *Myriopteris wootonii*) is found in the Southwestern United States and Northern Mexico. The Navajo-Ramah of New Mexico call the fern "life medicine" and used cold infusions externally on gunshot wounds (Moerman 1986). Ramah is the English-Biblical name for the reservation. The Navajo call the land *tl'ohchini* meaning "onion grass."

CHRISTELLA

Downy Maiden Downy Wood Fern

Downy maiden or downy wood fern (*Christella dentata*) methanol extracts exhibit antihyperglycemic and antinociceptive activity (Tanzin et al. 2013).

Christella dentata fern is edible but hyperaccumulates arsenic, suggesting potential use in the phytoremediation of contaminated sites. The fern is a traditional skin remedy.

A guinea pig study found feeding the shade-dried fern for 285 days resulted in proliferative urocystica (bladder cancer) and adenoma. Not a surprise!

On the other hand, a study by Chai et al. (2015) found a water extract as toxic as 5-fluorouracil (5-FU) against human chronic myelogenous leukemia (K562) cell lines.

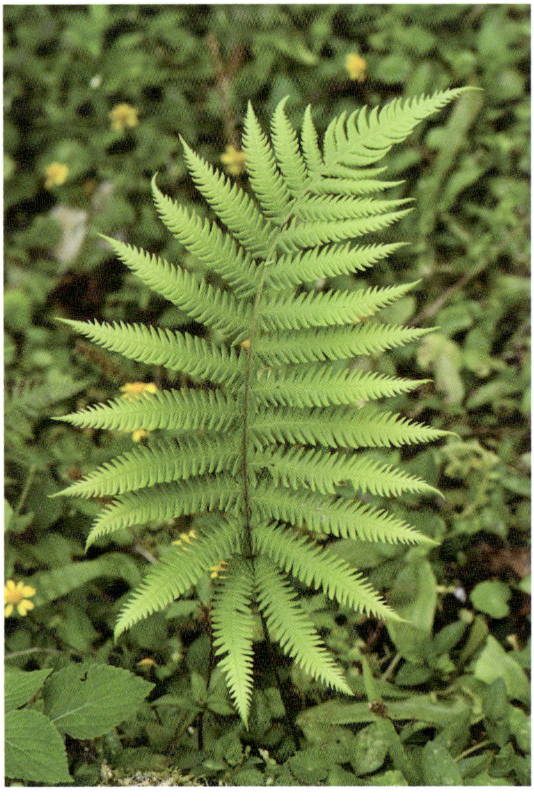

Christella dentata (Downy Fern)
Photo by Alan Rockefeller

CIBOTIUM

Chain Fern
Golden Chicken
Man Fern
Scythian Lamb
Woolly Fern

Geographic Range: China, Indonesia, Malaysia, Taiwan, Thailand, Vietnam, West Indies

Habitat: desert-like environments, dry and sunny areas, forested regions, tropical climates

Practical Uses: cosmetics

Medicinal Applications: antibacterial, anticonvulsant, anti-inflammatory, antioxidant, apoptosis promotion in glioblastoma, blood circulation, bones, cartilage degeneration, cytotoxicity, dysuria, gastric protection, hemorrhage prevention, hepatoprotective, lower back pain, menstruation, neuralgia, osteoarthritis, osteoporosis, peptic ulcers, rheumatism, sarcopenia, sciatica, smooth muscles, tendons, wounds

Warning: Wooly contraindicated in certain cases of dysuria. Listed as an endangered species according to the Convention on International Trade in Endangered Species (CITES).

Woolly fern, Scythian lamb, or chain fern (*Cibotium barometz*) is native to Eastern Asia, including Taiwan, Thailand, and China, and is considered an endangered species.

The genus derives from the Greek *kibotion*, meaning "little chest," or "little box."

The woolly rhizome may have inspired the mythical "Vegetable Lamb of Tartary." *Barometz* may be a Tartar word meaning "lamb," but this is uncertain.

Herodotus, the Greek historian, wrote of trees in India with fruiting wool that the natives used to make clothing.

The myth spread when Sir Hans Sloane found a specimen in a Chinese cabinet in 1698 and surmised the "lamb" was discovered by removing leaves from the woolly rhizome, which, when inverted, appeared as a woolly lamb with legs. The lamb's flesh was said to taste like fish, and the blood tasted like honey.

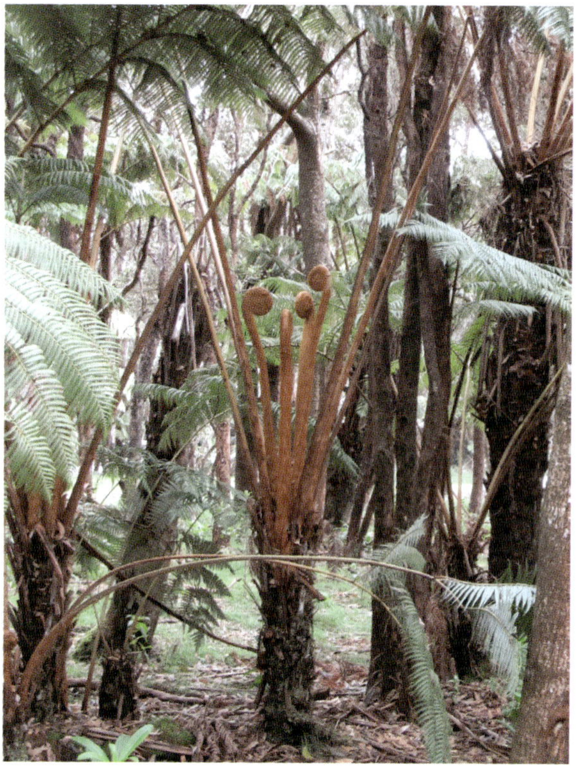

Cibotium sp. (Man Fern)
Photo by Drew T. Henderson

However, the history goes back much further. The myth was first known in the 11th century and appeared on the title page of John Parkinson's famous gardening book *Paradisi in sole paradisus terrestris* (1629), where the vegetable lamb is depicted grazing in the Garden of Eden. John Parkinson was the personal physician to the King of England, but even he was fooled by the ridiculous myth. He notes, "the pulp or meat underneath which is like the flesh of a Creville or Lobster, having as it is said blood also in it."

Jewish folklore called it *yeduah*. The "lamb" was used in predicting the future in several cultures.

Various poems were written of barometz, include Erasmus Darwin's *The Loves of the Plants* (1781) and Gillaume de Salluste du Bartas (1587). Demetrius de la Croix contributed the following verses in *Connubia florum Latino carmine demonstrata* (1791).

For in his path he sees a monstrous birth,
The Barometz arises from the earth
Upon a stalk is fixed a living brute,

A rooted plant bears quadruped for fruit,
. . . It is an animal that sleeps by day
And wakes at night, though rooted in the ground,
To feed on grass within its reach around.

GILLAUME DE SALLUSTE DU BARTAS

The rhizomes of golden chicken or woolly fern (*Cibotium barometz*), known as *gou ji*, are used in TCM to strengthen bones and tendons, when combined with other yang tonic herbs. The fern is part of a formula called The Root of Pregnancy, for infertile women with lower back, knee, or ankle pain, fatigue, and menstrual issues. It is, however, contraindicated in cases of dysuria with scant, yellow or brown-tinged urine, a bitter taste in the mouth, or a dry tongue.

The dried frond powder is used as a styptic for prevention and treatment of hemorrhage from dental extractions. In Malaysia, the fern has been traditionally used for various ailments, including peptic ulcers. In Indonesia and Malaysia, the golden-yellow hair on the rhizome is used in ointments to staunch bleeding. In the West Indies, the ferns are used to stop bleeding (Hare 1916). In Malaysia, a frond infusion is said to cure fainting. In Vietnam, the rhizome is prized for neuralgia, sciatica, lumbago, and rheumatism.

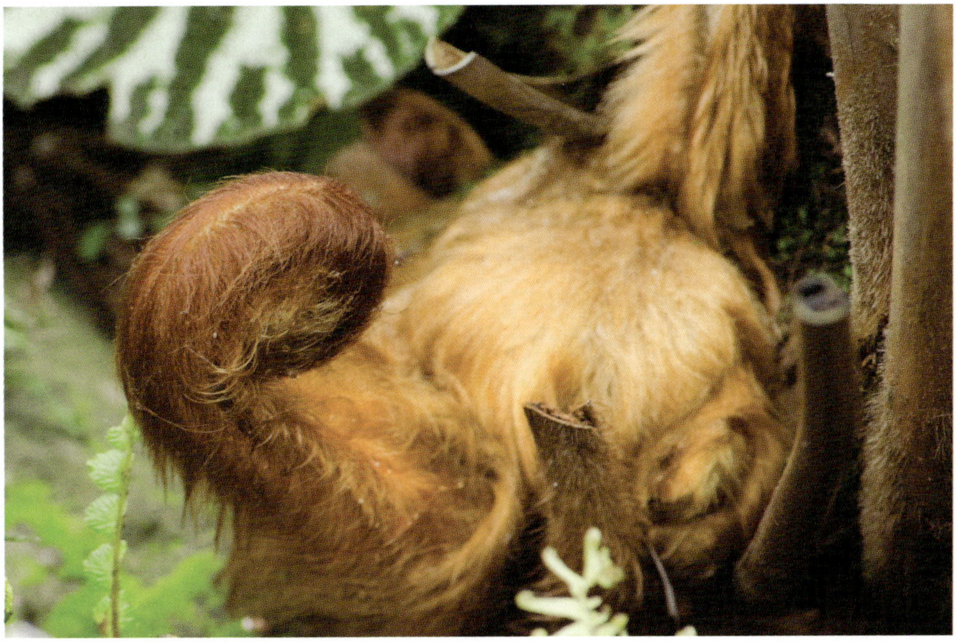

Cibotium barometz (Woolly Fern)

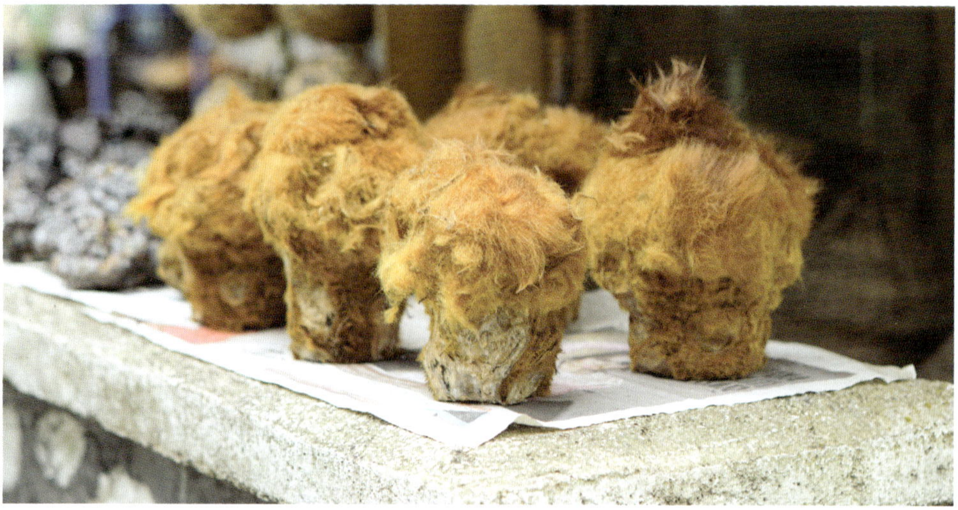

Cultivated *Cibotium barometz* in an Asian Market

The fern rhizome contains two rarely phenolic acid-substituted alloses (glycoses), glucosides and glycoside compounds, β-sitosterol, caffeic acid, daucosterol, alternariol, 5-hydroxymethyl-2-furancarboxaldehyde, (3R)-des-O-methyl lasiodiplodin, protocatechuic acid, n-butyl-β-D-fructopyranoside, palmitic acid, 1-monopalmitin, d-glucose and 30% starch.

Work by Li et al. (2019b) identified four compounds protective against induced HepG2 (hepatic) cell damage, stronger than the positive control, bicycol. Two compounds reduced PC12 (neuroplastic) cell death by serum deprivation. Cuong et al. (2009) identified cibotiumbarosides A and B, and the glycoglycerolipid cibotiglycerol. Three compounds showed inhibition of osteoclasts, suggestive of benefits in treating osteoarthritis and other bone-related conditions. Osteoclasts dissolve old and damaged bone tissue so it can be replaced by newer, healthier tissue created by osteoblasts.

Raw rhizome slices of the fern contribute to osteoblast proliferation in vitro (Xu et al. 2014). Both protocatechuic acid and protocatechuic aldehyde provide similar benefits. It is worth noting that retinoic acid, widely used in female cosmetics, reduces osteoblast mineralization in vitro. A female rat study found that ovariectomy-induced bone loss was prevented in the femur, accompanied by a significant decrease in skeletal remodeling. Once again suggestive of benefits for postmenopausal osteoporosis (Zhao et al. 2011). In vivo experiments reveal the fern can prevent cartilage degeneration, benefiting osteoarthritis by inhibiting the inflammatory response (Chen et al. 2022b).

Various extraction methods have been studied for the optimal benefit in growing osteoblasts with the traditional method of wine extraction likely being optimal.

The fern rhizome and seeds of *Astragalus complanatus* increase bone formation by stimulating osteoprotegerin expression and downregulating RANKL expression in osteoblasts and bone marrow stromal cells (Liu et al. 2013).

Cibotiumbarosides F and I, two hemiterpene glycosides, are hepatoprotective against induced acute liver damage, again proving more effective than bicycol (Xie et al. 2017).

Onychin, found in this fern, inhibits the proliferation of vascular smooth muscle cells through the G1 phase cell cycle by decreasing tyrosine phosphorylation of ERK1/2, the expression of cyclin D1 and cyclin E, and sequentially inhibiting Rb phosphorylation (Yang et al. 2005).

Excessive proliferation of vascular smooth muscle results in remodeling and plays a role in vascular disorders such as restenosis, atherosclerosis, and pulmonary hypertension. After injury to arteries, platelets can release platelet-derived growth factor, which can penetrate the vascular wall. Multisystem smooth muscle dysfunction syndrome is a serious genetic disease.

Sarcopenia is a progressive muscle disease associated with loss of muscle mass (atrophy), strength, and physical performance. In vitro studies on dexamethasone-induced muscle atrophy in a cell model suggest possible benefits of rhizome ethanol extracts in C2C12 myotubes (Kim et al. 2023b). The rhizomes promote hemorheology in mice with adjuvant arthritis by promoting blood circulation and removing blood stasis (Li et al. 2008a), with sand-processed rhizomes proving even more effective.

Glioblastoma is a malignant nervous system tumor with poor outcomes. Temozolomide has been the go-to drug for over a decade, but its efficacy is limited by acquired resistance. Polysaccharides from the rhizome (both raw and processed) significantly increase the drug's toxicity to U87 (glioblastoma) cell lines, promote apoptosis, enhance cell cycle change, and arrest cells in the S phase. Polysaccharides derived from raw rhizome showed better results than those derived from drugs (Shi et al. 2020).

Fractions from the rhizome exhibit hormonal influence on LNCaP and PC-3 prostate cancer cell lines (Bobach et al. 2014). The medicinal fern is, unfortunately, on the Convention on International Trade in Endangered Species (CITES) list of endangered species but is now undergoing cultivation.

Early work by Creasey (1969) identified antitumor activity in the related Mexican tree fern (*Cibotium schiedei*).

CONIOGRAMME

Bamboo Ferns

Japanese bamboo fern (*Coniogramme japonica*) can grow to almost a meter tall and wide. The fern possesses plastic-feeling dark green fronds and is popular among landscapers and fernophiles. The genus name derives from the Greek *konios* meaning "dusty" and *gramme* meaning "line."

In Japan, the fern has been traditionally used for ulcerated sores, mastitis, and inflammation. The rhizomes contain pterolactam, 5-hydroxymethylfurfural, methyl linoleate, trilinolein, dehydrovomifoliol, and butyl-2-formyl-5-butoxymethyl-1H-pyrrole-1-butanoate.

Pterolactam-designed amides possess antifungal activity against five strains with reduced susceptibility to commonly used antifungal drugs (Dascalu et al. 2020). Trilinolein (a triacylglycerol) inhibits neuronal apoptosis and may prove efficacious in the prevention of cerebral ischemia and cardiovascular disease (Chen et al. 2022f). Trilinolein also inhibits proliferation of A549 (non-small cell lung) carcinoma and induces apoptosis (Chou et al. 2011). The compound is also present in the widely used TCM herb *Panax notoginseng.*

Dehydrovomifoliol mitigates non-alcoholic fatty liver disease via regulation of the AKT/mTOR signaling pathway (Ma et al. 2023). The compound is an active ingredient in *Artemisia frigida*, widely found and gathered for medicine throughout Northern Canada.

Bamboo fern (*Coniogramme maxima* syn. *C. serrulata*, contains ten sesquiterpenoids, including (3S)-pteroside D, epi-pterosin L, peterosin D, onitin, pterosin z, onitisin, onitisin-glucopyranoside, onitin-15-O-β-D-glucopyranoside; as well as uracil, β-sitosterol, and daucosterol (Chen et al. 2012b).

Onitin is an antioxidant, liver protectant, and smooth muscle relaxant. Uracil is a naturally occurring base of RNA and plays a role in antiviral immunity. It can also be incorporated into DNA during genome replication, but fortunately, our cells have evolved enzymatic pathways to detect and remove it, thereby protecting the genome. Uracil derivatives include the chemotherapy drug 5-fluorouracil (5-FU). Ongoing research for novel antimicrobial and antiviral drugs involves uracil derivatives.

CRYPTOGRAMMA

Parsley Fern Slender Cliff Brake

Species of *Cryptogramma* are commonly known as parsley ferns, due to their shape and color.

Parsley fern (*Cryptogramma crispa* syn. *Osmunda crispa*) is a small, delicate plant living in rock crevices. The Nlaka'pamux, living near the Fraser and Thompson rivers of British Columbia, infused the fern and used it externally as an eyewash and internally to treat gallstones (Turner et al. 1990).

Slender cliff brake (*Cryptogramma stelleri*) lives on limestone in cool, damp areas. The fern is cold hardy and has been found near Coppermine River in Western Nunavut, Canada. The genus name derives from the Greek words *crypto*, meaning "hidden" and *gramme*, meaning "line," referring to the lines of sori being hidden by the curled pinnae margins. Today, the term crypto refers to hidden or chain-blocked currency, for instance Bitcoin.

CULCITA

Woolly Tree Fern

Woolly tree fern (*Culcita macrocarpa* syn. *Dicksonia culcita*) is a large fern, up to two meters tall and wide. It is endemic to Portugal, Spain, and the Azores Islands.

The fern is critically endangered in Portugal due to eucalyptus plantations. On the Azores, the fern hairs were once used as packing material. The genus name derives from the Latin meaning "mattress" or "stuffing for pillows or cushions."

CYATHEA

Silver Fern Tree Ferns

Geographic Range: Australia, Brazil, Central America, Chatham Islands, China, Guianan highlands, Madagascar, New Caledonia, New Zealand, Panama, Tanzania

Habitat: dry environments, forests, jungles, rock crevices, tropical regions, woodland areas

Practical Uses: food

Medicinal Applications: antioxidant, antiviral, anthelmintic, apoptosis induction, blood sugar regulation, cancer, cytotoxicity, diarrhea, gastrointestinal issues, heart health, hyperventilation, liver protection, neuroprotection, vasodilation, vasorelaxant properties, wound healing

Warning: Possible skin irritation may occur from bristly fronds and stems; caution is advised due to potential toxicity in livestock; the species is listed as endangered under CITES.

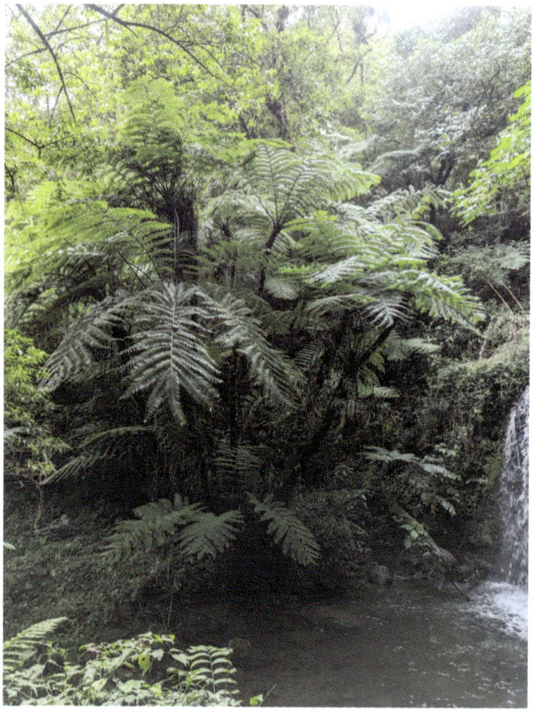

Cyathea sp. (Tree Fern)
Photo by Alan Rockefeller

Tree ferns (*Cyathea* spp.) are huge. The genus name derives from the Greek *kyatheion*, meaning "little cup," in reference to the cup-shaped sori on the underside of the fronds.

In the early 1970s, I was traveling through the jungles of Panama. The sight of giant tree ferns, up to twenty meters tall, took my mind back to the age of dinosaurs.

There are about 500 species worldwide, with more than forty in Panama alone.

Four species have been traditionally cooked for food: *Cyathea canaticulata* in Madagascar, silver tree fern (*Cyathea dealbata*) in New Zealand, black tree fern (*Cyathea medullaris*) in Australia, and *Cyathea viellardii* in New Caledonia (Uphof 1968).

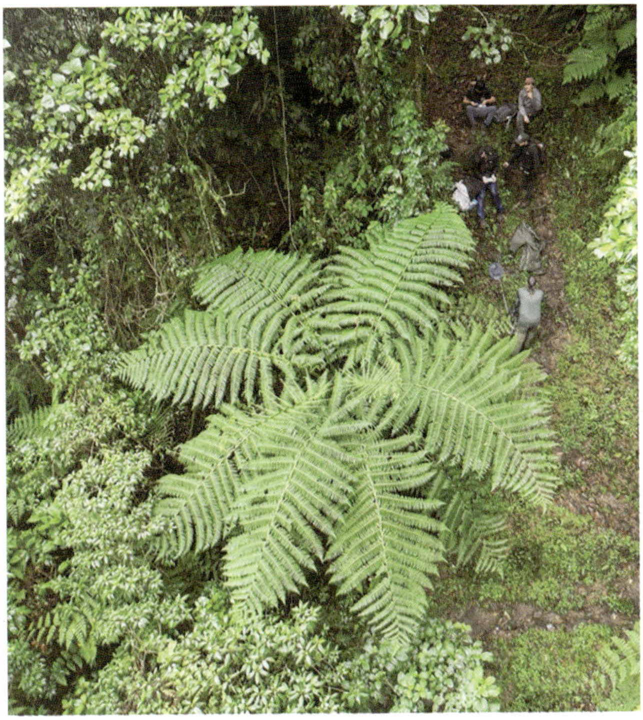

Cyathea sp. (Tree Fern)
Photo by Alan Rockefeller

An unidentified *Cyathea* tree fern extract, derived from a Guianan highlands species, exhibits medium cytotoxicity against HT29 (colon), A549 (lung), and MDA-MB-231 (breast) cancer cell lines (Guil-Guerrero and Campra 2009).

Australian tree fern (*Cyathea cooperi* syn. *Sphaeropteris cooperi*) can grow to over nine meters tall with a 30-centimeter-wide trunk. The fronds and stems are bristly and can irritate the skin.

Three species, hairy tree fern (*Cyathea crinita*), *C. nilgirensis*, and giant tree fern (*C. gigantea*) were extracted with ethanol and found to decrease cell viability and exhibit cytotoxicity against MCF-7 (breast) cancer cell lines (Janakiraman and Johnson 2016).

Lupeol has been extracted from *Cyathea crinita* and *Cyathea gigantea* and stigmasterol in all three ferns mentioned above. Lupeol is an androgen receptor inhibitor that enhances sensitivity in prostate cancer cells to anti-androgen enzalutamine-based treatment both in vitro and in vivo (Khan et al., 2023).

Silver tree fern (*Cyathea dealbata*) is a living fossil, found in New Zealand and the Chatham Islands. The Māori call it *ponga* or *kaponga*. According to a legend, silver fern formerly lived in the ocean, and Māori hunters would angle the white underside towards the moon to illuminate their way home.

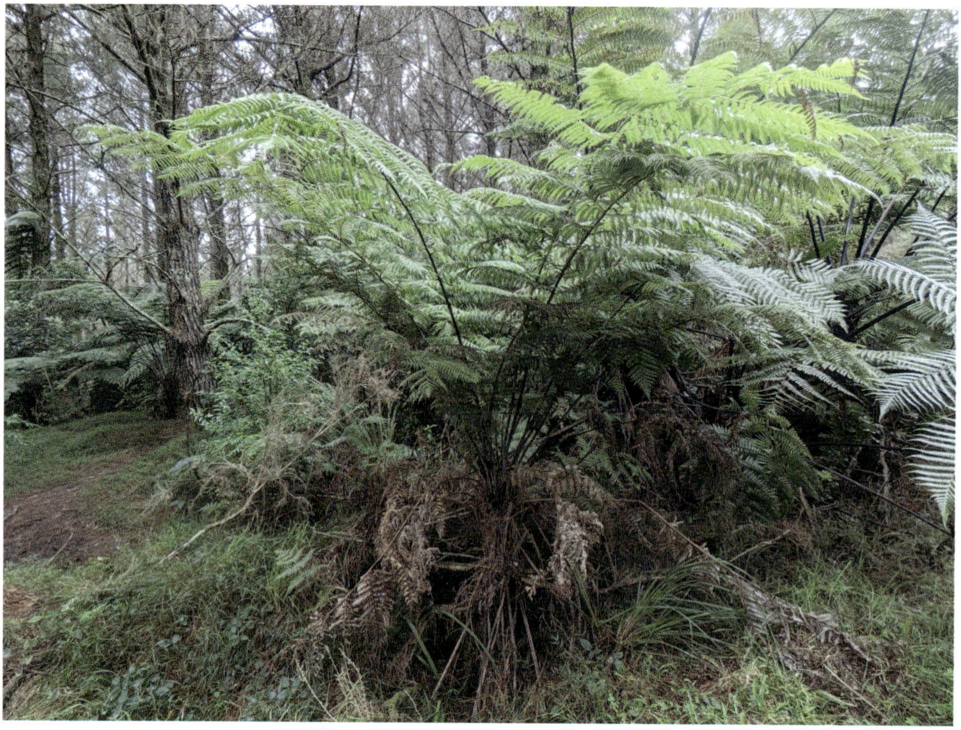

Cyathea dealbata (Silver Tree Fern)
Photo by Alan Rockefeller

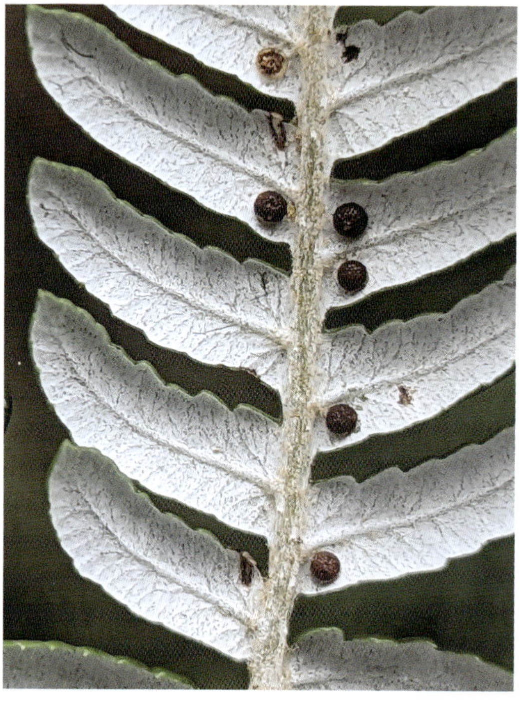

Underside of *Cyathea dealbata* (Silver Tree Fern)
Photo by Alan Rockefeller

Silver fern, so named for the silver-white underside of fronds, appears on the coat of arms of New Zealand and the logo of the New Zealand Labour Party. The uncoiled frond is known to the Māori as *koru*, meaning "loop" or "coil." The fiddlehead spiral shape is a symbol of their arts, carvings, and tattoos, and represents new life, growth, strength, and peace.

The aged fronds of silver tree fern (*Cyathea dealbata* syn. *Alsophila tricolor*), exhibit the highest level of 20:5n-3 (eicosapentaenoic acid) (Nekrasov et al. 2019). This omega-3 fatty acid (EPA) is usually found in cold-water fish, along with docosahexaenoic acid (DHA). EPA has numerous health benefits, including preventing blood clots, reducing triglyceride levels in the blood, and reducing inflammation, pain, and swelling. EPA helps balance emotional moods, while DHA is vital to cognitive function.

SILVER FERN ESSENCE

This essence of *Cyathea dealbata* facilitates inner healing, peace, and stillness at the soul level, particularly after experiences of heartfelt trauma or deep sorrow that have impacted the soul and are locked into cellular memory. It serves as an excellent antidote for hatred and jealousy. It helps those who have "heart issues" who feel they "can't breathe" or who feel "suffocated," claustrophobic, or prone to hyperventilation. Find as First Light Flower Essence of New Zealand No. 40 Silver Fern.

Cyathea dichromatolepsis exhibits significant antioxidant activity (Johnson, M et al. 2023).

The related tree ferns *Cyathea delgadii* and *Cyathea phalerata* exhibit inhibition of MAO-A at 70.3% and 74%, respectively (Andrade et al. 2014). MAO inhibitor drugs were an early attempt to treat depression, albeit with significant side effects, especially involving tryptamine-rich food and drinks.

Extracts of common tree fern (*Cyathea dregei*) proved cytotoxic as a possible anthelmintic to livestock but were also identified as toxic to the animals. It is widespread in southern Africa and known as *gewone boomvaring* in the Afrikaans language.

Crude extracts of *Cyathea gigantea* exhibit activity against *Staphylococcus aureus* (gram-positive bacteria), *Escherichia coli*, and *Pseudomonas aeruginosa* (gram-negative bacteria). Significant synergistic activity was shown with ciprofloxacin, tetracycline, ampicillin, and oxacillin, in descending order. This suggests possible adjunctive use against multidrug-resistant bacteria (Nath et al. 2019).

Methanol extracts of the fronds exhibit significant benefit on paracetamol (acetaminophen)-induced hepatoxicity in rats. This treatment reduced the elevated levels of SGOT, SGPT, ALP, TB, and reversed the liver damage (Kiran et al. 2012).

Brush pot tree (*Cyathea lepifera*) fronds contain p-coumaric acid, 3-hydroxy-β-ionone, nicotinic acid N-glucoside, and trigonelline. The compound 3-hydroxy-β-ionone inhibits progression of SCC15 (squamous carcinoma) cell lines and induces apoptosis (Luetragoon et al. 2020). Head and neck cancers, typically treated with chemotherapy and radiation, often develop drug resistance and have severe side effects.

Spirulina (*Arthrospira platensis*, formerly *Spirulina platensis*) is a widely cultivated functional food, known for its anti-inflammatory, antihypertension, antioxidant, and anti-atherosclerosis properties.

The apocarotenoid 3-hydroxy-β-ionone in spirulina has been shown to significantly suppress the expression of IL-1b and IL-6 in macrophages, indicating anti-inflammatory activity (Tan et al. 2021). It also inhibits the proliferation of MH7A synovial fibroblast cells, suggesting benefits for rheumatoid arthritis (Zhao et al. 2021b).

Trigonelline is found in fenugreek seeds and plays a role in reducing blood sugar levels. Trigonelline is a methylation product of niacin (vitamin B3) and is sometimes referred to as methylated niacin. It exhibits hypoglycemic, hypolipidemic, neuroprotective, sedative, anti-migraine, memory-enhancing, antibacterial, antiviral, and antitumor properties (Zhou et al. 2012).

Nearly twenty years ago, I was commissioned by the government department of Alberta Agriculture to identify crops with commercial market potential. I identified rose root (*Rhodiola rosea*) as the number one herb, which has since become a thriving industry worldwide. Due to overharvesting, this valuable adaptogen is now on the CITES list.

Number five on my list was fenugreek (*Trigonella foenum-graecum*).

Spiny tree fern (*Cyathea manniana* syn. *C. usambarensis*) frond and its inner core is used by the Chagga people of Tanzania and South Africa for treating parasites (Usher 1971; Watt and Breyer-Brandwijk, 1962).

In New Zealand, another black tree fern, *Cyathea medullaris*, is known by the Māori as *mamaku*. The fronds contain an unusual shear-thickening,

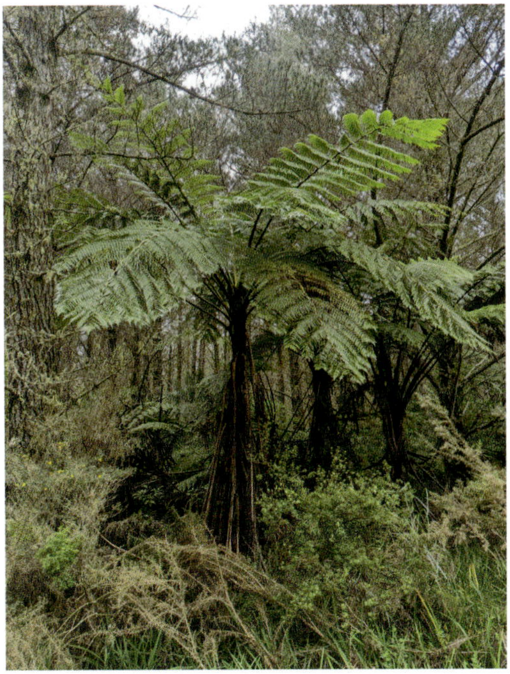

Cyathea medullaris
(Black Tree Fern)
Photo by Alan Rockefeller

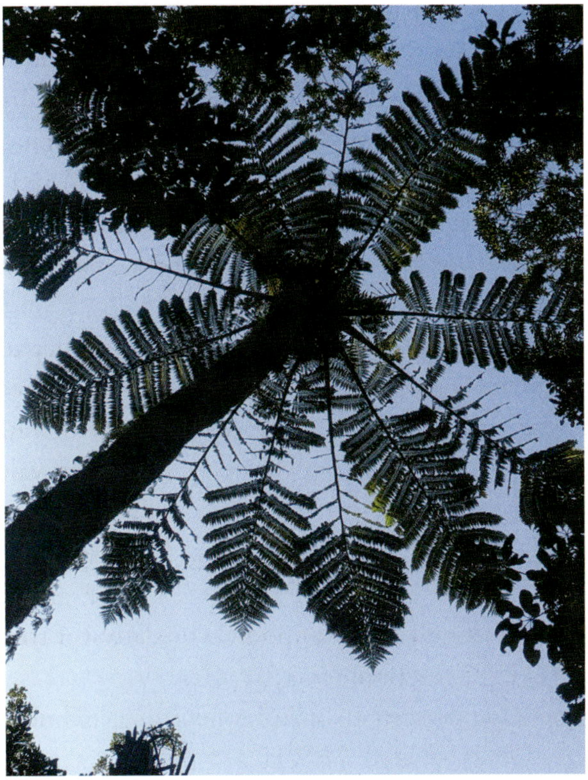

Underside of *Cyathea medullaris* (Black Tree Fern)
Photo by Alan Rockefeller

water-soluble polysaccharide gum resin. The Māori have used this extract to coagulate blood from wounds, combat skin conditions, and treat diarrhea and other gastrointestinal disorders.

The gum resin may modulate gut function by reducing enzyme activity, binding bile acids, and altering the microbiome towards healthier bacteria, and producing short-chain fatty acids (Bisht et al. 2023). The gum may also offer palliative benefits for patients suffering from dysphagia. In India, an unidentified *Cyathea* fern, possibly this species, has been used for major skin wounds and quickly staunching excessive bleeding.

The maquique fern can be up to ten meters tall, with fronds up to four meters in length. In some parts of Central America, the frond scales are used to staunch bleeding from external skin wounds (Usher 1971).

The stem of the Brazilian tree fern (*Cyathea phalerata*) contains cyathenosin A. In Brazil, the fern is known as *xaxim*.

Ethyl acetate extracts from this fern possess vasodilation and vasorelaxant properties, based on an animal study (Hort et al. 2019). The authors suggest the activity mainly involves the NO-cGMP pathway, hyperpolarization, and prostanoids. An ethyl acetate extract also protects from oxidative stress-induced liver damage by CCl4 in mice studies, probably related to its antioxidant properties (Hort et al. 2008).

The fern contains kaempferol 3-O-neohesperidoside, which enhances glucose uptake in the L6 cell line, suggestive of possible benefits for managing blood sugar disorders (Yamasaki et al. 2010). This glucoside also exhibits antiviral activity against SARS-CoV-2 (Rahayu and Timotius 2022).

The fresh fronds of *Cyathea podophylla* syn. *Gymnosphaera podophylla* contain dryocrassyl formate, sitostanyl formate, 12α-hydroxyfern-9(11)-ene, and ten triterpenoids, three derivates of phytol, and β-tocopherol.

The extraction of brush pot tree fern (*Cyathea spinulosa*) with ethanol revealed eight compounds: stigmast-4-ene-3,6-dione, stigmast-3,6-dione, ergosterol, protocatechuic aldehyde, 1-O-β-D-glucopyranosyl-(2S,3R,4E,8Z)-2-[(2-hydroxyoctadecanoyl]-4,8-octadecadiene-1,3-diol, (2S,3S,4R)-2-[(2'R)-2'hydroxytetracosanoylamino]-1,3,4-octacecanetriol, β-sitosterol and daucosterol (Jiang et al. 2012).

Stigmast-4-ene-3,6-dione was one of six compounds isolated from *Amaryllidaceae* extract. Five of them exhibit neuroprotective effect on SH-SY5Y neuroblastoma cells, suggesting possible benefits in treating neurodegenerative conditions like Parkinson's disease (Ibrakaw et al. 2020).

The compound also exhibits moderate antioxidant and lipid peroxidation inhibition. Its activity against the COX-1 enzyme was weak (Dissanayake et al. 2022). This compound is found in the roots of black pepper (*Piper nigrum*) and cattail (*Typha latifolia*).

CYCLOSORUS

Hottentot Fern
Parasitic Maiden Fern
Parasitic Tri-vein Fern
Striated Maiden Fern
Swamp Shield Fern

Geographic Range: Australia, Argentina, Assam (India), Hawaii, Ivory Coast, Mexico, New Zealand, Polynesian Islands, South Asia

Habitat: swamps, subtropical forests, tropical regions

Practical Uses: beer preservative

Medicinal Applications: anti-inflammatory, antiaging, antibacterial, antidiabetic, antifungal, antioxidative, antispasmodic, apoptosis induction, blood sugar regulation, blood infections, cancer, diarrhea, exercise enhancement, gastric ulcers, malaria, fatty liver disease, urination, pneumonia, radioprotective, skin sores

Warning: *Cyclosorus parasiticus* poses an invasive plant threat.

The fern *Cyclosorus acuminatus* syn. *Thelypteris acuminata* is used in Traditional Chinese Medicine (TCM) for inflammation and pyretic stranguria (slow, painful urination). It is known as *jian jian mao ju*.

A flavonoid fraction from the fern has been found to reduce inflammation chronic non-bacterial prostatitis in rats by modulating prostatic expression of PPAR-γ and eventually reducing the NFκB-dependent inflammatory response. The extract was given orally to rats once daily for four weeks and it was shown to ameliorate the elevated prostatic index as well as proinflammatory cytokine levels (Chen et al. 2014b). The rhizome of this fern contains acetylated flavanone glycosides with moderate activity against *Streptococcus pneumoniae* and *Haemophilus influenzae* (Fang et al. 2006). The latter gram-negative bacterium does not cause influenza and was incorrectly suggested in 1893 as the cause of an influenza pandemic.

However, it is an invasive bacteria that can cause pneumonia, meningitis, and bloodstream infections. It is highly resistant to penicillin medications. The Hib vaccine has reduced incidence rate by over 90% in countries that routinely administer the vaccine to children under five.

In Assam, India, the fronds of jeweled maiden fern (*Cyclosorus extensus* syn. *Thelpteris opulenta*) are used to prepare rice beer. Various extraction methods, including temperature and time of fermentation, were trialed by Das et al. (2016). Ethyl acetate extracts showed the highest activity against *Escherichia coli* bacteria.

When tested as a preservative for rice beer, the kaempferol, luteolin, quercetin, and other flavonoid content kept the beverage stable when stored at 32°C/89.6°F for eight weeks (Das et al. 2019a).

Swamp shield fern or Hottentot fern (*Cyclosorus interruptus*) is native to tropics and sub-tropics from Mexico to Argentina, and throughout South Asia, Australia, New Zealand, and Hawaii. It was first collected by Joseph Banks and Daniel Solander in 1770 during James Cook's first voyage. The species name *interruptus* derives from the Latin, referring to the sori, which are in zigzag rows or V-shaped patterns along the leaf margins. This fern has been traditionally used for liver disease, gonorrhea, coughs, malaria, and skin sores (Oyen 2010).

Coumarin derivatives exhibit antibacterial activity, with two newly identified derivatives showing cytotoxicity to the KB (human epithelial carcinoma) cell line (Quadri-Spinelli et al. 2000). The striated maiden fern *Cyclosorus interruptus* var. *striatus* has been traditionally used as a decoction in the Ivory Coast for liver ailments (Bouquet 1974).

The parasitic maiden fern or parasitic tri-vein fern (*Cyclosorus parasiticus* syn. *Christella parasitica*) is widespread throughout tropical Asia and found on some Polynesian Islands. The fern is not parasitic in the usual sense, but is so named for its invasive nature, which poses a potential threat to native plants.

The orange-colored epidermal glands of parasitic maiden fern have been researched for bioactive compounds. An extract of the shade-dried fronds of glandular morphophytes was soaked in acetone. The extract exhibited antibacterial activity but was also toxic to mosquito larvae and tadpoles (Paul et al. 2011).

Parasiticin C and 2',4'-dihydroxy-6'-methoxy-3',5'-dimethylchalcone (DMC) exhibit substantial cytotoxicity against six human cancer cell lines, particularly HepG2 (human liver) cells. Wei and colleagues (2013b) demonstrated that the two compounds could induce apoptosis, which may contribute to their cytotoxicity.

Earlier work by the same team found diaporthichalasins D and H cytotoxic to all cancer cell lines, except MCF-7.

DMC induces apoptosis and G1 cell cycle arrest in BEL-7402/5-FU (drug-resistant hepatoma cancer cells) Ji et al. (2019). An earlier study found that combining DMC with 5-fluorouracil (5-FU) significantly increased hepatoma tumor inhibition by over 72%.

Other research suggests potential benefits in MCF-7 (human breast), C-33A, HeLa and SiHa (all three human cervical), HCT116 and LOVO (both human colorectal) and K562 (human leukemia) cancer cell lines.

Tamoxifen is perhaps the most commonly used antiestrogen adjuvant treatments for estrogen receptor-positive breast cancer. Despite its success, it carries an increased risk of serious side effects such as uterine cancer, stroke, and pulmonary embolism. Dimethyl cardamonin (DMC), a potent estrogen receptor alpha inhibitor, has proved to be a good alternative.

Pancreatic cancer diagnosis has a very low survival rate. Work by Tuan and colleagues found that DMC exhibited cytotoxicity against PANC-1 and MIA PACA2 (human pancreatic) cancer cell lines (Tuan et al. 2019). DMC also enhances exercise performance, improves glucose tolerance, ameliorates gastric ulcers, and exhibits antispasmodic and calcium antagonistic activity in cases of diarrhea.

The endophytic fungus *Nodulisporium*, derived from the parasitic maiden fern, contains nodulisporisterone B, which exhibits potent inhibition of nitric oxide production in LPS-stimulated RAW264.7 macrophages. Along with two ergosterol derivatives (dankasterone A, and demethyllincisterol A_3), these compounds display cytotoxicity against A549 (lung), HeLa (cervical), HepG2 (hepatoma), and MCF-7 (breast) cancer cell lines (Yang et al. 2023).

Dankasterone A exhibits potent inhibition against P388 (murine lymphoma) cancer cell lines (Amagata et al. 2007).

The biological transformation of the medicinal mushroom lion's mane (*Hericium erinaceus*) and sweet annie (*Artemisia annua*) in 75% ethanol yielded dankasterone, which exhibited activity against *Helicobacter pylori*, a bacterium associated with gastric and duodenal ulcers (Zhao et al. 2022b).

Dankasterone A also shows moderate antifungal activity.

Interruptin B, isolated from *Cyclosorus terminans*, has been shown to stimulate brown adipocyte differentiation and increase glucose uptake in adipose-derived stem cells. This involves binding to peroxisome proliferator-activated receptor alpha (PPAR-α) and gamma (PPAR-γ). This strongly suggests benefits in the treatment of diabetes (Kaewsuwan et al. 2016). In TCM the fern is known as *ding yu mao jue*.

Both interruptin A and B exhibit antidiabetic, anti-inflammatory, and anti-oxidative effects. In a study of high-fat-diet-induced obese rats, an extract containing interruptin A and B ameliorated insulin resistance and non-alcoholic fatty liver disease via improved insulin signaling pathways, reduced inflammatory responses, improvement of lipogenesis and fatty acid oxidation (Songtrai et al. 2022).

Interruptin C, also derived from *Cyclosorus terminans*, is radioprotective, reducing toxicity to normal tissues during radiation therapy. Pre-treatment with interruptin C increased the survival rates of irradiated MCF-10A (normal breast cells) and HaCaT (normal skin cells), without promoting the survival of MDA-MB-231 and Hs578T breast cancer cells (Chumsuwan et al. 2022).

Interruptins A and B, but not C, are highly effective reactive oxygen species (ROS) scavengers, particularly in human dermal fibroblasts. This suggests they are potent natural antioxidants and show potential for antiaging cosmeceutical products (Chaiwong et al. 2023).

CYRTOMIUM

Fortune's Holly Fern
House Holly Fern
Japanese Holly Fern
Large-leaved Holly Fern

Geographic Range: China, United States, Japan, Africa, and Pacific Ocean islands

Habitat: rich, moist, well-drained soils

Practical Uses: phytoremediation (mercury)

Medicinal Applications: antidepressant effects, antidiabetic, anthelmintic, antiviral, cardiovascular disease potential, cholesterol reduction, cytotoxic, immune modulation, memory improvement, neuroprotection, skin depigmentation, skin inflammation, wormicidal against liver flukes, wound healing

The genus contains about thirty-five species.

Japanese holly fern, also known as house holly fern, (*Cyrtomium falcatum* syn. *Polystichum falcatum*) has been traditionally used as an anthelmintic against intestinal parasites, including tapeworms. This hardy, perennial fern

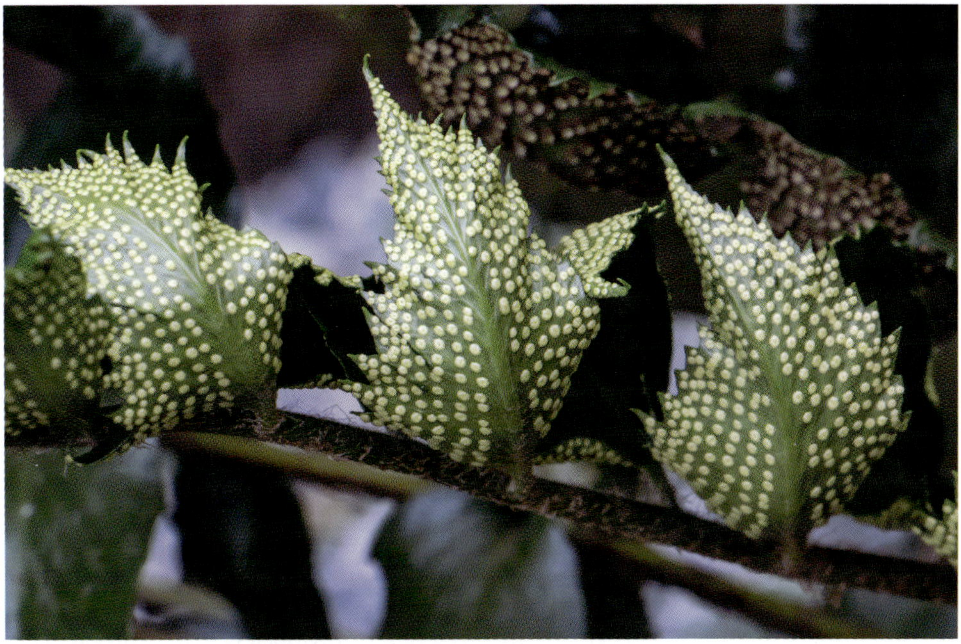

Cyrtomium falcatum (Japanese Holly Fern)

has escaped cultivation and is now found around the world. The term "holly" refers to the waxy holly-shaped leaves.

A novel RNA mottle virus has been identified infecting the fern. Honey mushroom (*Armillaria mellea*) mycelial mats have also been identified on Italian fern roots.

Fortune's holly fern (*Cyrtomium fortunei*) was named in honor of Robert Fortune, a Scottish botanist and horticulturalist who collected and shipped plants from China in the 1800s. This fern has escaped from gardens in Oregon and has naturalized in some states in the United States, including in the Deep South.

The fern, known as *guan zhong* in TCM, was formerly used externally for disinfection and prevention of infectious disease pandemics.

Cyrtomium rhizomes show potent antiviral activity, potentially stronger than the drug peramivir. Water extracts of this fern contain neoechinulin A and phellopterin, both of which exhibit significant cytotoxicity against a panel of human cancer cells. Neoechinulin and another compound identified and tested by Yang et al. (2013c) exhibit significant cytotoxic activity against MGC-803 (gastric carcinoma), PC3 (prostate), and A375 (melanoma) cancer cell lines.

Neoechinulin A has been shown to improve memory function in LPS-treated mice and exert antidepressant-like effects through changes in the 5-HT system (Sasaki-Hamada et al. 2016). Neoechinulin A also exhibits potent inhibition against SARS-CoV-2, comparable to the reference standard GC376 (Alhadrami et al. 2022).

The fern contains neoechinulin derivatives or stereoisomers. A review of diketopiperazine-type indole alkaloids by Sharifi-Rad et al. (2021) notes that neoechinulin A is a promising anticancer and anti-neuroinflammatory compound.

Neochinulin B shows potential against the hepatitis C virus. It is worth noting that these compounds are also found in prickly pear cacti and *Cannabis sativa*.

Yang et al. (2013b) identified pimpinellin as potent cytotoxic compound against MGC-803 (gastric carcinoma) cells, as well as PC3 (human prostate), and A375 (human melanoma) cancer cell lines.

Phellopterin cream helps attenuate chronic inflammation and promote new skin growth through SIRT1 upregulation, and lCAM-1 downregulation in in vitro and in vitro studies on diabetic wound healing (Zou et al. 2022). The compound activates GPR119 and increases active GLP-1 and insulin secretion in vitro and enhances glucose tolerance in both normal and diabetic mice.

Phellopterin also alleviates atopic dermatitis-like inflammation, suggesting a possible topical therapy for this persistent type 2 cause of skin lesions. A reduction in serum immunoglobulin E (IgE), and infiltration of eosinophils and mast cells in skin lesions was observed in studies by Chen et al. (2022e).

The compound acts as a partial agonist of benzodiazepine receptors in vitro and also serves as a neuraminidase inhibitor. Work by Takomthong et al. (2020) showed that phellopterin inhibits acetylcholinesterase and prevents neural cell damage caused by hydrogen peroxide and amyloid-$\beta_{1\text{-}42}$ toxicity, thus inhibiting the pathogenesis of Alzheimer's disease.

In a diabetic animal model, phellopterin significantly reduced blood sugar, triglycerides, and total cholesterol. This suggests enhanced insulin sensitivity and possible application for human metabolic diseases, including diabetes and cardiovascular conditions.

Phellopterin and vancomycin exhibit significant synergy against multidrug-resistant *Staphylococcus aureus*. Among the four coumarins and eight antibiotic combinations tested, the combination of phellopterin and chloramphenicol also proved highly effective (Zuo et al. 2016).

Water extracts of the fern inhibit activity of Coxsackie virus B3 by interfering with its inactivation, adsorption, and replication. In my own clinical practice, three cases of endocarditis associated with viral infections were noted, and all three clients obtained benefit from *Astragalus* root decoctions. The extracts also show activity against the related Coxsackie virus B5, polio virus 1, and echoviruses 9 and 29 (Guo et al. 2006).

Decoctions of the fern may be useful in reducing the ill effects of influenza and measles, the latter by expelling the toxins outward and speeding up recovery.

An essential oil has been produced from the fronds through carbon-dioxide extraction. Twenty-six compounds were identified. This essential oil demonstrated significant antitumor activity against MGC-803 (human gastric), Bcap-37 (breast) and A549 (human lung) cancer cell lines (Yang et al. 2015a).

A methanol extract of the rhizome appears to inhibit tyrosinase activity and melanin production in melan-a cells and exhibits depigmenting effects on UV-induced hyperpigmentation in brown guinea pig skin (Choi 2013).

Water extracts of the rhizome are effective wormicidals against the Chinese liver fluke (*Clonorchis sinensis*) (Rhee et al. 1981).

The large-leaved holly fern (*Cyrtomium macrophyllum*) has been used in traditional medicine to treat various infections, including tapeworm, colds, and viral diseases.

The fern contains polysaccharides that overcome induced immune suppression in mice by elevating nitric oxide production, TNF-α secretion, and iNOS protein levels in RAW264.7 cells. These polysaccharides also strongly increase NF-κB levels, suggestive of immune modulation (Ren et al. 2014a).

An in vivo study on mice followed, where an ethanol extract of the fern improved immune function after exposure to cyclophosphamide (Ren et al. 2014b).

The fern also shows promise to phytoremediate mercury-polluted soils (Xun et al. 2017).

CYSTOPTERIS

Bulblet Fern Fragile Bladder Fern Mountain Bladder Fern

Bulblet or mountain bladder fern (*Cystopteris bulbifera*) is found on moss-covered limestone boulders and cliff ledges. The genus name is derived from the Greek *kystos*, meaning "bladder" and *pteris*, meaning "fern," referring to the bladder-like indusium. The species' name *Cystopteris* refers to the ball-like bulblets growing along the mid-stem on the underside of the frond. These bulblets are tiny, functional rhizomes that quickly root and send up new fronds when they fall off due to rain.

The fern is native to Eastern North America, with disjunct populations growing on limestone in Southwestern regions. It will hybridize regionally with the fragile bladder fern and other species.

The fern, known to the Gitxsan of British Columbia as *ax*, has a one to two centimeter rhizome that tastes and looks like a woody sweet potato. When first dug up, the rhizome is black, but it turns orange when cooked, similar to a red turnip. It was generally baked in steam pits and then peeled as a survival food.

Fragile bladder fern (*Cystopteris fragilis*) is found on moist slopes and rocky edges. The species name refers to the fragile or brittle thin petioles. The Cherokee considered this fern a febrifuge and included it in fern combination infusions for chills. The Ojibwa drank the fern tea for stomach disorders. The Navajo used cold compound infusions as a fomentation for skin injuries (Moerman 1986).

Antimicrobial activity is higher in ferns collected before sporulation.

In North Carolina, the fern was formerly considered a pectoral, mucilaginous, expectorant, and refrigerant tonic (Jacobs 1958).

The fern contains various xanthone derivatives: 1,2-dihydroxy-5,6,7-trimethoxy-xanthone, and 1,6-dihydro-3,5,7-trimethoxyxanthone, isomangiferin 3-methyl ether, mangiferin, isomangiferin, 1,3,6,7-tetra-hydroxyxanthone and flavonoid compounds including astragalin, kaempferol-3,4'-O-bis-glucoside, kaempferol-3-O-(glucoside-3,6'-sulfate), caffeolyglucose 6'-sulfate and 3'-sulfate.

The fern has a distinct bitter almond scent, suggesting dietary avoidance and possible presence of hydrocyanic acid.

DAVALLIA

Hare's Foot Ferns
Rabbit's Foot Fern
Squirrel's Foot Fern
White Paw Fern

Geographic Range: Canary Islands, Eastern Asia, Fiji, Japan, Korea, Taiwan

Habitat: epiphytic, tropical, subtropical

Practical Uses: biofiltering, outdoor plant

Medicinal Applications: anti-inflammatory, arthritis, bone fractures, cancer, diabetes, diarrhea, dyslipidemia, gout, osteoporosis, pain, rheumatoid arthritis, uric acid

Several Davallia species are known as squirrel's foot fern or rabbit's foot fern. Worldwide there are around forty species, most of them epiphytic.

The most popular commercially available fern for outdoor gardening is *Davallia fejeensis*, a native of Fiji.

Hare's foot fern (*Davallia canariensis*) is highly prized as a house plant. The species name refers to the Canary Islands.

A number of *Davallia* species called *gu sui bu* (GSB) in Traditional Chinese Medicine (TCM) are used to relieve diarrhea. Six species with this common name were chosen for an examination of their benefits in cases of enterotoxigenic *Escherichia coli* diarrhea. Four members of the genus inhibited heat-labile enterotoxin-induced diarrhea while *Drynaria fortunei*, also known as gu sui bu, showed no antidiarrheal effect (Chang et al. 2014).

Rabbit's foot fern (*Davallia bilabiata*) is also referred to as gu sui bu and is used as a substitute for *Drynaria fortunei*, to treat rheumatoid and degenerative arthritis in China.

Work by Liu et al. (2017a) found that the fern's rhizome inhibits in vivo angiogenesis in a chorioallantoic membrane assay, decreased MMP-2 activity through the upregulation of TIMP-2 and RECK and inhibits the gene expression of VEGF-A through D, and VEGFR-1 through 3. This explains the mechanism of action in rheumatic and arthritic pain relief.

Research by Yang et al. (2014a) further identified the anti-inflammatory pathways of this fern, suggesting an alternative or adjunct therapy for conditions such as rheumatoid arthritis and osteoarthritis.

Some ferns, including the Boston fern (*Nephrolepis exaltata*), have the ability to purify household air by removing pollutants such as formaldehyde. Squirrel's foot fern (*Davallia bullata* syn. *D. cylindrica*) has been found to exhibit similar benefits as an ornamental biofiltering plant.

Flavonoids show similar or higher free radical scavenging than rutin, exhibit cytotoxicity against A549 (human lung) cancer cell lines, and inhibit acetylcholinesterase in a dose-dependent manner, which is associated with brain health (Cao et al. 2014).

Davallia divaricata has been traditionally used in Taiwan for the treatment of lung cancer and known as *da ye gu sui bu*. This fern contains davallic acid, a compound known to repress A549 (human lung) cancer cell line growth and induce apoptosis (Cheng et al. 2012).

Lacy hare's foot fern (*Davallia formosana*) is used in TCM to treat osteoporosis, bone fractures, and other bone-related diseases, including arthritis.

Bone metabolism was studied in ovariectomized female rats, using ethanol extracts of *Davallia formosana*. A twelve-week study found that the ethanol extract ameliorated bone loss via inhibition of bone resorption, identifying (-)-epicatechin 3-O-β-D-allopyranoside (ECAP) as the active ingredient in the rhizome (Ko et al. 2012).

ECAP, which has been isolated from the fern's stems and rhizomes, was shown to also significantly decrease blood glucose, triglycerides, and insulin levels in high-fat diet mice. Leptin levels decreased and adiponectin levels increased, suggestive of benefits in management of type 2 diabetes and dyslipidemia (Shih et al. 2015).

Recent work by Hsiao et al. (2019) confirmed that ECAP effectively suppressed inflammation, pain, and adjuvant-induced arthritis, indicating therapeutic potential in treating rheumatoid arthritis. *Davallia formosana* is specifically cultivated in Taiwan for its benefits in bone fracture, arthritis, and osteoporosis.

An ethanol extract of the fresh rhizome inhibits osteoclast differentiation by inhibiting NF-κB activation and effectively relieves ovariectomy-induced osteoporosis. This suggests benefits in treatment of bone disorders associated with excessive osteoclastic activity, such as rheumatoid arthritis and osteoporosis (Lin et al. 2013).

ECAP also ameliorates the diabetic and dyslipidemia condition in streptozotocin (STZ)-induced diabetic mice (Lin et al. 2017).

The fern shows promise in reducing serum uric acid levels in vivo. Several flavonoid glycosides may be responsible for the xanthine oxidase inhibition, which is associated with gout (Chen et al. 2014a). Ethanol extracts suppressed the proliferation, migration, and invasion in PCa (human prostate) cancer cell lines, and to decrease androgen receptor and prostate-specific antigen expression in cancer cells (Hsieh et al. 2020).

Squirrel's foot fern (*Davallia mariesii*) is an epiphytic fern native to Japan and Eastern Asia. The common name derives from the soft, furry brown rhizomes. The fern contains epicatechin derivatives and procyanidin B5, a condensed tannin compound that inhibits angiotensin-converting enzyme. Other sources of this compound include hawthorn flowers and fruit, as well as grape seeds. The fern has been used in traditional Korean medicine for cancer treatment.

The rhizome has also been traditionally used for inflammation, arteriosclerosis, and bone injuries. Recent work suggests it may benefit both acute and later allergic responses, particularly with IgE-induced reactions (Do et al. 2017).

Water extracts of the rhizome contain two identified compounds that significantly increase alkaline phosphatase activity and mineral deposition in a study on female mice without ovaries (Lin et al. 2021). The fern also contains the tetrameric proanthocyanidin davallin.

The neuroblastoma (B35) cell line is protected from oxidative damage by extracts of this fern through various pathways (Wu et al. 2018a).

The whole fern of hare's foot fern (*Davallia solida*) has been traditionally used to treat dysmenorrhea and leucorrhea (Ho et al. 2011). It contains the novel benzophenone glycoside, 4-O-β-D-glucopyranosyl-2,6,4'-trihydroxybenzophenone.

White rabbit's foot or white paw fern (*Davallia tyermanii* syn. *Humata tyermanii*) contains a unique hydroxynitrile lyase (enzyme) that exhibits selective synthesis of cyanohydrins.

DENNSTAEDTIA

Boulder Fern Hay-scented Fern

The genus name honors the German botanist and physician August Wilhelm Dennstaedt (1776–1826). Worldwide, there are about 270 species in the family *Dennstaedtiaceae.*

Hay-scented or boulder fern (*Dennstaedtia punctilobula*) has been traditionally used by the Lenape and Iroquoians of the Delaware River Valley region for chills and bloody expectoration. The Cherokee and Mahuna prepared the ferns for similar uses (Moerman 1986). Indigenous tribes in California used the nodules at the crown of the root for bloody hemorrhages of the lungs (Romero 1954), although this fern is primarily found in the Eastern and Midwestern United States.

The common name *hay-scented* fern derives from the scent of fresh mown grass or hay when crushed by hand. This fern exhibits allelopathic properties, discouraging the growth of northern red oak (*Quercus rubra*) seedlings and arresting forest succession in oak-transition hardwood-hemlock forests. It is also no friend of black cherry seedlings.

Conversely, white-tailed deer (*Odocoileus virginianus*) avoid browsing on this fern, making it a favorable choice for those who love their fern gardens.

Dennstaedtia scabra syn. *D. zeylandica* ethanol extracts contain onitioside A and B, onitisin, pterosin A, pinocembrin, pinocembrin 7-rutinoside, kaempferol, nicotiflorin, and galangin.

Onitinoside A and B and onitisin inhibit the contraction of isolated guinea pig ileum, suggesting they may act as a smooth muscle relaxant. Pinocembrin is

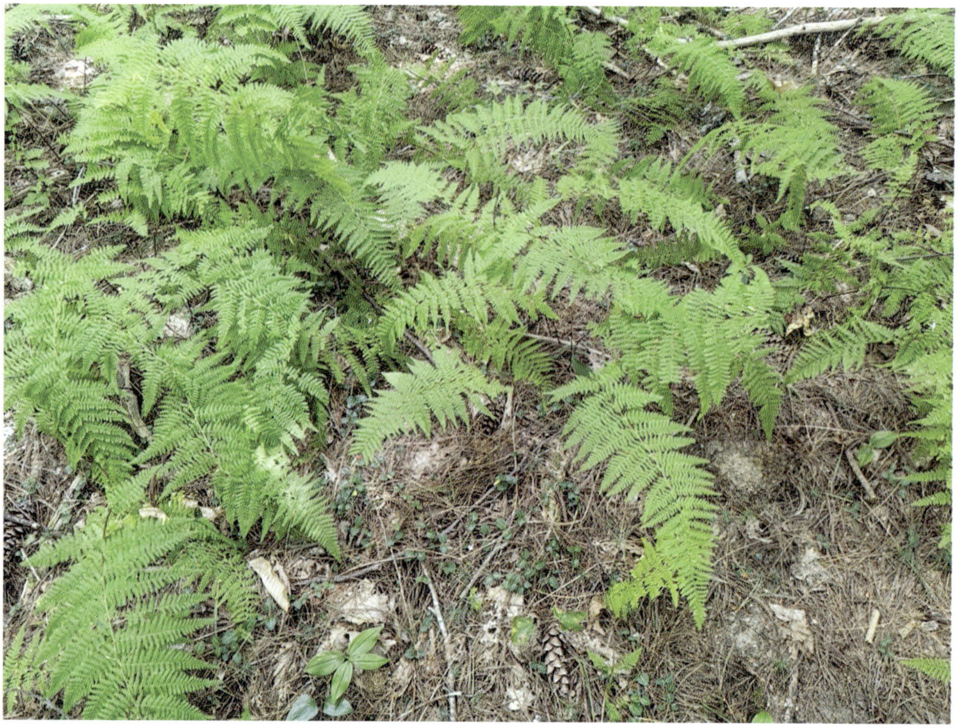

Dennstaedtia punctilobula (Hay-Scented Fern)
Photo by Alan Rockefeller

an important compound found in numerous and various plants, possessing cardiac benefit in atrial fibrillation. The compound ameliorates depression, inhibits microglial activation alleviating morphine tolerance and inhibits melanoma cells, in vitro. The fern also contains dennstoside A, an analogue of ptaquiloside.

Nicotiflorin shows potential in inhibiting coronavirus, ischemia, kidney impairment, liver complications, memory dysfunction, and myocardial infarction. It also shows potential to inhibit α-glucosidase and α-amylase, multiple myeloma cells, and promoting insulin secretion (Patel 2022). Nicotiflorin, also found in safflower petals, exhibits neuroprotection in neural cultures and potential benefits in cerebral ischemic illness (Li et al. 2006).

Pterosin A reverses increased serum insulin and insulin resistance in a diabetic mouse model (Hsu et al. 2013). Galangin is a flavonoid with potent antitumor activity. Work by Kong et al. (2019) found galangin induces apoptosis, pytoptosis, and autophagy in U251, U87MG, and A172 (human glioblastoma multiforme, GBM) cancer cell lines. Galangin inhibits neural degeneration of dopaminergic neurons via the Nrf2/Keap1 pathway, suggesting potential as treatment for Parkinson's disease (Chen et al. 2022d).

DEPARIA

Silvery Spleenwort Fern

The American botanist and horticulturist William Cullina uses humor to explain the complex taxonomic classification of silvery spleenwort fern (*Deparia acrostichoides*). He points out that this fern has been reclassified multiple times, moving from one genus to another, including *Asplenium*, *Athyrium*, and *Diplazium*, much like a child might move between different households after a divorce. In this analogy, the maidenhair fern (*Adiantum* sp.) is the popular child, full of life and most likely to succeed. Meanwhile, the silvery spleenwort fern (*Deparia* sp.) is more like the polite student with good grades and makes no impression. Cullina also amusingly critiques the fern's name, noting that it is "about as silvery as a gold brick" (Cullina 2008). I highly recommend reading his book. He uses the analogy of movie producers pitching a new script in which the lady fern attracts the New York fern, and in turn meets ostrich fern.

DICRANOPTERIS

False Staghorn Fern Forked Ferns

Geographic Range: China, Fiji, Hawaii, India, Indonesia, Java, Malaysia, New Guinea, Philippines

Habitat: forests, subtropical regions, tropical regions

Practical Uses: activated biochar, ash fertilizer, hats, hyperaccumulation of rare earth elements, lithium-ion battery anode material, phytoremediation, against citrus red mite, cigar cases

Medicinal Applications: analgesic, anthelmintic, antidiabetic, antioxidant, antinociceptive activity, antiviral, asthma, biofilm disruption, cancer, cell repair, hepatoprotective, hypotension, liver protection, wound healing, wormicide

In Fiji, the fern referred to as *beki ni sina* (*Dicranopteris caudata*) is used in traditional medicine to treat type 2 diabetes. Work by Mala et al. (2022) found that methanol extracts of the fern exhibited a higher total phenolic content compared to vanillic acid, the control.

The forked fern (*Dicranopteris dichotoma* syn. *D. pedata*) contains a range of tetranorclerodanes and clerodane-type diterpene glycosides, as well as aylthonic acid and (6S,13S)-cleroda-3,14-diene-6,13-diol. The latter compound exhibits modest anti-HIV-1 activity (Li et al. 2007). Earlier work by the same research team identified dichotomain B, which also exhibits weak anti-HIV-1 activity.

Forked fern (*Dicranopteris pedata*) contains afzelin and quercitrin. Afzelin is present in a number of fern species. The compound inhibits triple-negative breast cancer, gastric cancer, and prostate cancer cell lines. It relieves asthma, inhibits aldose reductase, reduces hypertension, and inhibits the growth of pathogenic bacteria. PubMed lists a total of 145 studies, too numerous to include all of them here.

A clerodane-type diterpene glycoside, derived from the fern, exhibits weak inhibition against SMMC-7221 (human hepatoma), MCF-7 (breast), and SW480 (colon) cancer cell lines (Gao et al. 2021).

Quercitrin has been widely researched for its benefits in bone metabolism, gastrointestinal, cardiovascular, and cerebrovascular diseases. More human clinical trials would be welcome, as quercitrin is a widely available dietary supplement. One interesting study found that quercitrin stimulates hair growth (Kim et al. 2020). The expression of Bcl2, an essential marker for anagen hair follicle and cell survival, was increased by quercitrin treatment.

Alcohol extracts of this fern repel and reduce oviposition of citrus red mite (*Panonychus citri*) (Cen et al. 2004).

False staghorn or Old World forked fern (*Dicranopteris linearis* syn. *Gleichenia linearis*) is known as *uluhe* in Hawaii, and *dilim* in the Philippines.

The fern's long leaf stalks are woven into hats and cigar cases in Java, Indonesia (Benedict 1915), and the rhizome is used to treat intestinal worms in India and China, as well as skin ulcers in New Guinea and fevers in Malaysia.

In India, the fronds, known as thicket fern or *rajhans*, are decocted in warm milk to improve fertility in women (Vasudeva 1999).

The fern is a potential phytoremediator for abandoned nickel mines. In uncontaminated areas, the cooked fern serves as a vegetable. In Malaya, the stems are used for making pens, mats, walls of huts, fishing nets, traps, and chairs (Uphof 1968). The fern has also been applied externally to wounds.

Dicranopteris linearis contains flavonol 3-O-glycosides. Three varieties of this fern species have been noted and contain different compounds: *Dicranopteris linearis* var. *brevis* contains afzelin and quercitrin, *Dicranopteris linearis* var. *tenuis* contains quercetin and isoquercetin, and *Dicranopteris linearis* var. *sebastiana* is rich in astragalin, isoquercetin, rutin, and a glucopyranoside.

The wound healing properties are probably due to the fern containing polyphenols, which induce proliferation of selected fibroblast cells, enhance cell migration, and promote cell repair (Ponnusamy et al. 2015). Chloroform extracts have been shown to reduce pain and inflammation in an animal model (Zakaria et al. 2006).

Various extracts (water, chloroform, methanol) exhibit in vitro activity against several cancer cell lines, including MCF-7 (breast), HeLa (cervical), HT-29 (liver), HL-60 (myeloid leukemia), K562 (chronic myelogenous leukemia), and MDA-MB-231 (ductal breast) (Zakaria et al. 2011).

The leaves of the fern, extracted with ethyl acetate, were found to provide antioxidant and hepatic protection in rats with paracetamol-induced liver intoxication (Zakaria et al. 2020a). It reduced the levels of liver enzymes, perhaps due to content of rutin, gallic acid, quercetin, methyl palmitate, and shikimic acid, among other compounds.

Water extracts from the same fern also exhibit hepatoprotective activity in paracetamol and carbon tetrachloride-induced liver toxicity in mice (Ismail et al. 2014). Similarly, the water portion of a methanol extract from the fronds protects against liver damage induced by paracetamol (acetaminophen) (Zakaria et al. 2019).

Hexane extracts of the fern have been shown to disrupt biofilms formed by *Staphylococcus aureus*. This disruption is linked to the presence of α-tocopherol, which does not affect the cells within the biofilm but rather the biofilm matrix, suggesting potential benefits of adding α-tocopherol in treating other biofilm-associated infections (Mawang et al. 2017).

A methanol extract shows inhibition against MDA-MB-231 (breast) cancer cell lines by inducing apoptosis and S-phase cell cycle arrest (Baharuddin et al. 2018). Methanol extracts of the fronds also exert opioid/NO-mediated antinociceptive activity, suggesting its potential as a novel analgesic (Zakaria et al. 2020b).

Ethanol extracts of the fern exhibit anthelmintic activity against the adult *Gastrothylax crumenifer*, a common parasitic trematode in goats (Kalpana et al., 2020; Rajesh et al. 2016). The fern is also known to be a hyperaccumulator of rare earth elements, making it an effective phytoremediation tool for contaminated soils.

A *Dicranopteris*-like Fe-Sn-Sb-P alloy has been explored as a promising anode material for lithium-ion batteries (Zheng et al. 2012). To my knowledge, no further research has been done on this topic.

At the same time, the fern may be a source of activated biochar for possible use as an electric double-layer capacitor electrode in tropical and subtropical regions (Trinh et al. 2020).

DICKSONIA

Man Fern Soft Tree Fern

Tasmanian fern, soft tree fern, or man fern (*Dicksonia antarctica* syn. *Cibotium billardierei*) is an evergreen tree fern found in Eastern Australia. It grows to 5 meters in height, although some can reach up to 15 meters, with a canopy up to 6 meters in diameter. This fern begins to sporulate at around twenty years of age. The spore extracts damage K562 (human premyeloid leukemia) cells (Simán et al. 2000).

The inner pith and the top of the trunk have been traditionally used as source of starch. The latter was split open, and the center, said to resemble a turnip, was removed and either roasted in coals or eaten as a bread.

Soft tree fern has been traditionally eaten like breadfruit in Hawaii (May et al. 1978).

DIDYMOCHLAENA

Mahogany Fern

Mahogany fern (*Didymochlaena truncatula*) is endemic to the Madagascar rainforest. Unlike most ferns, it enjoys more sunshine and, of course, high humidity if brought into one's home. The name *mahogany* refers to the initial frond color, which later becomes bronze and finally dark green with red-brown stipes.

One study by Cao et al. (2006) found that the fern contained camptothecin and 9-methoxycamptothecin, lignan derivatives didymochlaenone A and B, and (-)-wikstromol, a (E)-3-methoxy-5-hydroxystilbene.

In a subsequent study of a second fern collection, no camptothecin derivatives were found due to a coding error. Confirming their presence in future studies would be valuable, given their significance as cytotoxic agents.

Further work by Andrade et al. (2014) found that the fern exhibits high antichemotactic activity (93.41%), at a concentration of 10 μg/mL and inhibits MAO-A (82.61%). MAO-A encodes the key enzyme for the degradation of serotonin and catecholamines. Congenital deficiency is linked to a higher risk of antisocial behavior, and low MAO-A activity in the brain is strongly associated with increased aggression, potentially explaining the impact of prenatal smoke exposure on antisocial behavior. Today, MAO-A inhibitors are considered a third-line class of antidepressants compared to selective serotonin reuptake inhibitors (SSRIs).

DIPLAZIUM

Molokai Twinsorus Fern   Vegetable Fern

Geographic Range: Assam, Brunei, Hawaii, Himalayan and sub-Himalayan regions, India, Japan, Malaysia, Papua New Guinea, Philippines, Sub-Himalayan regions

Habitat: tropical forests

Practical Uses: food, decoration, indoor plant

Medicinal Applications: analgesic, anaphylactic, anti-inflammatory, antibacterial, antifungal, anthelmintic, antioxidant, bone fractures, constipation, diabetes, diarrhea, dysentery, fever, glandular swellings, headaches, high blood pressure, labor pains, liver bile acid metabolism, measles, nerve regeneration, pain, rheumatism, smallpox, spermatorrhea, toothache, wounds

Warning: Consumption of vegetable fern may cause erythrocyte damage and immune suppression.

The genus *Diplazium* contains about 400 species worldwide. Diplazium derives from the Greek *diplό* meaning "double," alluding to the indusia lying on both sides of the vein.

Diplazium donianum syn. *D. lineolatum* contains makisterones A and D, an unidentified stereoisomer of makisterone B, and several unidentified phytoecdysones.

Makisterone A was shown to alleviate cholestatic liver injury and dysregulation of hepatic bile acid metabolism in a mouse model. Cholestasis is a buildup of bile acids in the liver due to impaired bile formation, secretion, and excretion due to infection, drugs, and metabolic and genetic diseases. At the present time, there is only one drug (ursodiol) approved by the FDA for the treatment of primary biliary cholangitis, but nearly 40% of patients do not respond well to it. In June 2024 the FDA approved Iqirvo (elafibranor) to treat primary biliary cholangitis. Makisterone A targets the farnesoid X receptor, which plays a key role in bile acid metabolism (Kang and Li 2022).

Vegetable fern (*Diplazium esculentum*) frond, root, and rhizome are consumed in Himalayan and sub-Himalayan regions, as well as in Brunei, where the frond is used in the traditional dish *budu pakis* and prepared as a pickle condiment.

The fern has been traditionally used for preventing or treating diabetes, smallpox, asthma, diarrhea, rheumatism, dysentery, headache, fever, wounds, pain, measles, high blood pressure, constipation, bone fractures (fresh leaf poultice), and glandular swellings. Its rhizomes, shoots, leaves, and fronds possess analgesic, anaphylactic, antioxidant, antifungal, antibacterial, anti-inflammatory, and anthelmintic properties. The tincture of the leaves is used for sarcoptic mange (scabies).

Young fronds are used by pregnant women to ensure protection against a difficult childbirth (labor pains) (May 1978). A broth of young fronds is also effective for toothache and dental caries. In the Philippines, the rhizome and fronds are made into a decoction for treating coughing with blood (Quisumbing 1951).

This fern has numerous common names depending on the region. In India, it is *dung-kek* or *dhekia*, in Japan *kuware-shida*, and in Papua New Guinea, *sigogo*. Among the Semai of Malaysia, the fern is known as *snegoh*, and in Hawaii it is called *warabi*.

Among the Mishing community of Assam, the fern is used in religious ceremonies associated with funerals.

The fern contains ascorbic acid, eriodictyol 5-O-methyl ether 7-O-β-D-xylosyigalactoside, tannins, phytates, α-tocopherol, hopan-triterpene lactone, lutein, the toxic ptaquiloside, pterosin, phenol compounds, and three ecdysteroids (amarasterone A1, makisterone C, and ponasterone A). The protein content is notably high.

Ponasterone A induces and boosts HEK-293 cells to release higher levels of bioactive nerve growth factor. This may lead to improvement of peripheral nerve regeneration and functional recovery and may be superior to nerve isografts (Scholz et al. 2010).

The fresh fronds of this fern are cooked in water for consumption and to treat various health conditions. In Malaya the green tips are cooked and eaten. A project in 1932 attempted to domesticate the fern because the supply was so large (Copeland 1942).

The root and rhizome are decocted for spermatorrhea (premature ejaculation), macerated for dysentery and infection, and crushed into a poultice for rheumatism and smallpox. However, even when boiled, the fern may induce infertility by altering male reproductive function, based on a lengthy mice study by Roy and Chaudhuri (2017).

Consumption of the fern may cause erythrocyte damage even after cooking and may evoke immune dysfunction and suppression (Roy et al. 2013). Various extracts of the fronds show weak to moderate activity against a variety of bacteria.

The World Health Organization (WHO) estimates that melanoma kills around 48,000 people worldwide each year. Makisterone C shows promise in modulating signaling involved in development of this deadly cancer (Bhattacharya et al. 2023).

The fern possesses modest antioxidant activity, but hydro-ethanol extracts exhibit high α-amylase (92%), and α-glucosidase (70%) inhibition. Junejo et al. (2018) found that giving an extract to STX-induced diabetic rats for three weeks, reduced blood glucose and lipids, and regeneration of pancreatic beta cells.

One mouse study (Roy et al. 2013) found the extracts to be immunosuppressive, but when boiled and given to mice for up to six months, the fern decreased the concentration of Th1 and Th2 cytokines, compared to the control. This suggests it may affect innate and cell-mediated immune responses via modulation of these levels (Roy and Chaudhuri 2015b).

A cognitive study of 132 middle-aged adults consuming an average of 15.1 $\pm$ 8.2 grams of this fern per day found protective effects (62.9%) against mental decline (You et al. 2020). Inhibition of anticholinesterase and NADH oxidase with a methanol extract was reported by Roy and Chaudhuri (2015a).

Recent in vitro work by Kunkeaw et al. (2021) found that the fern extract inhibits acetylcholinesterase, suggesting possible benefits in Alzheimer's disease (AD). An ethanol extract administered to *Drosophila* models of Ab-mediated toxicity contributed antioxidant and inhibitory activity against AD-related enzymes. The extract acted as a BACE-1 blocker and reduced amyloid beta

42 peptides in the fruit fly models, resulting in improved locomotion. More research is required to confirm these findings. The effective inhibition of beta-secretase may be involved (Sirichai et al. 2022).

The chikungunya virus (*Togaviridae alphavirus*) is carried by mosquitoes and poses a significant health risk for humans. Symptoms include fever, joint pain, headache, muscle pain, and rash lasting up to two weeks. The virus has a mortality rate of 12% and there is no vaccine or specific biomedical treatment. Extracts of this fern possess virucidal effect and reduce viral loads compared to a control group (Chan et al. 2021).

No cytotoxicity against several human cancer cell lines has been observed. Ethanol extracts of this fern show significant antiparasitic activity against *Trypanosoma brucei* (Norhayati et al. 2013).

Recent work isolated stigmasterol and ergosterol 5,8-endoperoxide. The latter is a steroid and shows strong inhibition against the *Plasmodium falciparum* 3D7 (chloroquine-sensitive) strain, likely due to the inhibition of endoplasmic reticulum calcium-dependent ATPase (Safar et al. 2022).

The essential oil of this fern contains α-(10.5%) and beta-pinene (17.2%), caryophyllene oxide (7.5%), sabinene (6.1%) and 1,8-cineole (5.8%).

Semwal et al. (2021) wrote a comprehensive review article on this fern, which I recommend for those interested in further research.

Diplazium maximum is traditionally consumed in parts of Western Himalayas, and known as *dhaunte ningro*. The dried, young fiddleheads are rich in dietary fiber (38/100g) and protein (25/100g) with branched-chain essential amino acids and fatty acids, including the unique di-mono-γ-linolenic acid (ω-5 poly-unsaturated fatty acid, PUFA). Phenolics include epicatechin, myricetin, catechin and protocatechuic acid (Sareen et al. 2021).

Molokai twinsorus fern (*Diplazium molokaiense*) is one of the rarest ferns in the world. It is endemic to Hawaii and is only found on Maui, where fewer than seventy ferns remain.

Nyama idim (*Diplazium sammatii*) fronds are edible and slightly differ in health benefits whether young and tender or more mature. Young fronds contain more zinc and copper, while older fronds contain more iron. Oxalate levels are slightly higher in young leaves, while tannins increase with age (Bassey et al. 2001).

Diplazium subsinuatum syn. *Deparia lancea* contains a number of acetylated glycosides such as hopane-triterpene glycosides. Diplazioside III is unique as a naturally occurring bisdesmoside with a hopane aglycone.

DOODIA

Kunth's Hacksaw Fern   Rasp Fern

Kunth's hacksaw fern (*Doodia kunthiana*) is known in Hawaii as *okupukupu*, *okupukupu lauii*, or *pamoho*. It is perennial with long fronds, and its stems are used for ornamental plaiting.

RASP FERN ESSENCE

This essence of *Doodia media* facilitates inner healing, peace, and stillness after experiences of emotional or sexual trauma or deep sorrow that has impacted the soul and become locked into cellular memory. It helps the unconscious mind release the memories that it is not safe to let one's emotional guard down. This fern is helpful for those who have emotional fears or who feel emotionally scarred by life. Find as First Light Flower Essences of New Zealand No. 38 Rasp Fern.

DRYMOGLOSSUM

Dragon Scale Fern   Penny Fern

Drymoglossum carnosum syn. *Lemmaphyllum carnosum* syn. *Lepisorus microphyllus* and *Drymoglossum subcordata* are both epiphytic ferns growing in temperate zones of Eastern Asia. Their fronds and young shoots were eaten in China (Read 1946).

Leaves of dragon scale fern or penny fern (*Drymoglossum piloselloides*) inhibit nucleation, growth, and aggregation of calcium oxalate stones associated with kidney stones (Hewagama and Hewawasam 2022). The Malay name is *paku sisek naga* meaning dragon scales, due to the pale, star-like hairs on the fronds.

The small fern exhibits activity against athlete's foot, other fungi, and common pathogenic bacteria (Somchit et al., 2019).

DRYNARIA

Basket Ferns

Geographic Range: Celebes (Sulawesi), China, Indonesia, Korea, Taiwan, Tibet, Vietnam

Habitat: epiphytic, trees, rocks, forests
Practical Uses: food, ornamental plant
Medicinal Applications: anti-inflammatory, antibacterial, antidiarrheal, antioxidant, back pain, bone density, cognitive function, cancer, cytotoxicity, diabetes, gangrene, hair loss, hearing loss, kidneys, teeth, bones, ototoxicity prevention, pain, rheumatoid arthritis, tinnitus, traumatic brain injury, vitiligo
Warning: Oakleaf basket fern may induce uterotonic activity with antifertility effects and could act as an abortifacient. It also shows potential hepatoxicity in combination with certain medications.

Drynaria baronii extracts inhibit prostaglandin E(2) production by LPS-stimulated RAW264.7 cells and inhibit cyclooxygenase COX-2 expression at both protein and mRNA levels. This suggests potent anti-inflammatory activity (Chu et al. 2009b). This fern is native to China and Tibet, and its rhizome is one of several known as gu sui bu (GSB).

The rhizome is used in TCM for kidney deficiency associated with back pain, tinnitus, hearing loss, loose teeth, bone fractures, alopecia areata and vitiligo. The rhizome exhibits weak anti-HIV activity and induces apoptosis in HL-60 (human promyelocytic leukemia) cell lines (Chu et al. 2009b). Early work by Zhou (1987) confirmed the rhizome's benefits on experimental osteoporosis.

In Vietnam, the rhizomes of *Drynaria bonii* syn. *Aglaomorpha bonii* are used to treat bone fractures, osteoporosis, stimulate hair growth, and remedy tinnitus. Methanol and hexane extracts proliferate MG-63 (human osteoblast-like) cells. Trinh et al. (2016) identified a new compound, drynaether A, and five known compounds, uracil, 4-hydroxy-7-methoxyflavan, kaempferol, indole-3-carboxylic acid, and protocatechuic acid. Previous work also identified drybonioside, α-tocopherol, 24-methylenecycloartan-3β-ol, triphyllol, and ethyl β-D-fructopyranoside, the latter of which exhibits positive antitumor metastatic activity (Wang et al. 2011).

Tinnitus, the perception of sound in the absence of external noise, is influenced by the alteration of auditory perceptions, particularly involving muscarinic acetylcholine receptors, with the M1 type playing a key role.

Synthetic drynaran analogues, derived from this fern, may be useful in treating chronic tinnitus. Specifically, the 1b and 1g lignans are competitive agonists to the antagonist tiotropium and act in synergy with bromazepam (da Rocha et al. 2023).

Drynaria fortunei syn. *D. roosii* syn. *Agiaomorpha fortunei* is an important fern in Traditional Chinese Medicine (TCM). The latter is the latest taxonomic binomial. The fern grows basket-like on trees or rocks.

The fern rhizome is commonly known as gu sui bu (GSB), here meaning "mender of shattered bones." Other common names for the rhizome in Chinese are *mao chiang* "hairy ginger," *shih pan chiang* "stone plate ginger," *wang chiang* "monkey ginger," and *p'a shan hu* "mountain-climbing tiger." In Korea it is known as *gol se bo*.

The rhizome was used as hemostatic for gangrene of the fingers in earlier times (Roi 1955). In Taiwan, formerly known as Formosa, the rhizome was decocted for rheumatism (Usher 1971).

The species name honors Robert Fortune (1812–1880), a Scottish botanist and plant hunter. He traveled to China and Japan, introducing Chinese tea (*Camellia sinensis*) to neighboring India, controlled at the time by the English East India Company, breaking the tea monopoly formerly held by China.

Fortune also illegally shipped some 250 ornamental plants back to England, Australia, and the United States. He disguised himself by shaving his head and wearing Mandarin attire. Fourteen species and one genus of plants are named in his honor.

The rhizome's energy is warm, and its taste is bitter. In TCM, it is considered to influence the kidney and liver systems. Herbal practitioners use the rhizome for cases of Kidney Yang deficiency syndrome.

Drynaria roosii rhizomes contain liglaurates A through E, as well as methyl and glyceryl 12-caffeoyloxylaurates. Liglaurates A through D possess significant cytotoxicity against HeLa (human epithelial/cervical) cancer cell lines (Wufuer et al. 2022).

The hairy rhizome, commonly referred to as GSB, is most noted for its ability to improve bone density, but numerous human clinical trials have demonstrated its benefits in various health conditions. Water extracts contain protocatechuic acid, caffeic acid 4-O-D-glucopyranoside, 5,7-dihydroxychromone-7-O- rutinoside, neoeriocitrin, and naringin.

Both GSB and naringin (the compound) inhibit the binding of bone morphogenetic protein (BMP-2) and BMPR-1A, thereby controlling cell differentiation by blocking BMPR-1A and enhancing BMPR-1B signaling. This suggests both compounds are natural BMP regulators for bone tissue engineering by inducing osteogenic differentiation in bone marrow mesenchymal stem cells (Dong et al. 2020).

Neoeriocitrin has shown higher activity than naringin in promoting proliferation and osteogenic differentiation in MC3T3-E1 (*preosteoblast*) cells (Li et al. 2011a). Naringin promotes proliferation and differentiation of human periodontal ligament cells (Hu et al. 2010).

Drynaria methanol and ethanol extracts inhibit SP2 (myeloma) cancer cell lines (Li et al. 2013a). Myeloma in humans is known as multiple myeloma, a cancer of the white blood cells. This condition leads to the rapid growth of abnormal cells, which crowd out normal cells in the bone marrow that produce red blood cells, platelets, and normal white blood cells.

Drynachromosides C and D, along with one other chromone isolated from the rhizome, exhibit inhibitory activity on triglyceride accumulation (Han et al. 2015).

In a year-long clinical trial of eighty post-menopausal (40 in the active group and 40 in the placebo group) with osteoporosis and high lipid profiles, Lu et al. (2022) found that the rhizome supplement effectively improved both bone density and lipid profiles. The fern rhizome also suppressed the NLRP3 inflammasone and associated cytokines by either increasing SIRT1 or decreasing Notch1 expression.

In an in vivo zebrafish model of glucocorticoid-induced osteoporosis, GSB showed osteogenic effects. The bone resorption activity was retained after treatment, suggesting benefits in maintaining normal bone remodeling (Peng et al. 2022a).

Rhizome flavonoids increase bone trabeculae and bone mineral density by promoting bone formation and inhibiting bone absorption, thereby alleviating diabetic osteoporosis in a rat model. The activation of the BMP2/Smad signaling pathway is likely responsible for these benefits (Fang et al. 2023).

Flavonoids may also help in the treatment of rheumatoid arthritis by inhibiting Th17 differentiation and reducing the inflammatory response of synoviocytes (Chen et al. 2022b).

GSB may regulate stem cells, osteoblasts, osteoclasts, and immune cells through various pathways, potentially playing a role in osteonecrosis of the femoral head (ONFH) and possibly avoiding hip joint replacement.

The rhizome selectively exerts estrogenic activity differently from the drug tamoxifen. Although similar in effect, GSB, at clinical dose, dramatically ameliorated changes in bone and dopamine metabolism in ovariectomized rats.

However, unlike tamoxifen, GSB did not induce uterine and breast tissue growth (Zhou et al. 2022).

A chloroform fraction of the fern exhibits antibacterial activity against periodontic pathogens *Porphylomonas gingivalis* and *Prevotella intermedia*. Strong synergistic activity was found when combined with ampicillin or gentamycin, suggesting potent effects against oral bacteria (Cha et al. 2017).

GSB flavonoids also promote the differentiation and proliferation of dental pulp stem cells, indicating potential applications in dental tissue engineering and bone regeneration (Huang et al. 2012).

The fern extract has been found to help treat aminoglycoside-induced ototoxicity (Chen et al. 2021b). Ototoxicity, a serious concern associated with aminoglycoside antibiotics like streptomycin, gentamicin, and neomycin, can lead to hearing loss in young children, but can also cause deafness, tinnitus, balance problems, and dizziness in adults. An estimated 466 million people worldwide suffer from hearing loss, and untreated hearing loss costs approximately $750 billion per year. Aminoglycoside drugs damage hair cells in the inner ear, causing permanent hearing loss (Fu et al. 2021).

An in vivo study by Long et al. (2004) found that a flavonoid fraction from the rhizome protected against gentamicin-induced ototoxicity.

The use of glycocorticoid drugs can induce osteoporosis. A deep dive into the various flavonoids by Zhang et al. (2022a) identified 191 flavonoid compounds in vitro and forty-eight compounds in vivo, which may play a role in addressing this issue. Tartrate-resistant acid phosphatase has been suggested as a key player in both adipose and bone metabolism and may be a novel approach to the prevention and treatment of cortisone-induced osteoporosis.

The drug alendronate is used clinically to prevent or treat osteoporosis after menopause or long-term use of cortisone. The drug is effective but also comes with side effects including esophageal ulcers and in rare cases, jaw issues. Alendronate in combination with rhizome extracts given to osteopenic rats promoted fracture healing and callus formation significantly better than therapy alone (Chen et al. 2018).

Extracellular vesicles (EVs) are nano-sized membrane vesicles released from plant cells. In GSB, seventy-seven proteins have been identified in EVs, with 47% being enzymes. Work by Cao et al. (2022) found that most of these proteins, including NAD(P)H-quinone oxidoreductase (NQO1), are enriched in the oxidative phosphorylation pathways in humans with Alzheimer's, Huntington's, and Parkinson's diseases.

This suggests that rhizome EVs could potentially alleviate these neurological conditions with NAD(P)H playing a critical role.

A study by Wen et al. (2022) identified a potential mechanism by which the rhizome may alleviate lower back pain via numerous pathways. The rhizome flavonoids inhibit extracellular matrix (ECM) degeneration by increasing the expression of aggrecan and collagen type 2 and preventing the upregulation of collagen types 1 and 3. This suggests possible benefits in difficult-to-treat cervical spondylosis (Zhao et al. 2021a).

Aggrecan is also known as chondroitin sulphate proteoglycan I, a protein encoded by the ACAN gene. It is an integral part of ECM in cartilage tissue, helping cartilage withstand compression. Aggrecan aggregates with hyaluronan to ensure adequate load-bearing capacity in articular cartilage of joints. Matthew Wood (2021), a noted herbalist, wrote an excellent book on ECM from a balanced and holistic perspective.

In the brain, aggrecan provides mechanical buffering and contributes to the formation of perineural nets, which regulate synaptic plasticity. Aggrecan is also found in cardiac jelly, developing heart valves, and blood vessels (Koch et al. 2020). However, when present in excess, it is involved in atherosclerosis, aortic aneurysms, vascular restenosis after injury, and varicose veins.

Drugs and herbs containing quinone derivatives, such as mitomycin C, RH1, E09 (apaziquone), and b-lapachone, induce cell death by NQO1 reduction of two electrons. NQO1 is overexpressed in several cancers, including breast, lung, cervix, pancreas, and colon cancers, compared to normal human cells (Preethi et al. 2022).

GSB water constituents, including (2S)-neoeriocitrin and caffeic acid 4-O-glucoside, have shown significant axonal elongation and regeneration in an Alzheimer's disease (AD) model, reversing atrophy in cultured cortical neurons of mice (Yang et al. 2015b). The fern also contains eight acetylcholinesterase-inhibitory flavonoids that may be helpful in preventing or treating AD.

The fern may also have potential in treating traumatic brain injury (TBI). Research by Wang et al. (2015) identified eriodictyol in the fern extract, which may protect the brain in a rat study. They found that post-treatment with the fern rhizome decreased brain lesion volume, improved neurological and cognitive function, and reduced anxiety and depression-like behavior. Reduced blood levels of IL-6 and increased levels of IL-10 were also noted.

Eriodictyol is a natural flavonoid that ameliorates ischemic stroke in animal studies. The benefits are thought to result from the inhibition of inflammation, oxidative stress, autophagy, and apoptosis. However, a well-designed clinical trial would be needed to validate its benefits in humans (Guo et al. 2023b).

The flavonoid fraction of the fern prevents nephrotoxicity, improves kidney function, and promotes the regeneration of kidney primary epithelial tube cells in a guinea pig study of acute renal failure (Long et al. 2005).

The dry rhizomes of the oakleaf basket fern (*Drynaria quercifolia*) contain friedelin, epifriedelinol, β-sitosterol, β-sitosterol 3-β-D-glucopyranoside, and naringin. The compounds have been used in traditional medicine in India, China, and Southeast Asia.

In ayurvedic medicine, the *Ashwakatri* rhizome is boiled, and the decoction is consumed for its antipyretic properties, as well as for treating tuberculosis, diarrhea, cholera, and typhoid fever, syphilis, and skin conditions. In the Philippines, the rhizome was used for its astringent properties, and the whole fern was used to treat hectic fever, cough, and bacterial infections (Chopra et al. 1956; Quisumbing 1951).

An extract of the fern inhibits multidrug-resistant bacteria such as *Neisseria gonorrhoeae* and *Streptococcus beta-haemolyticus* (Tan and Lim 2015).

Friedelin, a triterpenoid also found in cannabis, is known for its analgesic, antipyretic, and anti-inflammatory properties without binding to opioid receptors. The compound shows significant antioxidant and liver-protective effects. There are nearly 350 studies on its health benefits cited on PubMed.

Epifriedelinol ameliorates induced breast cancer in mice, induces apoptosis in human cervical cancer cell lines, and may be useful as adjuvant therapy in prostate cancer (Zhang et al. 2022b). Specifically, the compound induces apoptosis on C33A and HeLa (human cervical) cancer cell lines (Yang and Li 2017).

Epifriedelinol also protects against neuropathic pain associated with spinal cord injury by downregulating the N-methyl-D-asparate (NMDA) receptor function (Guan et al. 2022).

The fresh rhizomes were traditionally used for birth control in parts of India. Both methanol (87%) and water (68%) extracts possess uterotonic activity with relatively low toxicity. Methanol extracts showed higher efficacy as an abortifacient and anti-implantation agent and also affected hormone release levels. These findings suggest significant antifertility activity (Das et al. 2014).

The fronds have been traditionally used to alleviate rheumatic and arthritic pain. Ethanol extracts of fertile fronds have traditional use for edema, pain, inflammation, swellings, liver protection, and fevers. The flavanone glycoside naringin (1.2%) and its aglycone naringenin (0.02%) may be partially responsible for their analgesic and anti-inflammatory effects.

Work by Modak et al. (2021) prepared methanol extracts of the rhizome and found potent anti-inflammatory and antiarthritic activity, using both in vitro and in vivo rat models of rheumatic arthritis. Various compounds were identified in the extract, including squalene, γ-tocopherol, n-hexadecanoic acid, which showed potent inhibition of COX-2, TNF-α, and IL-6 markers.

When acetone extract treatment was combined with paracetamol (acetaminophen), it significantly reduced hepatoxicity in mice. This benefit is attributed to the increased protein and mRNA expressions of the transcription factor Nrf2 and its target genes (Chatterjee et al. 2022). Earlier work by Saravanan et al. (2013) also found significant in vivo benefits, including reductions in reactive oxygen species, lysosomal enzymes, TNF-α and IL-1b; and increased levels of anti-inflammatory cytokine IL-10.

In vitro studies of the fern's rhizomes and fronds have shown they stabilize cell membranes and exhibit antioxidant and thrombolytic potential. Specifically, crude methanol extracts of the rhizome and its aqueous fraction exhibited noticeable clot lysis (Chaity et al. 2016).

Rhizome extracts have also been shown to attenuate liver fibrosis in a rat study (Anuja et al. 2018). Additionally, an extract showed inhibition of sexually transmitted *Neisseria gonorrhoeae* isolates and World Health Organization (WHO) strains, especially against multidrug-resistant strains (Shokeen et al. 2005). Water extracts of the fern have been found to inhibit acetylcholinesterase activity and reduce oxidative stress in memory-impaired mice, suggesting possible benefits in neurological disorders, including Alzheimer's disease (Ferdous et al. 2024).

The basket fern (*Drynaria rigidula* syn. *Aglaomorpha rigidula*) is an epiphytic fern whose fronds were once used as a vegetable in Celebes (Sulawesi), Indonesia (Usher 1971). The spores are surrounded by rust-colored sterile fronds that resemble a basket or large bird's nest.

The fronds are up to 1.2 meters in length. The rhizomes have been used in traditional medicine and possess antioxidant, antidiarrheal, and anti-gonorrhea properties (Tam and Lim. 2015; Usher 1971).

The fronds and fertile fronds of lobed basket fern (*Drynaria sparsisora* syn. *D. linnei*) exhibit tyrosinase inhibition and antioxidant activity (Tam and Lim 2015). The rhizomes have been traditionally applied to snakebites. Unspecified parts of the fern were used for eye complaints.

DRYOATHYRIUM

False Spleenwort

Dryoathyrium is found in wet, swampy tropical and subtropical regions of the Old World.

A variety of flavonoids derived from an extract of false spleenwort (*Dryoathyrium boryanum* syn. *Deparia boryana*) exhibit antioxidant activity, although the extract showed no effect on acetylcholinesterase (Cao et al. 2013a).

DRYOPTERIS

Autumn Fern
Bear's Paw Root
Borrer's Scaly Male Fern
Buckler Ferns
Deceptive Fern
Dwarf Male Fern
Golden-scale Fern
Goldie's Fern
Grassland Fern
Hay-scented Fern
Indian Male Fern
Mountain Fern
Male Fern
Narrow Spinulose Shield Fern
Oak Leaf Ferns
Scaly Male Ferns
Shaggy Field Fern
Wood Ferns

Geographic Range: Asia, Canada, China, Eastern North America, Europe, Himalayas, Japan, Korea, South Africa, Sub-Saharan Africa, Tibet, Western Himalayas

Habitat: damp shaded areas, forests, grasslands, rocks near water, sinkholes, temperate climates, woodlands

Practical Uses: bedding for livestock, decorative baskets, deodorizing meat, hair wash, food, insulation, ornamental plant, perfume ingredient, scent masking for hunting

Medicinal Applications: anthelmintic, antibacterial, antiviral, appetite stimulant, cancer, cognitive impairment, Crohn's disease, diarrhea, edema, gonorrhea, intestinal parasites, liver health, neuralgia, pain relief, rheumatism, skin conditions, stomach issues, sweating (diaphoresis), tapeworm treatment, tuberculosis, uterine congestion, vermifuge

Warning: Male fern root should not be consumed by individuals with anemia, heart disease, liver or kidney issues, or diabetes. It is also unsafe for children, pregnant women, and the elderly. An overdose can cause serious nervous system problems,

including spasms, paralysis, vision issues, and blindness. In severe cases, seizures or respiratory failure may occur, requiring benzodiazepines and oxygen for treatment.

Over 450 species of *Dryopteris* ferns are found in Asia alone. Many of them are commonly known as wood ferns, male ferns, or buckler ferns.

Wood ferns are prolific producers of spores, with some species releasing up to seven million spores annually. Some wood fern species contain up to 6% oil in their green rhizomes. The fatty acids contain more than 90% monoethenoid acids, and 30% of total fatty acids consisting of 9-hexadecenoic acid (Eckey 1954).

Dryopteris rhizomes have been traditionally used as a vermifuge against flatworms. Compounds such as flavaspidic acid, aspidin, desaspidin, and methylene-bis(aspidinol) are present in many species. These compounds have been shown effects on egg production and death of *Schistosoma mansoni* blood fluke parasites, similar to those of the drug praziquantel (Magalhães et al. 2010).

The World Health Organization (WHO) reported over 236 million people worldwide with schistosomiasis in 2021, most infections caused by *Schistosoma mansoni*. The species name honors Patrick Manson, a Scottish physician and parasitologist, who studied the parasite in a patient returning from the West Indies. The parasite was first identified by the Brazilian parasitologist Pirajá da Silva in 1907.

The hay-scented or buckler fern (*Dryopteris aemula*), the narrow scaly male fern (*Dryopteris cambrensis*), and the alpine lady fern (*Athyrium distentifolium*) have been tested and shown to possess compounds that are effective against drug-resistant helminths. The Finnish name for alpine lady fern, *tunturihiirenporras*, means "field mouse's stair."

The barber's pole worm is one of the most pathogenic nematodes affecting sheep and goats. The adult worm attaches to the abomasal mucosa and feeds on blood. The female can lay over ten thousand eggs a day. Both the larvae and adult worms cause anemia, edema, and death by sucking blood.

All three fern extracts tested were effective against these pathogenic worms, significantly decreasing the viability of female worms of both drug-susceptible and drug-resistant strains (Pavičić et al. 2023).

The golden-scale or scaly male fern (*Dryopteris affinis* syn. *D. borreri* syn. *D. pseudomas*) is notable for its fiddleheads, which are covered with bronze-yellow scales. The species name borreri honors William Borrer (1791–1862), a

19th century English botanist. The fern is native to Europe and parts of Asia and can grow up to 1.2 meters tall. It contains more than 10% propionyl filicinic acid and a sweet flower odor due to the presence of aristolene (28%).

Both the rhizome and fronds of this fern exhibit potent antibacterial activity against *Staphylococcus aureus* and *Escherichia coli* (Bahadori et al. 2015).

Grassland fern (*Dryopteris athamantica*) fronds were traditionally consumed in South Africa for parasites (Usher 1971). The rhizome of this fern has been used as a vermifuge in South Africa (May 1978; Watt and Breyer-Brandwijk 1962). *Dryopteris athamantica* syn. *Aspidium athamanticum* is found among rocks and sinkholes near water, but usually in open grass fields, widespread across sub-Sahara Africa. The fern is used as anthelmintic and considered by some authors to be more reliable than male fern. It has been traditionally used for treating gonorrhea. The Zulu use the whole fern as an anthelmintic and Sesotho people decoct or cook the rhizomes to remove retained placenta from cows after calving.

The species name *athamantica* is associated with the mythological Boeotian king, Athamas, associated with ferns. *Athamas* is also a genus of jumping spiders.

The coastal wood fern (*Dryopteris arguta*) fronds were infused by Costanoan people as a hair wash (Moerman 1986), and its leaves were used by the Yurok to clean meats and lay over meat to keep off flies (Moerman 2010).

The shaggy shield fern (*Dryopteris atrata*) rhizome contains dryatraols A (phloroglucinol derivatives). In vitro work by Zhang et al. (2023) found dryatraol C exhibited the strongest activity against both respiratory syncytial virus and influenza A virus (H1N1).

Dryatraols F through H showed considerable inhibition of herpes simplex virus type one. Further work determined dryatraol G may inhibit replication of the virus by interfering with the late stage of its life cycle.

Kawdead (*Dryopteris barbigera*) fronds, found in the Western Himalayas, are used for livestock bedding during winter (Khoja et al. 2022). *Hapat-daed (Dryopteris blanfordii* and *D. juxtaposita*) are used for the same purpose and both fern rhizomes were used traditionally for intestinal parasites (Chopra et al. 1956; Usher 1971).

Beaded wood fern (*Dryopteris bissetiana*) contains a variety of flavonoids, including juglanin, 6-hydroxyluteolin 7-O-laminaribioside, peltatoside, kaempferitrin, hyperoside, laminaribioside, and astragalin.

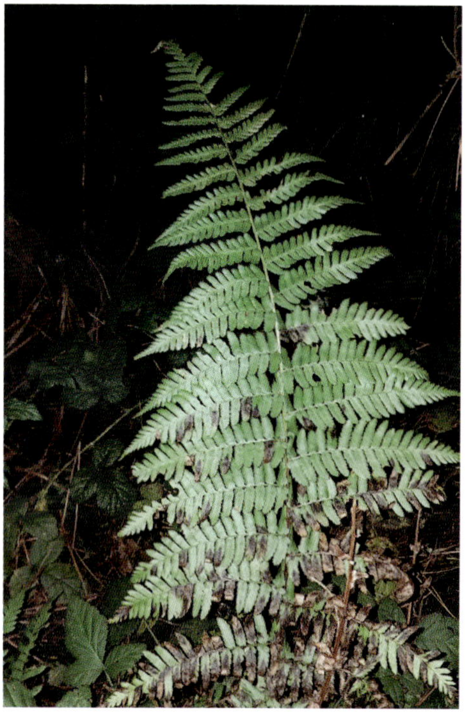

Dryopteris arguta
(Coastal Wood Fern)
Photo by Alan Rockefeller

Juglanin inhibits A549 (non-small cell human lung) cancer by inducing autophagy and apoptosis (Chen et al. 2017b) as well as human breast tumor growth in a mouse xenograft model (in vivo). Juglanin also offers neuroprotection against doxorubicin-induced cognitive impairment in an animal study (Wei et al. 2022b). Doxorubicin is a chemotherapy drug that, while effective, exhibits several side effects in human cancer patients, including diminished cognitive ability and cardiotoxicity.

This fern also exhibits activity against the gram-positive bacteria *Staphylococcus aureus* and *Streptococcus mutans* (Kim et al. 2022b). In Crohn's disease, higher levels of antibodies against laminaribioside are associated with small intestinal disease (Dotan et al. 2006).

Borrer's scaly male fern (*Dryopteris borreri*) contains significant amounts of filicinic acid and phloroglucinol derivatives including aspidinol (14.6%). The fern has some potential for fougère-type perfumes, containing more than 10% (E)-nerolidol. The fern contains the aromatic compound 4-hydroxy-3-methoxyacetophenone (12.6%) and the mushroom-like odor of 1-octen-3-ol results from 8.3% as the main lipid derivative.

The fronds of narrow scaly male fern (*Dryopteris cambrensis*, previously mentioned on page 132) contain various volatile oils including carota-5,8-diene (floral, woody, fresh bark note), (E)-nerolidol (floral and woody notes), and 4-hydroxy-3-methoxyacetophenone (20.6%). The organic compounds of this fern are also prized by perfumers and aromatherapists for use in fougère-type perfumes.

Mountain wood fern (*Dryopteris campyloptera* syn. *D. austriaca*) was taken internally by Lenape and Iroquoians of Eastern North America for diseases of the womb. The fern is thought to have derived from a hybrid between the diploid *Dryopteris expansa* and *Dryopteris intermedia* (Sessa et al. 2012), although this remains speculative. The Inuktitut people boiled the roots and added them to "ice cream" (Moerman 2010). Also known as Indian ice cream further south, this bitter, frothy saponin-rich foam was whipped up from the ripe fruit of Buffalo berry (*Shepherdia canadensis*). The Southern Kwakiutl cooked the rhizomes in steam pits or covered them with red ochre and roasted them on an open fire (Turner 1973).

The narrow spinulose shield fern or narrow spiny wood fern (*Dryopteris carthusiana*) is referred to by the Northern Cree as "raven's beak" or *ku(h) kuguwpuk*. In parts of the world, including the U.K., it is known as the narrow buckler fern. The Cree's generic name for all ferns is *masanahtik*. (See page 142 for the broad spiny wood fern (*Dryopteris dilatata*) and other synonyms.) The species name *carthusiana* honors the monks of the Carthusian Order of Grande Chartreuse in Grenoble, France. Chartreuse is an herbal liquor produced by the Carthusian monks since 1737, based on a recipe given to them in 1605. The liquor is composed of 130 herbs, and today, only two monks know the secret recipe. In 2022, worldwide sales exceeded $30 million, but a decision made in 2019 to limit supply has resulted in shortages.

Russell Willier, a Cree healer now deceased, taught me how to use this fern, which is recorded in a book written by David Young, Russell, and myself (Young et al. 2015).

Willier called this plant *wiyinohwask*, or fat root. The middle green part of the root is boiled and eaten, or the liquid is drunk to treat worms and to stimulate a strong appetite, helping people gain weight. Willier also used the fern in combinations for cancer treatment.

The pineapple-like rhizomes of fat root are dug up in fall when they are surrounded by the scaly fingers of next year's growth. They can be picked in the spring before the new ferns emerge, but this makes them harder to find. If dark and flat inside, the rhizome is not used for food, but if light colored and fleshy, it is steamed in pits or boiled over a fire, tasting similar to a sweet potato or yam. A traditional meal is made by peeling the rootstocks after cooking, and then smearing them with grease or fermented fish eggs. The roots are best for food in the spring or fall.

Various *Dryopteris* roots are used to treat toothache, worms, and other intestinal complaints. An ointment made from the root is used to heal ulcerous and cancerous tumors. This includes spiny wood fern, which was used medicinally as well as for food.

> Shield Fern is used to make infusions for dandruff. The roots are decocted and used as foot baths in treating varicose veins. Mature fronds are stuffed in linen bags for rheumatism. The root is thrown into the fire at the summer solstice as a power charm. Some indigenous tribes eat the uncurled fronds before a hunt, to help mask their scent. The curled shoots of Shield Fern are taken as part of a compound decoction as an appetite stimulant. The frond stipe bases have been traditionally decocted with other herbs for kidney pain, in other mixtures for skin washes, as cancer therapy, or smoked with other plants to treat "insanity" (Rogers 2014b).

The fiddleheads are also part of a decoction taken as appetite stimulant or treatment for cancer (Siegfried 1994). The Chipewyan know shield fern as *ts'elidher niteli ts'u choghe* meaning "muskeg white spruce." Another spelling I have seen mentioned is *nítélits' uchoghé*.

Moerman (2010) noted that Alaska natives ate the inner portion of the underground stem after roasting and peeling it. The young fronds were eaten as fiddleheads. Cooking the roots involves slow baking over coals or in a steam pit. When prepared in a steam pit, the root tastes similar to sweet potato or yam. The Kwakwaka'wakw of British Columbia would sometimes cover the rhizomes with red ochre and roast them on a hemlock spruce stick over an open fire. The finger-like spikes were then broken off, peeled like a banana, and eaten with fermented salmon eggs or grease. The Nuxalk, from Bella Coola, used the more bitter roots to lose weight or to cure sickness associated with eating shellfish infected with red tide toxin. They used the roots in a similar manner (Moerman 1986).

The Witsuwit'en call the fern *dieyin'*, and the Dakelh refer to the fern as *ʔah* or *dastan ʔah*. The Heiltsuk and Haisla call the fern roots *t'ibàm* and the fronds *t'ip'às*. The Kwak'wala, the edible root is known as *tsakkus* or *tsakus*, and the fronds as *telstelgw atluw'*. The Comox of Vancouver Island refer to the edible rhizome as *t'th ékw a* and the Sechelt further south on the island call the roots *stsawch*. Across the strait, the mainland Squamish know the roots as *ts'ékw a?*. The Klallam know the edible root similarly as *tsáqw a*. The Northern Lushootseed refer to fern as *k'lelk'aláts*, while the Southern Lushootseed use *ts'ekw í?*, *tsókwi* for edible rhizome. The Lower Cowliz refer to the fern as *ts'ekw í?* or *ts'kw ai* and the Stl'atl'imx of both the Pemberton and Fraser River regions use *s its' ekw a?* for this fern.

The Dena'ina of Alaska call the root *uh* or *ux*, baking them in pit fires for twenty-four hours (Usher 1971). They also prepare a type of ale called *uh biva*, which was probably learned from the Russians. The fern frond tea, *ux t'una*, was used as a form of eyewash and taken internally for tuberculosis, kidney trouble, and asthma.

The rhizomes, similar to those of male fern (*Dryopteris filix-mas*) (see page 144) contain oleoresins that paralyze intestinal worms, which can then be removed from the body when combined with a saline laxative. The rhizome contains albaspidin, filixic acids, aspidin, and other minor compounds. A number of present compounds exhibit anti-inflammatory activity (Li et al. 2023). (See *Dryopteris fragrans* later in this chapter for more information on aspidin.)

Caution: The fern root should not be administered in the presence of anemia, cardiac disease, liver or kidney disease, or diabetes. It is not advisable for children, during pregnancy, or for the elderly. Overdose can lead to central nervous system disorders such as spasms, paralysis, visual disturbances, and even blindness. In cases of seizure or respiratory failure, benzodiazepines and oxygen may be required (Young et al. 2015). It should be noted that the name *shield fern* also pertains to another genus (including *Polystichum*), but this name was given to us by Russell Willier.

Champion's wood fern (*Dryopteris championii*) has been extracted to yield six new acylphloroglucinols and their antibacterial activity was examined by Chen et al. (2017c) against *Staphylococcus aureus*, *Escherichia coli*, *Bacillus subtilis*, and *Dickeya zeae*. The latter is a destructive gram-negative pathogen that causes soft rot in rice, maize, banana, pineapple, and potato. The fern contains drychampones A through C (meroterpenoids), which possess antibacterial activity (Chen et al. 2016).

Dryopteris chrysocoma is used in India as a substitute for male fern in pharmacognosy. Ethanol extracts of the root, leaves, and stem inhibit inflammation in rats given formalin, reducing it by 51.19%, 41.66%, and 30.95%, respectively (Ahmad et al. 2011).

The rhizomes of Indian male fern (*Dryopteris cochleata*) rhizomes possess antioxidant and antimicrobial activity and were traditionally used to soothe skin sores and lesions, intestinal parasites, gonorrhea, muscle and rheumatic pain, and dog and snakebites. It is frequently used as a vegetable in the Western Himalayan region.

Locally known in India as *kakolisag* or *jatashankari*, extracts of the whole fern were used to cool the inflammation of gonorrhea (Vasudeva 1999). The fern is also used to treat mental health conditions. Water extracts are given to unconscious patients suffering from epilepsy in India.

Green-synthesized silver nanoparticles from the rhizome neutralize Indian Cobra (*Naja naja*) snake venom, significantly inhibiting phospholipase A_2 in vitro (Singh et al. 2020a). This snake is responsible for the highest fatality rate due to snake venom in Thailand and is commonly used by snake charmers. Although the venom has a wide range of medicinal uses, these are too numerous to cite in a book focused on ferns. For more information, see Rogers (2014a) *Sacred Snake Medicine Plants and Venom*.

Thick-stemmed or crown wood fern (*Dryopteris crassirhizoma*) is widely used in traditional medicine in Korea, Japan, and China to treat tapeworm infection, mumps, common colds, and cancer. The fern is non-genotoxic with an oral LD_{50} of > 2,000 mg/kg.

In Japan, the Ainu of Hokkaido used both the stipe and rhizome as a cure for stomach aches and to ease bruising (Mitsuhashi 1976). The rhizome contains filicin, which paralyzes intestinal parasites. In China the rhizome, known as *mianma guanzhong*, is widely available in the market.

In TCM the fern is considered to be slightly cooling and bitter energetically, with an affinity for the liver and stomach. It is used to clear internal heat, has antipyretic properties, and functions as an anthelmintic.

It is further used to treat intestinal parasites, uterine congestion, menorrhagia, leucorrhea, inflamed abscess due to excessive heat, and thyroiditis. While contraindicated during pregnancy, it is used postpartum to reduce hemorrhage after childbirth.

The fresh rhizome is used for skin abscesses, boils, sores, and carbuncles. Both the aerial parts and rhizomes contain phenolic acid and flavaspidic acid AB. The rhizomes are more potent, but the often under-utilized fronds also exhibit antioxidant activity (Wang et al. 2022d).

The fern contains various tocopherol (vitamin E) derivatives and acylphloroglucinol derivatives. Like many ferns, its water extracts support bone health.

The rhizomes contain drycrassirhizomamide A, drycrassirhizomamide B, (S)-(-)-N-benzolphenylalaninol, blumenol A, 8-C-glucosylnoreugenin, dryopteroside, and filmarone (Li et al. 2023), as well as various phloroglucinol derivatives, described in more detail below.

Trimeric acylpholoroglucinol meroterpenoids 7 and 8 exhibit significant activity against the fungus *Candida albicans*, and when combined with the antifungal medication fluconazole (FLC), exhibit strong antifungal activity against FLC-resistant *Candida albicans* (Hai et al. 2023).

Moderate antibacterial activity of this fern against *Micrococcus luteus* was also noted. This bacterium can cause severe outcomes in immunocompromised patients, including endocarditis and brain abscesses in those with lupus erythematosus, as well as exhibiting increased drug resistance in recent years.

Fatty acid synthase (FAS) is a therapeutic target for treating obesity and cancer. Work by Na et al. (2006) identified a series of acylphloroglucinols from the rhizome that inhibit FAS.

Phloroglucinol derivatives also possess potent xanthine oxidase inhibition, suggesting benefits in the treatment of gout. Four compounds, flavaspidic acid AB, AP, BB, and PB, were isolated and showed potent inhibition similar to the drug allopurinol, and superior to oxypurinol (Yuk et al. 2020). Flavaspidic acids AB and PB are highly active against gram-positive bacteria, including methicillin-resistant *Staphylococcus aureus* (MRSA), *Streptococcus mutans*, and *Bacillus subtilis* (Lee et al. 2009a).

Recent work by Bhowmick et al. (2023) identified potent anti-MRSA derivatives. Methanol extracts of this fern significantly eliminate *Streptococcus mutans*, a major cause of dental caries, by up to 99.9% after one hour of incubation. Ethanol extracts alleviate allergic inflammation by inhibiting the Th2 response and mast cell activation in a mouse model of allergic rhinitis (Piao et al. 2019). A later study found that an extract modulated Th1 and Th2 responses in an induced allergic asthma model.

Flavaspidic acids PB and AB exhibit potent antioxidant activity and inhibit lipid peroxidation (Lee et al. 2003). Flavaspidic acid BB, in combination with mupirocin, enhances antibacterial and anti-biofilm activity against antibiotic-resistant *Staphylococcus epidermidis* (Cai et al. 2022).

Extracts from the fern induce cell cycle arrest and apoptosis in PC3-MMC (prostate) cancer cells through both intrinsic and extrinsic pathways. They also exhibit a combined effect with TNF-related apoptosis-inducing ligand (TRAIL) in inhibiting cell proliferation, suggesting possible benefits in treating androgen-independent prostate cancer with minimal side effects (Chang et al. 2010).

The rhizomes contain water-soluble polysaccharides that exhibit antioxidant and immune-modulating activity. One fraction has shown antivirus activity with potential use in functional food, according to Zhao and colleagues (2019). Dryopteric acids A and B, derived from the rhizome, show potent inhibition against HIV-1 protease (Lee et al. 2008). The compound dryocrassin ABBA (a phloroglucinol derivative) exhibits inhibition of the avian influenza virus (H5N1) with low cytotoxicity (Wang et al. 2017a).

During the COVID-19 pandemic, numerous trials were conducted exploring natural products for potential cures. Dryocrassin ABBA and filixic acid ABA were found to inhibit influenza virus infection by targeting neuraminidase. Work by Jin et al. (2022) found that these compounds also inhibited the main protease of SARS-Cov-2 in Vero cells And were effective against SARS-CoV and MERS-CoV infections, suggesting broad-spectrum anti-coronaviral activity.

The stems of the fern are one of the main components of Lianhua-Qingwen formulation, traditionally used in TCM for heat-clearing and detoxification. Dryocrassin ABBA is a key antiviral component in the mixture. Synthesis of the compound showed better neuraminidase inhibition against the avian H7N9 virus, and moderate activity against highly resistant Shanghai N9 strain (Hou et al. 2019).

Among the thirty phloroglucinols isolated from methanol extracts of the rhizomes, three were found to significantly bind with the catalytic sites of protein tyrosine phosphatase 1B, suggesting potential use for treating type 2 diabetes (Phong et al. 2021). Several dimeric and trimeric phloroglucinols also inhibit β-glucuronidase, suggestive of antidiabetic benefits (Phong et al. 2022).

Dryocrassin ABBA significantly inhibits the coagulase activity of von Willebrand factor-binding protein (vWbp). This protein is secreted by *Staphylococcus aureus*, and activates prothrombin, converts fibrinogen to fibrin clots, and induces blood clotting. This is part of what makes the bacterium so problematic in cases of endocarditis, staph sepsis, and pneumonia. Research by Li et al. (2019a) found that dryocrassin ABBA interacts with vWbp without killing the bacteria or inhibiting its expression, as shown in a lung infection-induced mouse study. Lastly, dryocrassin ABBA induces apoptosis in HepG2 (human hepatic carcinoma) cells through a caspase-dependent mitochondrial pathway (Jin et al. 2016).

Nortrisflavaspidic acid ABB has been identified as the most potent α-glucosidase inhibitor (Phong et al. 2023). The research team also developed an optimal ultrasonic-assisted method for producing high-quality extracts.

Dryocrassin is a tetrameric phlorophenone compound that exhibits potent immunosuppressive potential for transplant rejection through the destruction of dendritic cell maturation and function. A study by Fu et al. (2014) was conducted on skin allograft transplantation and activated mouse bone marrow-derived dendritic cells, though further research is required to fully understand its implications.

Flavaspidic acid AB inhibits porcine reproductive and respiratory syndrome virus (PRRSV), which can be devastating to commercial pork producers. Research by Yang et al. (2013a) found that this compound significantly suppresses virus replication. PRRSV is estimated to cost pork producers almost $600 million annually in the United States alone.

In another study, carp immunized with a compound isolated from the fern exhibited maximum resistance against *Aeromonas hydrophila* infection (Chi et al. 2016). This gram-negative bacterium causes septicaemia, meningitis, and endocarditis in immunocompromised humans, with a fatality rate exceeding 50%. It is also associated with traveler's diarrhea, ranging from watery to dysenteric or bloody diarrhea. Fresh water fish are presently treated with Terramycin (oxytetracycline) or Remet-30 (a potentiated sulfonamide). This results, of course, in antibiotics entering the food chain.

Many years ago, while visiting our local botanical garden, I found myself walking across a low bridge over a koi (ornamental carp) pond. As I was standing there, my wallet fell from my pocket and lay on the surface of water. Several large carp began to nudge and move it around. To my amazement, they flipped it over the bridge to the other side, where more carp assembled. Before I knew it, the fish were passing it from one to another—there was carp-to-carp walleting!

Crested wood fern (*Dryopteris cristata*) rhizome has been traditionally decocted or infused by the Ojibwa for treating stomach and other digestive complaints (Moerman 1986). The rhizome tea taken hot was used to induce sweating (diaphoresis), clear lung congestion, and expel intestinal parasites.

This tetraploid fern has hybridized with the diploid goldie's fern (*Dryopteris goldiana*) resulting in the fertile hybrid Clinton's wood fern (*Dryopteris clintoniana*). Cullina (2008) suggests that 95% of fern species today are the result of past hybridization. He cites the example of crested wood fern

(*Dryopteris cristata*) and fancy wood fern (*Dryopteris intermedia*) creating the hybrid Boott's wood fern (*Dryopteris* × *boottii*), which is sterile.

Various kaempferol derivatives in shaggy wood fern (*Dryopteris cycanida*) inhibit α-glucosidase enzyme more effectively than acarbose, suggesting potential benefits in managing blood sugar dysregulation (Amin et al. 2020).

Earlier research investigated the analgesic effects of kaempferol-3,7-di-O-α-L-rhamnopyranoside. The compound appears to be mediated through antagonism of the cholinergic system, independent of calcium channel and opioid receptor involvement. Strong COX-2 inhibition was also noted (Ali et al. 2017).

The deceptive fern (*Dryopteris decipiens*) is a perennial found throughout temperate climates of Southeast Asia and Southern China. In Hawaii, the stems are woven into ornamental baskets and hats, though they are considered of poor quality.

The broad spiny wood fern (*Dryopteris dilatata* syn. *Dryopteris spinulosum* var. *dilatatum*) is known by the Yupik (Chugach) of Yukon/Alaska as *tseturqaaraat*. The rootstocks were eaten by numerous Indigenous groups in Northwestern North America. The fern is known to the Haida as *ts'aagul* or *saagwaal*. The rootstock of wood fern is known as *sk'yaaw*. Ethnobotanist Newcombe (1897) called the fern *sk!iaoxil* (Turner 2004).

The roots, which resemble clusters of fingers, are collected in the spring before new fronds emerge. They are traditionally cooked overnight in steam pits lined with skunk cabbage leaves. Swanton (1905) recorded a story in which the hero painted his face with a design of this fern to make himself appear more beautiful (Turner 2004).

The Saanich (Wsánec) of Vancouver Island call the fern *leqleqa*. The Northern Alberta Chipewyan name for it is *nítélits'uchoghé*, meaning "muskeg white spruce" or *ts'ëlidhér*. The Slave (also known as Slavey, Awokanak, or Etchareottine) of the Northwest Territories refer to it as *eya ha dala* (Marles et al. 2000).

In Washington state, the Cowlitz know the fern as *ts'kwai*, members of the Green River tribe as *taõ'kwî*, the Klallam similarly as *tsa'qwa*, and the Snohomish as *k!lalk!ala'ts*. The Cowlitz traditionally baked the rhizomes overnight in a steam pit and then scraped out the insides for food. Indigenous people of Puget Sound gather the rhizomes in the fall and early winter, when the fern goes dormant. The Klallam pound the rhizomes and apply the pulp to cuts (Moerman 1986) and the Snohomish soak the leaves in water as a hair rinse (Gunther 1945). In the West Indies, the rhizome was pounded and applied as poultice to cuts, and the fronds were infused as a hair wash (Lloyd 1964).

Broad buckler wood fern (*Dryopteris dilatata*) extracts have been shown to protect alloxan-induced diabetic rats from oxidative stress, and significantly ameliorate oxidative injury in the pancreas, liver, and kidneys (Ajirioghene et al. 2021).

The fern contains the volatiles (E)-2-hexenal and (Z)-3-hexenol, which contribute to a green odor in fougère perfumes and colognes.

Autumn fern (*Dryopteris erythrosora*) is native to Japan and Eastern Asia. It is oddly named, as its colors are more vibrant in spring. The spore-producing sori underneath the fronds are a bright red color. The fronds were used in traditional Asian medicine to treat hepatitis and protect liver health. When growing in full sunlight, the fern exhibits higher antioxidant activity.

Zhang et al. (2019) researched the optimal method for drying leaves to maximize flavonoid content and antioxidant activity. They found that drying leaves in the shade and then finishing in an oven at 75° Celsius yielded the best results. Twenty-two flavonoids were identified in the study. Earlier work by Xie et al. (2015) found that flavonoid content is significantly higher in stems (4.3%–12.5%) compared to leaves (2%).

The flavonoid content is lower in spring but increases through the summer onward, peaking in winter. Phenolic glycosides and flavonoids have been identified as key compounds (Yoo et al. 2017).

The flavonoid content follows a descending order from stems to roots, rachis, and then leaves, which also reflects their free radical scavenging activity (Zhang et al. 2012a).

These flavonoids exhibit cytotoxicity to A549 (lung) cancer cell lines and show dose-dependent inhibition of acetylcholinesterase (Cao et al. 2013b).

The fern root extract also exhibits antimicrobial activity against *Bacillus cereus* (Jun et al. 2013). Over 2,100 extracts were screened for use in infant cereals. The authors found that when this extract was combined with sand sedge (*Carex pumila*), it reduced the required efficacy dosage by 50% and 87.5% respectively, compared to the individual extracts.

The spreading wood fern, also known as northern buckler fern (*Dryopteris expansa*), plays a role in Tlingit mythology, where it was picked green and layered as food. In the myth, it is said that before "Raven's time the butts of ferns . . . were already cooked." Hunters were advised to watch out for "green fern roots" in areas where there are grizzly bears (Swanton 1909). The Tlingit call this fern *k^{w} álx*, the Haida know the edible rhizome as *sk'yaaw*, and the fronds as *saag^{w} aal* or *ts' aagul*.

The Gitxsan call the fern *ʔax*, and a ʻWii Ax crest appears on the totem pole of ʻWoosimlaxha at Kispiox Village. The root was a staple food. The Cowlitz baked the rhizomes in steam pits overnight and scooped out the insides. Indigenous Alaskans added the fiddleheads to soup after removing the covering, or boiled them and combined them with dried fish and seal oil for a meal. The Comox tell a story about a mountain goat hunter eating the fern roots, and women gathering the roots in winter during a famine (Boas 2002). The Dena'ina (Tanaina) kept is simple by naming the rhizome *ux*, and the leaf *ux t'una' ux*.

The Yupik name for rhizome is *kun'aq* and the Tahltan name for the fern may be *ch'ool*. *Ch' oh* is the term for porcupine quills.

The rhizome contains filicin, which paralyzes tapeworms. The fronds contain lipophilic compounds, including squalene, an unusual compound also found in olives and amaranth. Like other species of this genus, it contains apigeninidin and luteolinidin. Apigeninidin-rich extracts exhibit potent suppression of A549 (lung) cancer cells lines and prevent aflatoxin-related health issue in an animal study (Owumi et al. 2022). Luteolinidin blocks activity of the enzyme CD38, which is associated with ischemia/reperfusion of the heart, resulting in depletion of cardiac nicotinamide adenine dinucleotide phosphate NADPH(H) pool and preserving endothelial nitric oxide synthase (Boslett et al. 2017). Both compounds are plentiful in sorghum grain (*Sorghum bicolor*).

This fern is easily confused with *Dryopteris dilatata* (see page 142), but the fronds are smaller and contain half the chromosomes (2n = 82). The Clallam used the rhizomes for food, but this may have been *Dryopteris dilatata* (Moerman 2010).

Male fern, also known as bear's paw root (*Dryopteris filix-mas*) is a vermifuge, formerly recorded in the U.S. Pharmacopeia, making it the only fern ever included. The first recorded medicinal use in a Chinese materia medica dates back to 200 BC. Data collected from Romania between the 1860s and 1970s found that the fern was widely used in pediatric medicine. The fern has been mentioned in Russian pharmacopoeias since 1778, and its rhizome was known as a valuable vermifuge back in the times of Dioscorides and Theophrastus. The Greeks used the root as a lousing potion as far back as 100 AD.

About twenty years ago, I was scouting around a veterinary pharmacy and found a discounted one-ounce bottle of oleoresin extract. It was produced long ago by the Bush Company in Montreal and remains in my private collection.

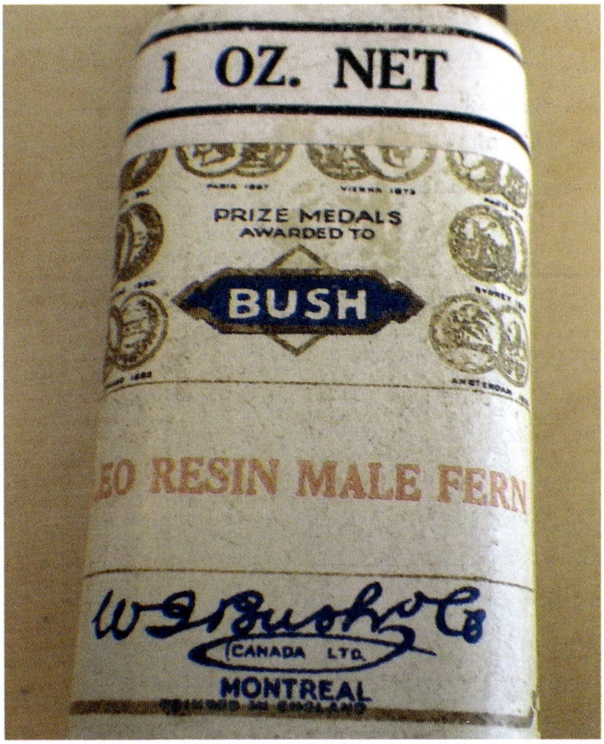

Oleo Resin from the Male Fern
Photo by Robert Dale Rogers

The rhizomes contain 6-15% oleoresins, with up to 24% filicin, composed of filicinic acid, filicylbutanone, aspidinol, albaspidin, paraspidin, and desaspidin; dryocrassin, butanon phloroglucides, filixic acid, filmarone, desaspidinol. Various triterpenes are also present, including 9(11)-fernene, 12-hopene, 11,13(13)-hopadiene, C29 and C31 n-alkanes, butanoic acid (butyric acid), and volatile oil.

"An oily extract that is sweet, woody, earthy and tenacious is made from the male fern root. . . . The oleoresin is made by soaking the powdered root in pure ether, filtering and then evaporating the ether from the tincture. . . . The resin is used as a fixative in Oriental perfume blends" (Rogers 2014b).

The fronds contain 2-4% filicin, including flavaspidic and filicinic acids, paraspidin and desaspidin. When mature, the deciduous male fern grows in damp, shaded areas up to 1.2 meters tall and wide. The common name *expansa* derives from its robust, vigorous growth and was at one time considered the male form of the lady fern.

The two can be distinguished by the shape of sori. Male fern sori are shaped like a kidney, and lady fern sori are more U-shaped. To be sure, cut the stalk and count the vascular bundles-seven for male fern and two for the lady.

The rhizome is best picked after the fronds have died down. The Bella Coola ate the rhizomes raw to lose weight (Moerman 2010) or to neutralize shellfish poisoning. John Gerard authored *The Herball* or *Generall Historie of Plantes* (1597). It is probably not original but a translation of *Stirpium historiae pemptades sex* (1583) by Rembertus Dodoens. A new, revised edition in five volumes was published by Thomas Johnson in 1633. Gerard notes as quoted by Grieve, "the roots of the Male Fern, being taken in the weight of half an ounce, driveth forth long flat worms, as Dioscorides writeth, being drunke in meade or honied water, and more effectually if it be given with two scruples, or two thirds part of a dram of scammonie, or of black hellebore: they that will use it, must first eat garlicke" (Grieve 1931).

The Swiss physician Dr. Louis Auguste Peschier introduced the root into medical practice in the 18th century. The rootstock was considered a good luck charm. It was cut to look like a hand with five fingers, then dried, and carried under names such as "lucky hand" or "dead man's hand." The young rolled fronds, known as "Saint John's Hand," were gathered on St. John's Eve (June 23) for protection from sorcery and the evil eye.

It was an important ingredient in love philtres during medieval times. An ancient Gaelic ballad goes:

> *T'was the maiden's matchless beauty, that drew my heart anigh:*
> *Not the fern-root portion, but the glance of her blue eye.*

The root was said to relieve rheumatic pain, with fronds sometimes sewn into clothing for this purpose.

In a clinical study, twenty-nine patients (12–60 years old) suffering from tapeworm infections, were treated orally with doses of 0.07 grams per kilogram body weight of a male fern extract, preceded by a solution of magnesium sulphate (Epsom salts) in water (15 grams/200 ml water). All patients had previously been treated with other anthelmintics without success. Twenty-five of twenty-nine were cured, with one woman expelling fourteen scoleces of pork tapeworm (*Taenia solium*), while 89% of all infections were attributed to beef tapeworm (*Taenia saginata*) (Mello et al. 1978).

The root's oleoresin helps expel tapeworms, hookworms, bandworms, and liver flukes, with roundworms being more resistant. For the expulsion of tapeworm, a full dose of 0.5 to 1 dram of the oleoresin should be taken while fasting, followed by a strong laxative like Epsom salts, but never castor oil.

This practice is not recommended but is noted here for historical reference.

Other herbalists note that the root is simmered in lard to create a wound ointment, and the powdered root is given orally for rickets in children, though this is no longer advised. The freshly grated root is also excellent for treating inflammation of the lymphatic glands and decoctions were useful in footbaths to treat fungal infections such as athlete's foot. The noted French herbalist Maurice Mességué used male fern in a combination for gout, used in footbaths (Mességué 1970).

Tinctures made from the fresh fronds involve chopping them finely and covering them with 60% alcohol in a glass jar, left to steep for a week in a warm, dark place. This tincture can be used externally as an embrocation, similar to eucalyptus oil. The key to reliable preparations is the use of fresh roots. The fern has demonstrated activity against both gram-positive and gram-negative bacteria.

In Norway, the uncurled fronds were traditionally boiled for food, mixed with flour for bread, and used to brew ales. The active compound in the fern is filicin, a mixture of phloroglucinol derivatives including flavaspidic and filic acids. Acylfilicinic acid (a polyketide) is also present. Aspidin and desaspidin, both present in the fern, exhibit significant in vivo inhibition of skin cancer (Kapadia et al. 1996).

In parts of Southern Nigeria, the fern is used to treat inflammation, rheumatoid arthritis, wounds, and ulcers. The fronds are beneficial for muscle pain, neuralgia, earache, and can be decocted for internal use against liver flukes and tapeworms, albeit having much weaker activity compared to the rhizome.

A study by Erhirhie et al. (2019) found that an ethanol extract of the fronds exhibited significant anti-inflammatory activity in mice. The active ingredient may be quercetin-3-O-α-L-rhamnopyranoside. The fern rhizome possesses antiviral activity against vesicular stomatitis, herpes simplex, and influenza virus type A.

A particularly intriguing study involved administering one drop of the fern extract, suspended in sunflower seed oil, to male mice and rats. It caused a spectacular enlargement of the penis, but no follow-up research has been conducted to this date (Kantemir et al. 1976). I am surprised that this finding hasn't attracted more attention.

The main volatile compound in the fern is (E)-nerolidol, which has a woody and fresh bark note. Solvent extracts of the rhizome are the main source of the "green note" used in fougère perfumes, mainly marketed toward—surprise, surprise—males.

It should be noted that this fern is toxic to horse and cattle.

Filix Mas (male fern) is a homeopathic remedy for worm infections, especially when accompanied by constipation. It is also used to relieve torpid inflammation of the lymphatic glands and to treat pulmonary tuberculosis in young patients, especially those with ulcerated lesions, formerly known as scrofula.

Indications

- The abdomen is bloated with gnawing pain, accompanied by an itchy nose, pale face, and blue rings around eyes.
- Painless hiccups ten minutes after consumption, lasting up to half hour.
- Trembling and cramping in hands and feet. Numbness in right shoulder, arm, and wrist.
- Mind is irritable and confused.
- Blindness, and yellow vision, especially in one eye.
- Increased menses, miscarriage, and sterility.
- Pain in bladder is associated with frequent urination.

Dose

Administer in the first to third potency. The mother tincture is prepared from the fresh rootstalk with the frond base, separated from the roots in autumn.

Compare with Panna (*Aspidium albamanticum*):

Administer three doses of two grams each, all within half an hour, while fasting, in a glass of milk. It is tasteless and will remove tapeworms.

Historical Notes

- The first fragmentary proving was conducted by Berridge with two females and one male at 101st and 102nd dilutions in 1876.
- Toxic effects from therapeutic anthelmintic use were observed by Allen and Clarke. Clinical observations were documented by Boericke (1927).
- Health Canada warning to stop use of Boiron's Filix Mas, 2015. Consider SBL for this particular remedy instead.

However, in my clinical practice, neither conventional treatments nor homeopathic remedies worked for an elderly woman who had survived both Nazi and Russian prisoner camps and had suffered from a tapeworm infection for nearly thirty-five years. Pomegranate tree bark tincture finally rid her of the parasite.

MALE FERN ESSENCE

This essence of *Dryopteris filix-mas* is made from the dark red "blossoms" (sori) that open around the summer solstice. It is useful for those desiring to know more about the nature of plants, and their metaphysical associations. A single drop of the essence is taken, along with the flower or mushroom essence of which you are requesting information, so that much clearer transmission can occur. Only one drop needs to be added to the mixture. The essences are taken under the tongue if you are sitting and while meditating with the plant or mushroom in question. This fern is part of my Prairie Deva Essences research line.

Fragrant wood fern (*Dryopteris fragrans*) is a circumboreal species, living on shaded cliffs, rocky regions, and limestone. The species' name derives from its fruit-like scent with some authors suggesting it is sickly-sweet or primrose-like. Aromatic glands on the surface of the fresh fronds release the beautiful fragrance, which becomes spicier as the fern dries. To me, the fragrance, which lingers for years as a bookmark, is a combination of raspberry and peach.

This fern has been traditionally used by Indigenous groups in North America for bedding and has also been prepared as a beverage.

It is a fern I know well, as it is common in the Rocky Mountains, west of my hometown.

In TCM, this fern is known as *xiang lin mao jue*. In China, it was used for various skin conditions, especially psoriasis, as well as rashes, dermatitis, ringworm, arthritis, and barbiers. Barbiers is a paralytic disease once very common in India. It may be a form of beriberi associated with vitamin B1 (thiamine) deficiency.

Some use fragrant wood fern as a cure for the ingestion of raw bracken fern (*Pteridium aquilinum*). The raw bracken can cause staggering or neurological problems due to thiaminase degrading thiamin, and can cause beriberi. This seems paradoxical to me but has been reported by some.

Research in Russia found that most fern extracts are more effective against *Staphylococcus* bacteria than fungi or protozoa. However, they found fragrant wood fern particularly active against *Trichomonas*, the protozoan involved in vaginal infections. Aspidin PB and albicanol are potent inhibitors of Epstein-Barr virus, suggesting potential in cancer prevention or treatment (Ito et al. 2000).

The fern contains aspidin PB, aspidin BB, dryofragin, albicanol, esculetin, isoscopoletin, flavaspidic acid BB, dryofracoumarin, fragranoside J and K, sesquiterpene glucosides including xianglinmaojuesides A through C, as well as three phloroglucinol derivatives and five terpenoids.

Ethanol extracts of the fern have shown significant cytotoxic effect against A549 (lung), MCF-7 (breast), and HepG2 (liver) cancer cell lines. (Zhao et al. 2014).

Four compounds, including esculetin and isoscopoletin, showed significant cytotoxic effect against A549 (human lung), MCF-7 (human breast), and HepG2 (human liver) cancer cell lines.

Dryofracoumarin A and aspidinol exhibit cytotoxicity against A549 (lung) and MCF-7 (breast) cancer cell lines. Albicanol exhibits cytotoxicity against the latter cancer line.

Esculetin shows potential therapeutic benefits for obesity, diabetes, cardiovascular diseases, kidney failure, cancer, and neurological issues due to its antioxidant, antiproliferative, and cytoprotective qualities (Kadakol et al. 2016).

Among various terpenes identified are 10-hydroxyl-15-oxo-α-cadinol, albicanyl acetate, α-cadinene, and albicanol. Phloroglucinol derivatives include aspidin PB, dryofragin, aspidinol, and aspidin BB.

Aspidinol displays significant anti-MRSA activity both in vitro and in vivo, comparable to the antibiotic vancomycin in a mouse study (Hua et al. 2018).

Aspidin BB inhibits the growth of *Propionibacterium acnes* (now reclassified as *Cutibacterium acnes*) by disrupting the membrane, DNA, and proteins, leading to cell death. This suggests aspidin BB as a treatment for acne vulgaris (Gao et al. 2016). Aspidin BB also induces S-phase cell cycle arrest and apoptosis in HO-8910 (human ovarian) cancer cell lines (Sun et al. 2013).

Aspidin PB exhibits inhibition on fibrogenesis in human keloid tissue. Keloids are a raised, overgrowth of scar tissue around wounds. In my clinical practice I noted some benefits from rosehip seed oil and homeopathic graphites (low potency). Individuals with darker skin form keloids twenty times more frequently than those with lighter skin. (Hellwege et al. 2018). Aspidin PB may be useful in preventing and treating keloids and perhaps other fibrotic diseases (Song et al. 2015).

Aspidin PB also induces cell cycle arrest and apoptosis in human osteosarcoma cell lines, and significantly inhibits tumor growth in U20S xenografts (Wan et al. 2015).

Compounds such as undulatoside A, frachromone C, and dryofracoulin A exhibit anti-inflammatory activity due to inhibition of nitric oxide production in LSP-induced RAW265.7 macrophages (Peng et al. 2016).

Plant extracts were tested against four human cancer cell lines by Liu et al. (2018c). One compound was cytotoxic to MCF-7 (breast) cancer cells and another against A549 (lung), MCF-7 (breast), and SGC-7901 (gastric) cancer cell lines.

Dryofraterpene A (a sesquiterpene) exhibits anti-proliferation against A549 (lung), MCF-7 (breast), HepG2 (liver), and PC-3 (prostate) cancer cell lines (Zhong et al. 2017).

Other derivatives, including dryofragone and dryofracoumarin show modest cytotoxicity against HeLa (cervical) cancer cell line (Zhang et al. 2018).

The compound dryofragin induces apoptosis in MCF-7 breast cancer cells through a reactive oxygen species (ROS)-mediated mitochondrial pathway (Zhang et al. 2012c).

Dryofragin inhibits U20S (osteosarcoma) cell migration and invasion by reducing the expression of MMP-2/9 and elevating the expression of TIMP-1/2 through two signaling pathways (Su et al. 2016).

Previous in vivo studies by Ito et al. (2000) found that aspidin B and albicanol suppressed two-stage carcinogenesis in the skin of mice.

Aspidin and dryofragin are also potent inhibitors of Epstein-Barr virus early antigen activation.

Desaspidin BB, is a phloroglucinol derived from an ethanol extract. This compound exhibits significant antibacterial activity against *Staphylococcus epidermis* (SEP), *S. haemolyticus* (SHA), and methicillin-resistant *S. aureus* (MRSA), including ceftazidime-resistant strains SEP1 through SEP4, SHA5 through SHA7, MRSA8, and MRSA9.

The sesquiterpenoid glycosides dryopteristerpene A and B were isolated from a water extract of the fern. Both show inhibition on nitric oxide production, suggesting anti-inflammatory properties (Peng et al. 2022).

Ethanol extracts possess antifungal activity through inhibition of ergosterol biosynthesis. Both *Trichophyton rubrum* (jock itch, athlete's foot, nail fungus) and *T. mentagrophytes* (ringworm) were tested in vitro. Synergistic activity with miconazole and terbinafine proved indifferent (Liu et al. 2018a).

Dihydroconiferyl alcohol, (E)-3-(4-hydroxyphenyl) acrylic acid, esculetin, and (4),5,7-dihydroxy-2-hydroxymethylchromone, found in this fern, exhibit antifungal activity against *Microsporum canis* and *Epidermophyton floccosum*

(Huang et al. 2014). Microsporum canis is a pathogen that attacks the skin of domestic cats and dogs and *Epidermophyton floccosum* causes skin and nail infections in humans. Ethanol extracts (95%) show the highest antifungal activity.

Genotype VII of sexually transmitted *Trichophyton mentagrophytes* has recently been reported among homosexual men in France (Jabet et al. 2023). Isoflavaspidic acid PB, extracted from aerial parts of the fern, not only inhibits *Trichophyton* biofilm formation but also reduces the metabolic activity of mature biofilms by 20–44%. It appears that the acid seriously destroys the hyphae (Lin et al. 2019).

Albicanol inhibits toxicity in fish caused by the insecticide profenofos, which was approved in the United States in 1982 mainly for application to cotton crops, but it is not approved in the European Union. Profenofos inhibits acetylcholinesterase and is toxic to birds, small mammals, bees, and fish, the latter usually affected through runoff into creeks and streams. Albicanol inhibits its hepatoxicity by regulating various pathways. Previous work found that albicanol exhibits antiaging and antioxidant properties, and counteracts the toxicity of heavy metals (Lihui et al. 2022). A mouse study found that albicanol can reverse D-galactose-induced aging by activating Nrf2 pathway-related genes (Chen et al. 2021b).

Flavaspidic acid BB exhibits activity against drug-resistant *Staphylococcus haemolyticus* and its biofilms. This pathogen is the cause of serious skin and soft tissue infections, especially associated with medical devices like catheters. *Staphylococcus haemolyticus* can produce enterotoxins, and infections can lead to endocarditis, sepsis, peritonitis, urinary tract infections, and bone and joint involvement. Strains resistant to vancomycin and teicoplanin are beginning to emerge.

Solvent-free microwave extraction yielded 0.33% essential oil with antioxidant activity. The fronds of *Dryopteris heterocarpa* syn. *Cyclosorus heterocarpus* syn. *Sphaerostephanos heterocarpus* were traditionally used in Malaya to treat leucodermia (vitiligo) (Usher 1971). In TCM the fern is known as *yi guo mao jue*.

The thin-stemmed forest fern (*Dryopteris inaequalis*) is native to South Africa and grows on stone or soil in deep shade. It is used as a vermifuge to kill parasites and induce diarrhea, that repels the dead worms. A decoction of the rhizomes is drunk for malaria, and the squeezed juice from fresh rhizomes is used as an eardrop for infections.

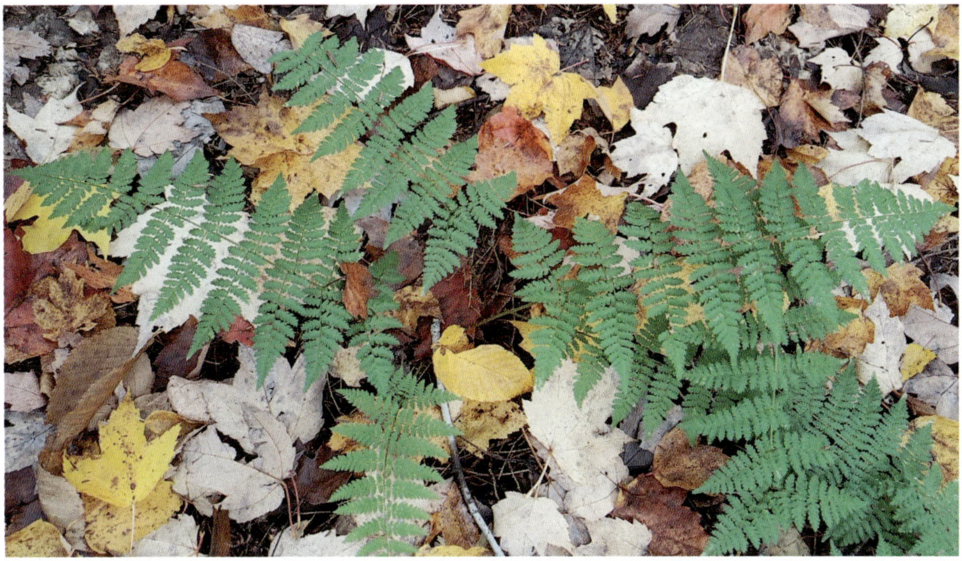

Dryopteris intermedia (Evergreen Wood Fern)
Photo by Alan Rockefeller

The diploid evergreen or glandular wood fern (*Dryopteris intermedia*) and tetraploid *Dryopteris carthusiana* fern (recall its mention on page 135) have created the hybrid *Dryopteris* × *triploidea* (Xiang et al. 2000).

The roots and shoots of *Dryopteris juxtapostia*, known in TCM as *cu chi lin mao jue*, were extracted with methanol and dichloromethane. The latter root extract proved superior in all ways: reducing inflammation, carrageenan- and formaldehyde-induced edema, brine shrimp mortality, and cytotoxicity against HeLa (cervical) and PC-3 (prostate) cancer cell lines. The extract showed the presence of albaspidin PP, 2-methylbutyryl-phloroglucinol, flavaspidic acid AB and BB, filixic acid ABA and ABB, tris-desaspidin BBB, tris-paraspidin BBB, tetra-flavaspidic BBBB, tetra-albaspidin BBBB, and kaempferol-3-O-glucoside (Rani et al. 2022).

The fern powder, fed to rats at 30% for eighty days, showed significant pathological and degenerative effects.

Dryopteris kirbi rhizome contains aspidinol B and P, as well as dryoptkirbioside. Crude extracts (methanol and hexane) and aspidinol B exhibit significant activity against *Staphylococcus aureus* and *Bacillus subtilis*, while aspidinol P exhibits moderate activity. Hexane extracts and fractions exhibit strong activity against A549 (lung), MCF-7 (breast), and HeLa (cervical) cancer cell lines (Matchide et al. 2023).

In Korea, leathery wood fern (*Dryopteris lacera*) is grown as an indoor plant and is similar to the more well-known Boston fern in air purification ability. The leathery wood fern reduces particulate matter in the atmosphere by 86.8% within eight hours (Jang et al. 2021).

Leathery wood fern (*Dryopteris lacera*) contains flavonoids, including juglanin (see pages 134 and 230), 6-hydroxyluteolin 7-O-laminaribioside (antioxidant), peltatoside (anti-inflammatory), kaempferitrin, hyperoside, and astragalin.

Peltatoside is an analogue of quercetin that inhibits pain through activation of peripheral cannabinoid (CB_1) receptors (Oliveira et al. 2017).

In vivo, the compound exhibits anti-inflammatory and immune-modulating properties in a manner similar to dexamethasone (Prata et al. 2020). The fern also shows activity against the gram-positive *Staphylococcus aureus* and *Streptococcus mutans* (Kim et al. 2022b).

Marginal wood fern (*Dryopteris marginalis*) has been traditionally used by Indigenous healers of Eastern North America to treat swellings and rheumatism (Moerman 1986). An infusion of its rhizome was used as an emetic, and a warm infusion was held in the mouth for toothaches. The common and species name derives from the location of its spore cases, found along the margins of the frond leaves. This wintergreen fern is easily damaged by frost, particularly in years with low snowfall. Historically, the rhizome was included in the U.S. Pharmacopeia and contains margaspidin, flavaspidic acid, paraspidin, and phloraspin. Notably, margaspidin is also found in wormwood (*Artemisia absinthium*), and flavaspidic acid is found in fragrant wood fern (*Dryopteris fragrans*, see page 149).

Stewart's wood fern (*Dryopteris odontoloma* syn. *D. stewartii* syn. *Lastrea odontoloma* syn. *Nephrodium odontoloma*) rhizome is used in the Himalayas as a vermifuge (Usher 1971). Water extracts of Stewart's wood fern (*Dryopteris stewartii*) show a higher antidiabetic potential than the ethanol extract. It decreased blood glucose levels 0.41-fold without affecting liver or pancreas tissue (Hanif et al. 2022). The young fronds, known locally as *kaw-daed* in the Western Himalayas, are consumed as a vegetable (Khoja et al. 2022).

Mountain or dwarf male fern (*Dryopteris oreades*) is native to the mountains of Eastern Europe, from Norway south to Spain and east to Pakistan. This species is one of several used for inflamed lymphatic glands, with a fresh, grated rhizome poultice.

Penther's wood fern (*Dryopteris pentheri*) is widespread in sub-Saharan Africa and is also used as an anthelmintic.

The Sesotho of Swaziland believe that inhaling the fern smoke helps protect them from danger.

The rhizomes and fronds of oak leaf ferns (*Dryopteris quercifolia*), *Drynaria rigidula* syn. *Amauropelta scalpuroides*, and *Drynaria sparsisora* have been analyzed for their antioxidant and tyrosinase inhibition. The fertile fronds of the former fern (say that fast three times!) exhibit the highest total phenolic content and antioxidant activity. The fronds of *Dryopteris quercifolia* and *D. rigidula* contain higher levels of phenolics and flavonoids than the rhizomes, even though the latter is more widely used in traditional medicine. The fronds of *Dryopteris quercifolia* exhibit high tyrosinase inhibition, but most *Drynaria* extracts, especially *Dryopteris sparisora* enhance tyrosinase activity (Tan and Lim 2015).

Branched wood fern (*Dryopteris ramosa*), known as *dead*, is a heavily traded plant in the Western Himalayas. It has been traditionally used for gastric ulcers, and as an antibiotic and laxative. The fronds are edible and sold at markets as a vegetable. The rhizome has been used in the past as a substitute for male fern.

The fern is rich in flavonoids, flavonoid-O-glycosides, isoflavone di-C-glycoside, flavanol, flavanone, rotenoid, phloroglucinol and coumarin derivatives, benzofuranone, abietic and phenolic acid, mangiferin, and isomangiferin.

Abietic acid is active against methicillin-resistant *Staphylococcus aureus* (MRSA) and methicillin-resistant *S. pseudintermedius* (MRSP). MRSA is a serious infection in humans, while MRSP is a concern in both human and veterinary medicine. Abietic acid is synergistic with oxacillin in increasing antibacterial activity and reducing biofilm formation (Buommino et al. 2021). MRSP is a serious concern in canines and can transmit to humans, often presenting as swelling, redness, and pain in infected skin. It is equally virulent as MRSA. Abietic acid also inhibits the viability of bladder cancer cells, but not normal cells, both in vitro and in vivo, and exhibits synergistic activity with various chemotherapy drugs (Xu et al. 2023).

Water extracts of this fern are used in Pakistan to treat bacterial gastrointestinal complaints. Work by Ishaque et al. (2022a) identified irflophenone-3-C-β-d glucopyranoside and compared its antibiotic activity with Cefixime, finding it more effective against *Klebsiella pneumoniae*, *Staphylococcus aureus*, and *Escherichia coli* than the standard drug. Extracts also exhibit cytotoxicity against HepG2 (liver) and PC-3 (prostate) cancer cells (Rehman et al. 2022).

Methanol extracts administered to mice showed mild to moderate sedation at higher tested doses, and showed significant anti-ulcer benefits, enhancing intestinal motility and increasing fecal volume. The laxative effect was similar to that of the standard drug Duphalac (Nazir et al. 2021).

An ethyl acetate crude extract inhibited the growth of *Pseudomonas aeruginosa*, similar to the standard drug Cefixime. Crude extracts exhibit calcium channel-blocking effects, equivalent to those of verapamil, and spasmolytic activity and muscarinic receptor-mediated activity in water extracts. The crude extract caused vasoconstriction in aortic tissue, which was completely blocked by an angiotensin II receptor antagonist. This suggests support of the traditional use for gastrointestinal activity (antidiarrheal) and possible benefits in asthma (bronchodilator) and cardiovascular conditions (Iqbal et al. 2023). The extract also inhibits α glucosidase by nearly 92%, while the methanol extract inhibits acetylcholinesterase by 58% and butyrylcholinesterase by 47% (Alam et al. 2021a).

Both mangiferin and isomangiferin have been isolated from the fern. Mangiferin, which is common in many plants, inhibits *Salmonella setubal* and *Bacillus subtilis*, and exhibits weak activity against *Escherichia coli*. Isomangiferin exhibited stronger antibacterial potential against all tested strains including *Escherichia coli* (Ishaque et al. 2022b). Isomangiferin also suppresses breast cancer growth, metastasis, and angiogenesis; and induces apoptosis in a xenograft mouse model (Wang et al. 2018).

Schimper's wood fern (*Dryopteris schimperiana*), a fern native to Eritrea to Malawi and south to Uganda as well as Northern Yemen, contains rhizomes with twice the filicin content (4.4%) of male fern, so caution is advised. The fern is named after Georg Heinrich Schimper (1804–1878) who collected plants, mainly in Ethiopia. The rhizome is known for its anthelmintic properties (Usher 1971).

Dryopteris sublaeta fronds contain several bioactive compounds, including 2(S)-5,7,3'-trihydroxy-6,8-dimethyl-5'-methoxyflavanone, matteucinol, demethoxymatteucinol and 5,7,2'-trihydroxy-6,8-dimethyl flavanone, piceid (resveratrol 3-glucoside), and various other glucosides.

Glioblastoma, a malignant brain tumor, is typically treated with chemotherapy using temozolomide (TMZ), but survival of patients averages only 15 months after diagnosis.

Research by Netto et al. (2022) found that a combination of TMZ and matteucinol inhibits glioblastoma proliferation, invasion, and progression, suggesting a synergistic effect. Matteucinol showed the strongest binding in docking studies with the cell death membrane receptor TNFR1 and the TNFR1/TMZ complex.

Piceid is the major resveratrol derivative in grape juice and wine and is easily converted to resveratrol by healthy probiotics and the microbiome.

The rhizome also contains sublaetentin A through D, matteuorienate A and C, arbutin, 3-methoxy-4-hydroxyphenyl-1-O-ß-D-glucopyranoside, and 3,4-dimethoxyphenyl-1-O-ß-D-glucopyranoside.

Matteuorienate A through C are potent aldose reductase inhibitors, also found in *Matteuccia orientalis* (see page 188). This suggests prevention of side effects associated with diabetes, including neuropathy and retinopathy.

Uniform wood fern (*Dryopteris uniformis*) contains over fifty endophytes that possess antibacterial activity against *Listeria monocytogenes*, *Salmonella typhimurium*, *Bacillus cereus*, *Staphylococcus aureus*, and *Bacillus psychrodurans* syn. *Psychrobacillus psychrodurans* (Das et al. 2017). The latter is a calcium carbonate-producing bacterium that shows promise for biocalcification as an eco-friendly biosealant in environmentally stressed concrete structures (Park et al. 2022). Human applications of this process have not yet been studied.

A diethyl ether extract of scales and rhizomes from alpine wood fern (*Dryopteris wallichiana*) contains albaspidin AA and AB, filixic acids ABA and ABB, as well as four unusual terpenylated aclyphoroglucinols. The latter compounds show moderate in vitro nematocidal activity against L4 stage larvae of *Nippostrongylus brasiliensis*, a gastrointestinal roundworm that infects rodents (Socolsky et al. 2012a). Previous work by Socolsky et al. (2011) identified three acylphloroglucinols from the fern that are active against the schistosomiasis vector snail *Biomphalaria peregrina*. Compounds isolated from the fern also exhibit inhibitory activity against coronavirus 2 (SARS-CoV-2) (Hou et al., 2022).

Albaspidin AA shows strong antibacterial activity against the vegetative form of *Paenibacillus larvae*, a spore-forming bacterial pathogen that causes lethal American foulbrood in beehives.

In a study by Hernández-López et al. (2014), albaspidin AA was one of six compounds isolated from *Hypericum* flower species. Hyperforin, derived from a lipophilic extract of Saint John's wort, incubated on *Paenibacillus larvae* spores, led to significantly fewer colonies. Although the herb is considered a noxious weed in many parts of North America, Saint John's wort has significant benefits for human health and offers protection for critically stressed and endangered honeybees.

ELAPHOGLOSSUM

Antilles Tongue Fern
Argentinian Fern
Deer Fern
Tongue Ferns

There are approximately 600 species of *Elapoglossum* species worldwide with over 450 found in tropical regions of the Americas.

The rhizomes of thick foot tongue fern (*Elaphoglossum crassipes*) contain nine terpenylated acylphloroglucinols; crassipins A–I.

Research by Socolsky et al. (2012b) identified crassipin A as the major acylphloroglucinol derived from an ethanol extract of this fern. A mouse study showed that the compound, given orally at 15 mg/kg, displayed antidepressant activity.

Phloroglucinols isolated from *Elaphoglossum gayanum* and Antilles tongue fern (*Elaphoglossum piloselloides* syn. *E. jamesonii*) exhibit moderate activity against the snail *Biomphalaria peregrina*, a vector in the transmission of tropical disease schistosomiasis (Socolsky et al. 2010b).

The Argentinian fern (*Elaphoglossum lindbergii* syn. *E. hydridum*) contains lingbergins E through I, with two compounds exhibiting in vitro leishmanicidal

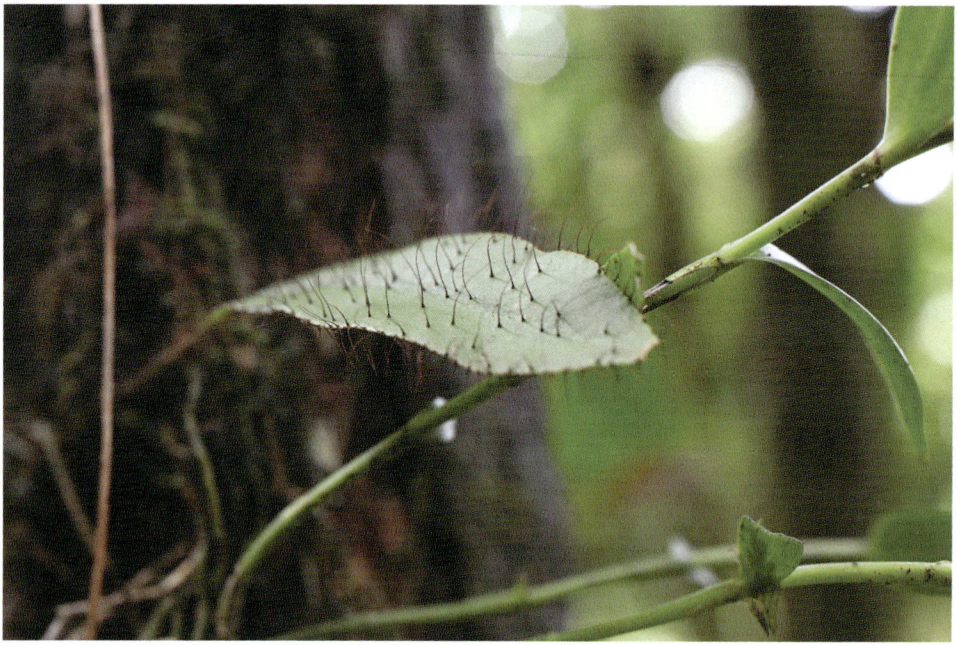

Close-up of *Elaphoglossum* sp. (Tongue Fern)
Photo by Alan Rockefeller

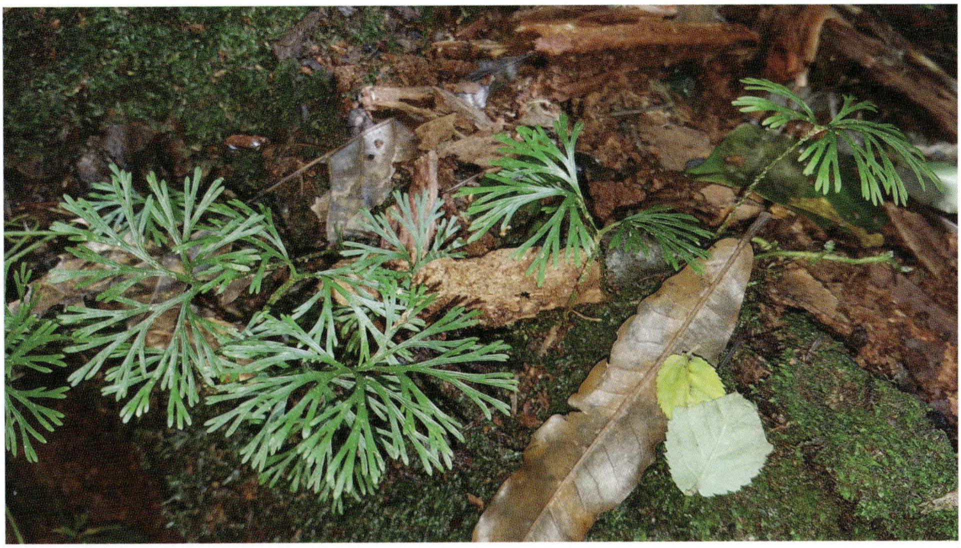

Elaphoglossum peltatum (Peltate Tongue Fern)
Photo by Alan Rockefeller

activity against promastigotes of *Leishmania braziliensis* and *L. amazonensis* (Socolksy et al. 2016).

Marginated tongue fern (*Elaphoglossum marginatum*) extract exhibits significant antioxidant activity (Seo et al. 2022).

The Mexican stag's tongue fern (*Elaphoglossum paleaceum*) contains paleacenins A and B. Extracts display inhibition of monoamine oxidase A (MAO-A) of 25% and 26.5%, and inhibition of MAO-B by 42.5% and 23.7%, respectively.

The extracts also exhibit cytotoxicity against a panel of prostate, cervical, colon, and breast cancer cell lines, with both compounds inhibiting nitric oxide production, suggestive of anti-inflammatory properties (Arvizu-Espinosa et al. 2019).

Rhizome decoctions of the graceful tongue fern, or Duss' tongue fern, (*Elaphoglossum petiolatum*) have been used as a gargle for sore throats (Watt and Breyer-Brandwijk 1962). Seven prenylated acylphloroglucinols, named yungensins A through G, have been isolated by the diethyl ether extract of the scaly rhizomes and roots of *Elaphoglossum yungense*.

The extract and yungensins A–F display antibacterial activity against *Staphylococcus aureus* and *Pseudomonas aeruginosa* and altered the biofilm production of both bacteria (Socolsky et al. 2010a).

GAGA

Lip Fern

The new genus *Gaga* is named in honor of Lady Gaga (Stefani Joanne Angelina Germanotta), the amazing musical popstar.

Gaga germanotta from Costa Rica is named after her family name and a Mexican species has been named *Gaga monstraparva*, meaning "monster-like," honoring her fans, whom she calls "little monsters."

This naming originated after she performed at the 2010 Grammy Awards, where she wore a green, heart-shaped Armani Privé costume with giant shoulders that Kathleen Pryer, biology professor at Duke University, thought looked like the bisexual gametophyte of ferns. A graduate student scanned the DNA of these newly discovered ferns and found "GAGA" spelled out in the DNA base pairs. Most of the other seventeen *Gaga* species were previously assigned to the genus Cheilanthes (Li et al. 2012).

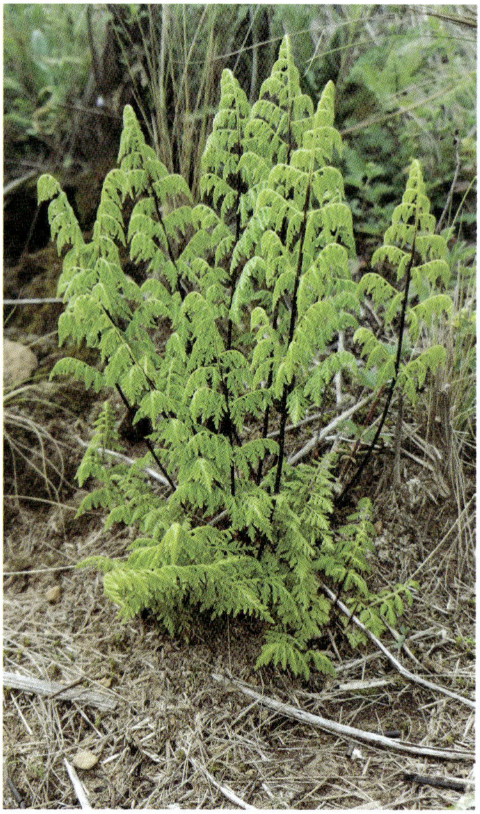

Gaga sp. (Lip Fern)
Photo by Alan Rockefeller

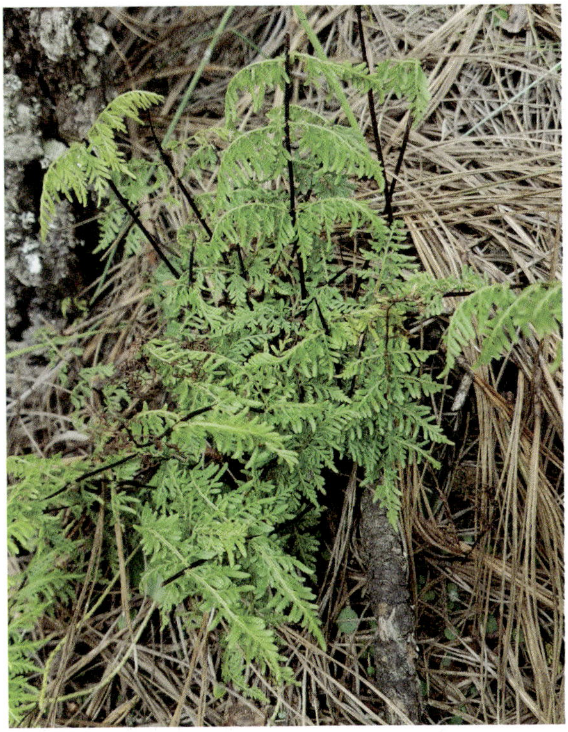

Gaga sp. (Lip Fern)
Photo by Alan Rockefeller

GLAPHYROPTERIDOPSIS

Glaphyropteridopsis erubescens young reddish fronds were decocted for gonorrhea and leucorrhea in the Deoprayag region of India (Gaur and Bhatt 1994).

GLEICHENIA

Bitter Fern
Comb-forked Fern
Split Fern
Umbrella Fern

The genus is named in honor of German botanist W. F. von Gleichen.

Split fern (*Gleichenia japonica*) is widespread throughout East to South Asia and forms large colonies due to allelopathic constituents exuded into its environment.

Comb-forked fern (*Gleichenia pectinata* syn. *Gleichenella pectinata*) has been synthesized with silver nanoparticles and exhibited excellent activity against *Pseudomonas aeruginosa*, *Escherichia coli*, *Klebsiella pneumoniae*, *Candida albicans*, and four multidrug-resistant pathogens (Femi-Adepoju et al. 2019).

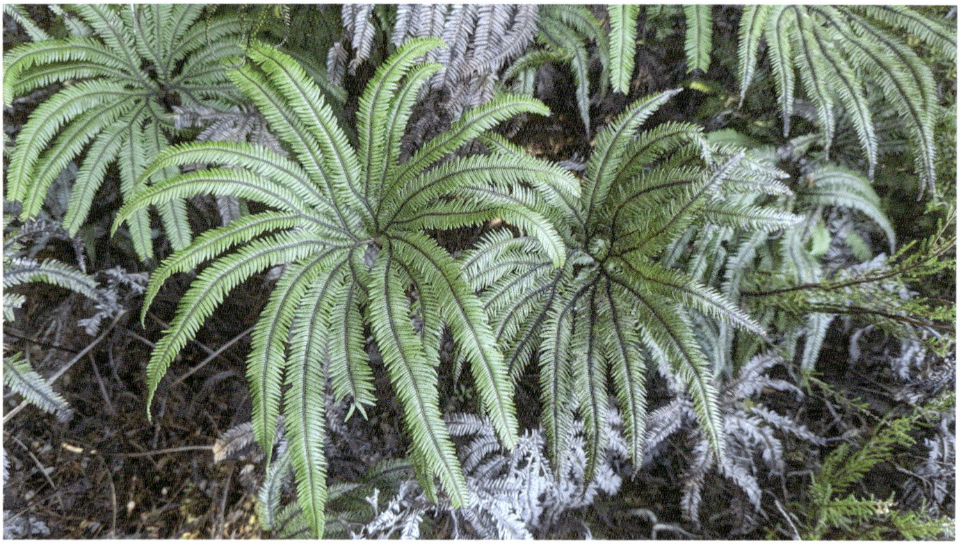

Gleichenia cunninghamii (Umbrella Fern)
Photo by Alan Rockefeller

Gleichenia quadripartita syn. *Sticherus quadripartitus*, native to Chile and locally known as *yerba loza*, *palmita*, *pata de cucho*, and *bi-iúl*, contains afzelin and fifteen diterpenoid glycosides. Afzelin exhibits antimetastatic potential and inhibits triple-negative breast cancer cell migration (Rachmi et al. 2020).

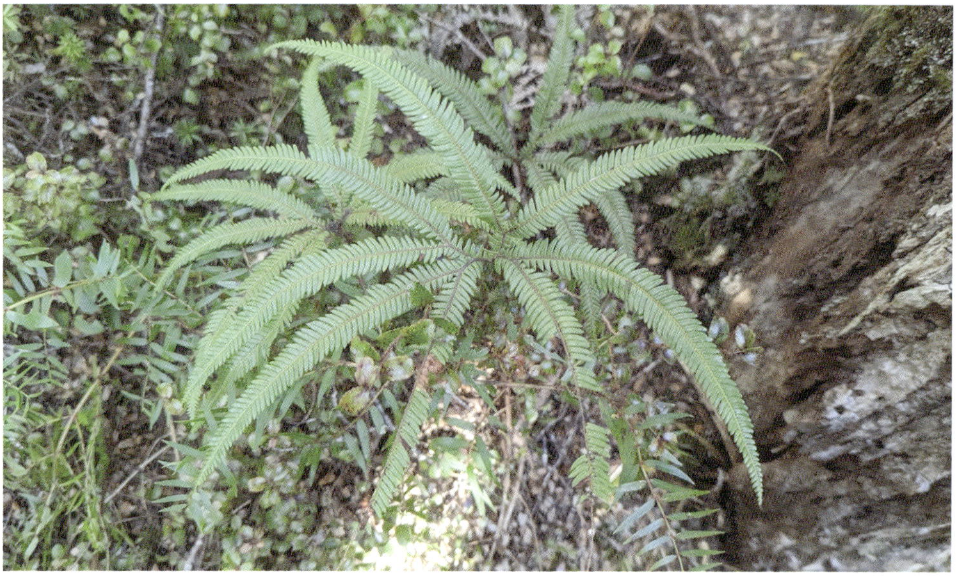

Gleichenia cunninghamii (Umbrella Fern)
Photo by Alan Rockefeller

Afzelin has also been found to exhibit possible benefits in aging and autoimmune diseases. A mouse study by Oh et al. (2021) found that afzelin improved neurocognitive and neuroprotective effects on synaptic plasticity and behavior by restoring the cholinergic system.

The tropical fern *Gleichenia truncata* syn. *Sticherus truncatus* is a highland fern traditionally used in parts of Asia to treat fever. In TCM it is known as *jia mang qi*.

The antimalarial and anti-inflammatory effects of the fern are mediated through the inhibition of glycogen synthase kinase-3, as observed by an in vivo mouse infection model (Suhaini et al. 2015).

The leaf extract also inhibits the growth of both gram-positive and gram-negative bacteria (Chai et al. 2013).

GYMNOCARPIUM

Common Oak Fern Northern Oak Fern Western Oak Fern

The common, Northern, or Western oak fern (*Gymnocarpium dryopteris* syn. *Dryopteris disjuncta)* is a slow-growing perennial found in the northern hemisphere. The common name makes no sense as it does not grow near oak trees (nothing does) and the fronds do not look like oak leaves. The genus name means "bearing naked fruit," referring to the absence of an indusium, which normally protect the sporangia.

Early uses of this fern involved crushing the fronds to repel mosquitoes or ease their bites. The fern is hardy, capable of surviving winters with temperatures as low as -46°C/-50.8°F.

The Haida call this fern *hlt' anʔanda*, the same name given to bracken fern (Newcombe 1897; 1901). Both elk and grizzly bears eat oak fern. The Nuu-chah-nulth call it *shishitlmapt*, and the Stl atl'imx refer to it as little bracken fern or *saqúuqw pzaʔ*.

The fern contains volatile compounds, including (E)-3-hexenoic acid and (E)-2-hexenoic acid, which have herbal and fruity notes. These volatiles are used in fougère absolutes in French perfumes.

It is believed that *Gymnocarpium dropteris* may be a fertile hybrid between the Eastern *Gymnocarpium appalachianum* and the Pacific oak fern (*Gymnocarpium disjunctum*).

HELMINTHOSTACHYS

Flowering Fern

Geographic Range: Ceylon (Sri Lanka), India, Indonesia, Malaysia, Malaya, Philippines, Taiwan
Habitat: tropical and subtropical regions, wetlands, woods
Practical Uses: braiding material, food
Medicinal Applications: anti-inflammatory, antioxidant, asthma, bones, brain, burns, catarrh, dysentery, edema, hyperglycemia, hyperlipidemia, impotence, lungs, malaria, melanogenesis, neuroprotection, nosebleeds, periodontitis, pneumonia, pulmonary edema, sciatica, sexual dysfunction, tranquilizer, whooping cough

Flowering fern (*Helminthostachys zeylanica* syn. *Osmunda zeylanica*) is found in Southeastern Asia and Australia. It is commonly known as *kamraj* and *tunjuk-langit*. In the Philippines, the fern is known as *túkod-langit*, *dhimraj* in India, and *tunjuk bumi* in Malay.

The genus name suggests benefits in treating helminths or parasitic worms, while *zeylanica* refers to Ceylon, the former name of Sri Lanka.

The leaf stalks of the fronds have long been used as braiding material. The rhizomes are harvested in the wet season and used in TCM, where they are known as *di wu gong*. In Taiwan, the rhizome, known as *daodi ugon*, is used to reduce inflammation, fever, burns, pneumonia, and edema associated with bone fractures. In Malaysia, the dried fronds are smoked to treat nosebleeds. In India, the fern is eaten like a cooked vegetable, and the rhizome is used to treat impotence. The rhizome is also used as a tonic in Malaya, for dysentery and catarrh in Indonesia, for sciatica in India, and for malaria in the Philippines (Quisumbing 1951; Uphof 1968).

The whole fern is considered an intoxicant, anodyne, and aphrodisiac (Baskaran et al. 2018).

In India, the rhizome is chewed with areca nut (*Areca catechu*) for whooping cough. The fronds serve as a sexual stimulant, euphoriant, and tranquilizer, and the rhizome is used to treat whooping cough (pertussis) and sexual disfunction. The fern is also used to treat sciatic neuritis due to sedative, pain-relieving, and anti-inflammatory properties (Singh and Singh 2012).

Various flavonoids have been identified in the rhizome, with some exhibiting anti-inflammatory activity more potent than the positive control pyrrolidine dithiocarbamate. Acetogenin and prenylated flavonoids inhibit superoxide anion generation and elastase release by human neutrophils (Huang et al. 2010b). Elastase inhibitors may help reverse pulmonary vascular disease, reduce airway hyperactivity, and help maintain skin elasticity associated with skin aging.

Ugonins E through L were isolated from the rhizomes. Ugonins J through L were shown to be more potent antioxidants than Trolox (Huang et al. 2003). The cyclized geranyl stilbenes ugonstilbenes A through C and neougonin A, also exhibit moderate antioxidant activity. Neougonin A inhibits LPS-induced inflammation (Cao et al. 2016).

Quercetin glucosides, derived from ethanol extracts of the rhizome, exhibit accelerated melanogenesis by 2.7 times in murine B16 melanoma cells, with no cytotoxic effects (Yamauchi et al. 2013). Conversely, ugonin J and K are potent inhibitors of melanin production, exhibiting much stronger activity than arbutin (Yamauchi et al. 2015). Ugonin J, K, and L are luteolin derivatives, with six ugonins showing significant neuraminidase inhibition. Ugonin J, in particular, blocks the biofilm formation of *Escherichia coli* without inhibiting the bacterium itself. The inhibitory potency was observed at a nanomolar level (35–50 nM), meaning the compounds were one hundred times more active than eriodictyol and luteolin derived from the fern (Shah et al. 2022).

Fern extracts given to mice on a high-fat diet for twelve weeks effectively protected them from hyperlipidemia and hyperglycemia. The extract prevented weight gain, adipose tissue expansion, and adipocyte hypertrophy, and reduced fat accumulation in the liver. The insulin sensitivity index was also restored (Chang et al. 2019).

Ugonins display significant inhibition against PTP1B and α-glucosidase, both of which are beneficial in blood sugar control (Shah et al. 2020a). PTP1B inhibition enhances insulin signaling, helping to monitor pancreatic function.

One flavonoid, ugonin K, exhibits strong inhibitory activity against RANKL-induced osteoclast differentiation, suggesting possible benefits in osteoporosis (Huang et al. 2017). This compound also promotes osteoblast differentiation and mineralization by inducing osteoid synthesis and bone nodule formation (Lee et al. 2011). This suggests that the traditional use of this fern to strengthen bones and cure bone fractures is well-founded.

Ugonin K also protects human neuroblastoma SH-SY5Y brain cells from hydrogen peroxide-induced apoptosis (Lin et al. 2009). A double-blind, randomized controlled study of 45 patients with ankle fractures requiring surgery was conducted by Su and colleagues (2022). One group (23 patients) received an oral extract of ugonin K, administered at one gram three times daily, the other group (22 patients) placebo for six weeks. The fern extracts increased serum PINP (propeptide of type 1 procollagen) levels and reduced radiographic healing time.

A rise of matrix metalloproteinase-9 (MMP-9) levels is found in blood of patients suffering from inflammatory diseases of the brain. Rhizome extracts of the fern significantly reduce MMP-9 levels induced by bradykinin in brain astrocyte cells, indicating a potential role in reducing brain inflammation (Hsieh et al. 2016).

Ugonin L has been found to inhibit osteoclast formation and promote osteoclast apoptosis, suggesting possible benefits in bone anti-resorption, osteoporosis, arthritis, periodontitis, and bone metastasis (Liu et al. 2023). Another flavonoid, ugonin M, has shown protective effects against LPS-induced lung injury in mice by reducing the severity of pulmonary edema (Wu et al. 2017b). Water extracts of the fern also reduced inflammatory responses in lung epithelial cells and ameliorated LPS-induced acute lung injury in mice (Liou et al. 2017).

Another study by Huang et al. (2020) found water extracts significantly decrease airway hyper-responsiveness, by suppressing Th2 cytokine production of asthma in a mouse model. Ugonin M, isolated from the fern, has shown potential to remediate acute liver injury induced by acetaminophen by reducing inflammation and oxidative stress. It also normalized lipid metabolism, including total cholesterol and triglycerides (Wu et al. 2017b).

Acetaminophen (Tylenol) overdose is the second most common cause of liver transplants worldwide. It is responsible for 56,000 emergency visits, 2,600 hospitalizations and over 500 deaths annually in the United States. The mortality rate for acute liver failure is around 28%, with one third of patients requiring a liver transplant. Acetaminophen is the most common cause of acute liver failure accounting for 50% of all reported cases and approximately 20% of liver transplant cases.

Ugonin U stimulates the NLRP3 (NOD-like receptor pyrin domain-containing protein 3) inflammasome by directly stimulating phospholipase, triggering superoxide release in human neutrophils. This ability, to trigger both human neutrophils and monocytes and to activate NLRP3 inflammasome, suggests ugonin U's great potential to treat various infectious diseases (Chen et al. 2017a).

Gastric cancer, the second most prevalent cancer worldwide, may also benefit from fern extracts. An ethyl acetate extract of the fern induced apoptosis in gastric cancer cells with little or no toxicity to healthy gastric epithelial (GES-1) cells. The extract also increased autophagy, exhibited antiproliferative effects through cell cycle arrest in G0/G1 and G2/M phases, and suppressed migration, suggesting a new adjunctive compound for the treatment of this widespread cancer (Tsai et al. 2021).

HEMIONITIS

Heart Leaf Fern

The fern *Hemionitis albofusca* grows in regions of China and has been mistakenly collected and used as silver cloak fern (*Aleuritopteris argentea*) to relieve menstrual issues.

Work by Pei et al. (2023) extracted and identified several diterpenoids from the fern and found various pathways that reduce inflammation. The fern has also been used in traditional Indian medicine to treat cancer (Santhosh et al. 2014).

Heart leaf fern (*Hemionitis arifolia*) is a traditional remedy for diabetes in parts of Asia. The heart-shaped, leathery green leaves do not look like those of most ferns. A fraction containing steroids and coumarins showed activity in alloxan-induced diabetic rats, based on serum glucose levels, influencing liver glycogen content and body weight (Ajikumaran et al. 2006; Kumudhavalli and Jaykar 2012).

Both crude and alcohol extracts of the aerial parts, including reproductive leaves, show considerable activity against gram-negative *Escherichia coli* (MTCC-739). The reproductive parts exhibit moderate activity against gram-positive *Bacillus subtilis* (Karmakar and Mukhopadhyay 2011).

HICRIOPTERIS

The stems of *Hicriopteris glauca* syn. *Diplopterygium glaucum* contain lunularic acid 4'-glucoside and 2,9-dihydroxy-4,7-megastigmadiene-3-O-β-glucoside. Various extractions were tested for cytotoxic activity by Fang et al. (2012). The butanol extract showed antitumor activity against A375 (human melanoma) cancer cell lines with an IC_{50} value of 0.80 μg/ml.

HYMENOPHYLLUM

Filmy Ferns Piripiri

The genus name *Hymenophyllum* means "membranous leaf" in reference to the very thin frond tissue. The common name filmy fern derives from this appearance, as the leaves are only one cell thick and lack stomata. These ferns survive only in very humid forests, mainly in South America (especially Ecuador), Asia, and New Zealand.

The Asian beard filmy fern (*Hymenophyllum barbatum*) contains several glycosides, including hemiterpene glycosides, hymenosides A through J, which possess a bitter or pungent taste, and perrottetin H, an acyclic bibenzyl derivative.

Tailed filmy fern *Hymenophyllum caudiculatum* can lose 60% of its water content, remain dry for a period of time, and recover 88% of photochemical efficiency after just half an hour of rehydration.

The rare protruding filmy fern (*Hymenophyllum exsertum* syn. *Medocium exsertum*) exhibits antimicrobial activity (Marisass 2009).

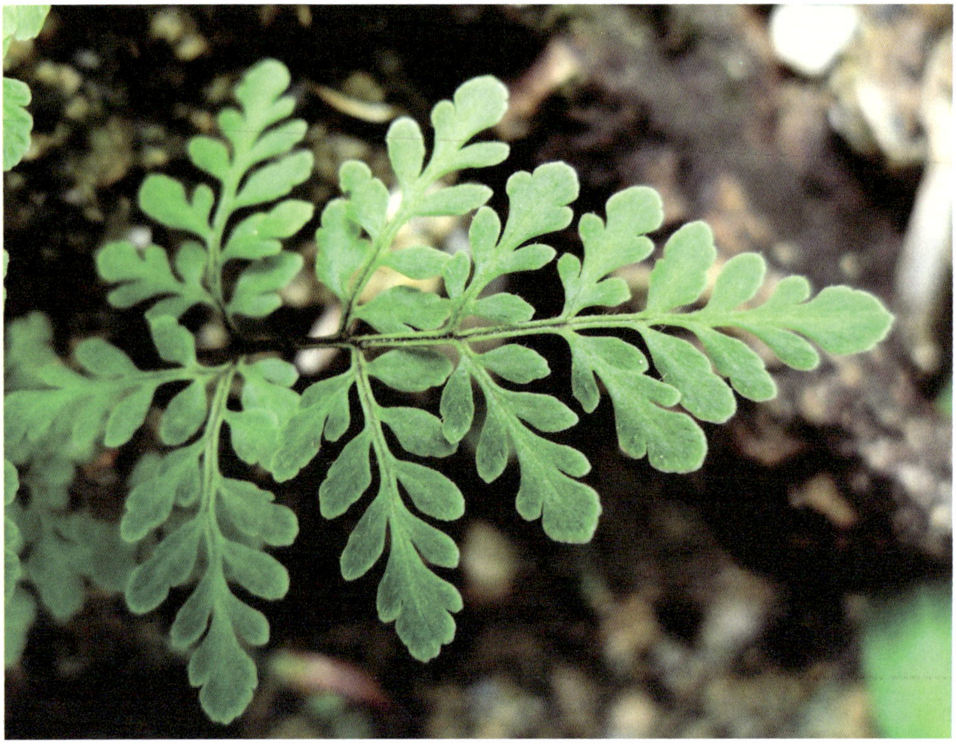

Hymenophyllum sp. (Filmy Fern)

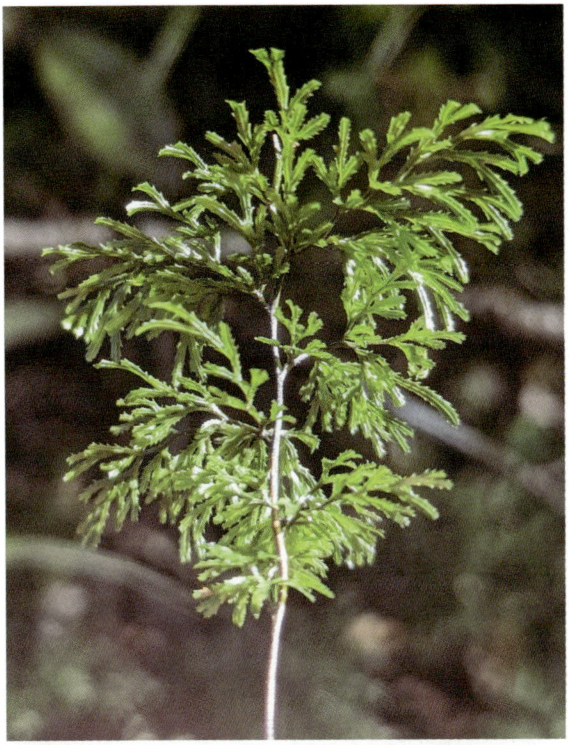

Hymenophyllum multifidum
(Much-divided Filmy Fern)
Photo by Alan Rockefeller

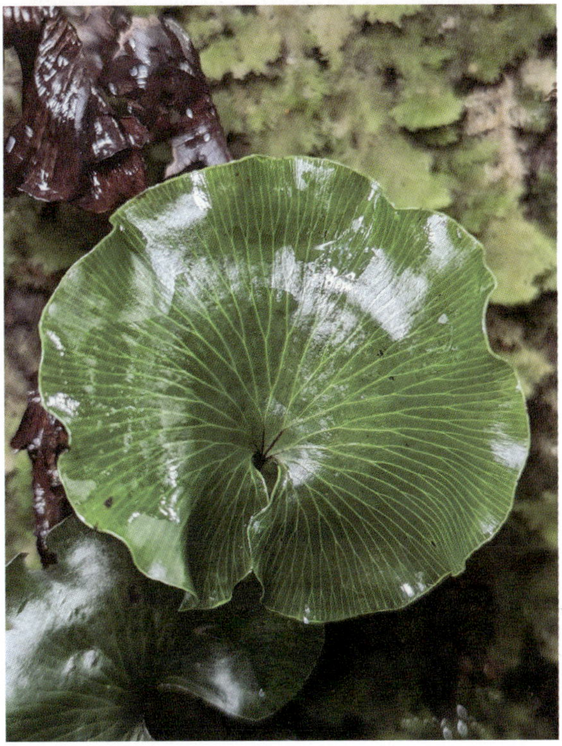

Hymenophyllum nephrophyllum
(Kidney Filmy Fern)
Photo by Alan Rockefeller

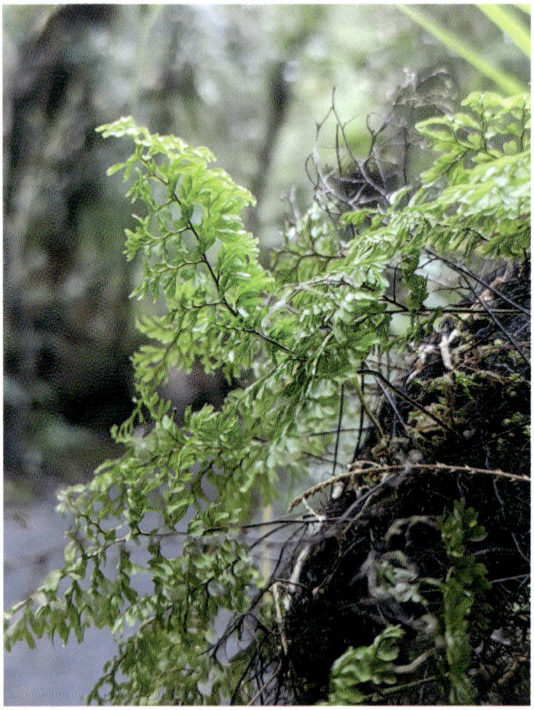

Hymenophyllum sanguinolentum (Piripiri)
Photo by Alan Rockefeller

The related Delicate filmy fern (*Hymenophyllum plicatum*) is even more tolerant, possibly due to the presence of more long-chain omega-3 fatty acids, enhancing membrane stability.

HYPODEMATIUM

Hypodematium crenatum is popularly known in India as *bhoot kesari* or *jaributti*. The TCM name is *zhong zu jue*.

The dry powder or paste of fronds is taken with cow's milk for five days after menstruation to help with conception (Vasudeva 1999).

Hypodematium squamuloso-pilosum is known in TCM as *lin mao zhong zu jue*, and in Korean traditional medicine as *huin geum teol go sa ri*, due to its resemblance to long white hair.

Beta-carboline alkaloids have been found in *Hypodematium squamuloso-pilosum*. Beta carboline and its derivatives influence brain function and possess antioxidant activity, with numerous examples in the plant and animal kingdom. The two alkaloids in this fern are 1-acetyl-8-hydroxy-ß-carboline and 1-acetyl-ß-carboline.

The latter exhibits synergistic activity against MRSA (methicillin-resistant) *Staphylococcus aureus* (Shin et al. 2010).

Clostridium difficile (*Clostridioides difficile*) is a bacterium that causes serious intestinal inflammation such as colitis. It poses a major health risk, and it often arises after patients take antibiotics, and can be acquired in hospitals, nursing homes, and long-term care facilities.

A population-based cohort study in Sweden included over 43,000 individuals and found that over 60% of those infected died during the study period, compared to 29% of the controls. The infection was associated with a three- to sevenfold increased mortality rate (Boven et al. 2023).

The related *Clostridium scindens* transforms primary bile salts into secondary bile salts and helps inhibit *Clostridium difficile* growth in vivo. The bile acid 7α-dehydroxylating gut bacteria *Clostridium scindens* secretes 1-acetyl-β-carboline, inhibiting the pathogenic bacteria (Kang et al. 2019).

HYPOLEPIS

Bead Ferns

Dotted bead fern (*Hypolepis punctata* syn. *Phegopteris punctata*) contains pterosin A and derivatives, which help regulate blood sugar homeostasis, protect pancreatic β cells by preventing their death, and reduce reactive oxygen species (Chen et al. 2015).

The fern exhibits a unique approach to self-defense. When the fern is damaged by the moth larvae *Bertula hadenalis*, it releases volatiles that attract the assassin bug *Sclomina erinacea*, ultimately sealing the larvae's fate.

Hypacrone, a sesquiterpene containing a reactive cyclopropane ring, has been isolated from the fern. It exhibits carcinogenic effects.

Young fronds of *Hypolepis* species are lightly boiled and incorporated in the diet of new mothers in Vanuatu (Bourdy and Walter 1992). The stems have been traditionally used for ornamental plaiting.

LASTREOPSIS

Shield Ferns

About forty-five species of *Lastreopsis* shield ferns are found in parts of Australia, Africa, and tropical regions of Asia.

The shield fern (*Lastreopsis amplissima* syn. *Filix-mas amplissima* exhibits high antioxidant activity (Andrade et al. 2014).

False shield fern (*Lastreopsis effusa* syn. *Parapolystichum effusum*) is available in potencies C12, C15, and C30.

The fern is commonly found throughout Central and South America, as well as various Caribbean Islands.

LECANOPTERIS

The genus name derives from the Greek *lekane* "basin" and *pteris* "fern." Fleshy basin fern (*Lecanopteris carnosa*) is a tropical epiphytic, myrmecophyte fern native to Borneo, Malaysia, the Philippines, and several Indonesian Islands.

Myrmecophyte means "ant plant" and refers to its mutualistic relationship with ants. This is not uncommon. Over one hundred plant genera offer food and shelter to ants, and in return, the insects aid in pollination, nutrient gathering, and spore dispersal. The ants live in frond or stem cavities, in facultative mutualism, meaning the ferns and ants can't survive without each other. The fronds are astringent, diuretic, pectoral, and used for rheumatism (Chopra 1956).

LEMMAPHYLLUM

Beard Fern

The fern *Lemmaphyllum diversum* syn. *L. intermedium* syn. *Polpodium diversum* syn. *Lepisorus carnosus* is used in TCM for inflammation, arthralgia, and bleeding due to trauma wounds or surgery. It is known as *pi zhen gu pai jue*.

LEPISORUS

Weeping Ferns

Lepisorus carnosus syn. *Lepidogrammitis drymoglossoides* syn. *Lemmaphyllum drymoglossoides* has been traditionally used in TCM for pharyngitis, pulmonary tuberculosis, rheumatism, arthritis, lymphadenitis, cholecystitis, urolithiasis, hypertension, and furunculosis.

The fronds contain lepidodromos A and B, which display moderate antiproliferative activity against HeLa (cervical) cancer cell lines (Guo et al. 2022a). They also contain ponasteroside B, β-ecdysterone, stigmasterol, physcion,

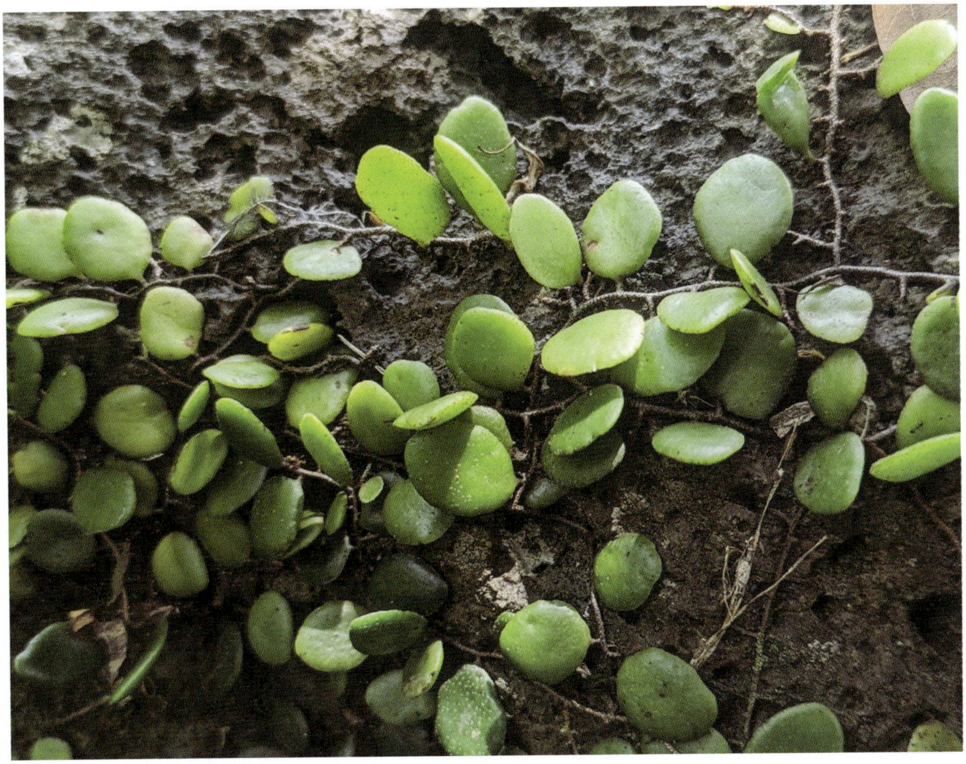

Lemmaphyllum microphyllum (Japanese Beard Fern)
Photo by Alan Rockefeller

emodin, umbelliferone, scoparone, aesculetin, caffeic acid, ferulic acid, protocatechuic acid, pyrocatechualdehyde, gallic acid, 4-hydroxybenzoic acid methyl ester, and docosanyl tetracosanoate.

The whole fern of *Lepisorus contortus* contains phenylethanoid glycosides, syringic acid, vanillic acid, phloretic acid, diplopterol, lutein, transilin and β-sitosterol. Quercetin-3-O-β-d-glucoside, derived from the fern, inhibits quinone reductase and demonstrates NF-κB activity. Four fern compounds exhibit aromatase activity, suggestive of benefits in hormone-sensitive cancers (Yang et al. 2011).

The Manchurian or Ussuri weeping fern (*Lepisorus ussuriensis*) contains dihydroquercetin, diosmetin, luteolin, transilin, baicalein, 7,8-dihydroxflavone, and 7-O-methylnaringenin-(4'>O>6"-scutellarein. Work by Luo et al. (2016) found that quercetin, diosmetin, and luteolin inhibited TNF-α-induced NFkB reporter gene expression on HeLa (human cervical) cancer cells up to 30μM and 100μM. The presence of baicalein and scutellarein remind me of the various skullcap species' constituents and their widespread benefits in numerous health conditions. Baicalein has over 2,500 citations in PubMed.

A good review of numerous benefits has recently been published by Gupta and colleagues (2022). In my book *Herbal Allies: My Journey with Plant Medicine* (Rogers 2017), I cover numerous health benefits of the North American marsh scullcap (*Scutellaria galericulata*) and blue scullcap (*Scutellaria lateriflora*).

Diosmetin has a wide range of anti-inflammatory, anticancer, cardiovascular, metabolic, neurological, and bone-protecting properties. Diosmetin induces apoptosis and enhances the drug paclitaxel in non-small cell lung cancer cells via Nrf2 inhibition, strongly suggesting its potential as an adjuvant treatment. Recent research suggests diosmetin protects neuroblastoma cells against advanced glycation end products (AGE) via multiple mechanisms and may be a potential option for the prevention and treatment of Alzheimer's disease. One target is the peroxisome proliferator-activated receptor gamma (PPAR-γ). Amyloid precursor protein upregulation, accompanied by an increase in production of amyloid-β caused by AGEs, was reversed by diosmetin (Lai et al. 2022).

LEPTOPTERIS

Common Crape Fern   Prince of Wales Feathers Fern

Prince of Wales Island or Muralag is a small rugged, woody island off the coast of Queensland, Australia. In 2021, sixty-two people inhabited the island.

PRINCE OF WALES FEATHERS FERN ESSENCE

This essence of *Leptopteris superba* facilitates inner healing, peace, and stillness at the soul level, particularly after experiences of trauma of humiliation or deep sorrow that have impacted the soul and are locked into cellular memory. It helps those who have communication issues and assists the unconscious mind to release memories that make it feel unsafe to relax, speak out, or let one's verbal guard down. Find as the First Light Flower Essence of New Zealand No. 41 Prince of Wales Feathers Fern.

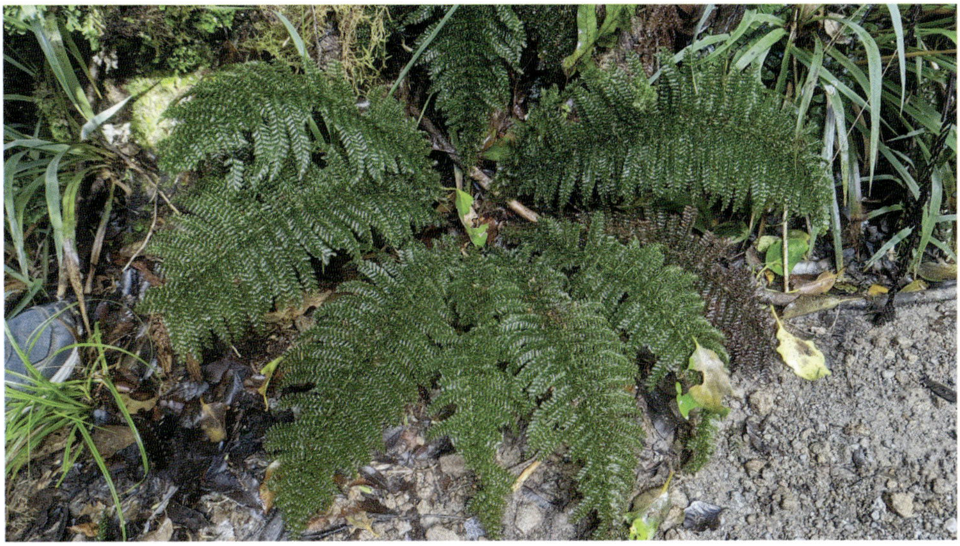

Leptopteris superba (Prince of Wales Feathers Fern)
Photo by Alan Rockefeller

LYGODIUM

Bushman's Mattress	Mangemange
Climbing Ferns	Octopus Flower
Hartford Fern	Red Finger Fern
Maidenhair Creeper Fern	Snake Fern

Geographic Range: China, India, Ivory Coast, Japan, Malaysia, Nepal, New Zealand, Papua New Guinea, Philippines, Southeast Asia, Southern United States, Thailand

Habitat: dense curtains of vines, moss-covered tree trunks, subtropical and tropical regions, wetlands, woodlands

Practical Uses: baskets, wreaths, eel traps, fishhooks, rope, roof thatch, sleeping material, weaving

Medicinal Applications: analgesic, antiandrogenic, anthelmintic, anti-inflammatory, antipyretic, antioxidant, antiproliferative, asthma, bones, cancer, cognitive function, contraceptive, diarrhea, dysmenorrhea, eczema, fertility treatment, fever reduction, gonorrhea, hair growth promotion, hiccups, jaundice, kidneys, liver, muscles, neuralgia, respiratory conditions, stomach pains, ulcers, viruses, wounds

Mangemange or bushman's mattress (*Lygodium articulatum*) is endemic to the North Island of New Zealand. It grows up to three meters tall and can create dense curtains that are difficult to navigate through.

The common name derives from the tough, springy vines, which were traditionally used as sleeping material, but was also used for making fishhooks, eel traps, rope, and roof thatching. The Māori made an infusion of the fronds for stomach pain. The dried leaves have a pleasing scent.

OCTOPUS FLOWER ESSENCE

This essence of *Lygodium articulatum* facilitates inner healing, peace, and stillness at the soul level and calls upon one's personal guardian and protector spirit/s of the infinite—the place of true cosmic limitlessness and original awareness. Anchors stellar light from the infinite into the eighth layer of the aura. Find as First Light Flower Essence of New Zealand No. 136 Octopus Flower.

Red finger fern (*Lygodium circinnatum* syn. *L. dichotomum*) is common to Southeast Asia. In the Philippines, it is known as *nitong-puti*, in China as *hai nan hai jin sha*, and in Malaysia as *ribu-ribu duduk*. In Malaysia, the creeping stem (vine) of the epiphytic fern can reach over thirty meters in length.

The fern is used in India to treat childhood illnesses, and the rhizome and stem are used in Papua New Guinea internally as a contraceptive (Blackwood 1935).

This species, along with maidenhair creeper fern (*Lygodium flexuosum*) and Japanese climbing fern (*Lygodium japonicum*), has been used for fiber. The epidermis of the stem is removed, and the rachises are sun-dried and then twisted into the rims and handles of baskets, as well as decorations. The root and leaves have traditionally been applied to wounds, and the stipe chewed and applied to venomous snakebites or insect bites (Quisumbing 1951).

Maidenhair creeper or flexible climbing fern (*Lygodium flexuosum*) is an epiphyte that grows on moss-covered tree trunks and branches. In India, it is found throughout the country, up to an elevation of 1,500 meters, and is locally known as *kalijar*. Juice from the frond rhizome has been traditionally used to treat gonorrhea, dysmenorrhea, menorrhagia, and female infertility (Nwosu 2002; Rout et al. 2009). In Nepal, the fern is used to great viral infections and traditional medicine used the fern for various ailments including carbuncles, inflammation, jaundice, dysmenorrhea, eczema, ulcers, respiratory conditions, muscle sprains, and wound healing (Baskaran et al. 2018). The fern is a rich source of alkaloids, saponins, flavonoids, coumarin, and the main constituent, lygodinolide, which is primarily used in wound healing.

A frond extract was formulated into an ointment and tested on excised wound models. Topical application increased the percentage of wound contraction, decreased epithelization time, and enhanced the breaking strength of wounds. Hydroxyproline levels also increased (Chandra et al. 2015).

Extracts of this fern exhibit antiproliferative activity and induce apoptosis on human hepatoma (PLC/PRF/5) and hepatic (Hep 3B) cancer cell lines (Wills and Asha 2009). This confirms the fern's use in Indian traditional medicine for liver disorders.

In rats treated for D-galactosamine-induced liver injury, similar benefits were observed as with silymarin derived from milk thistle seeds (Wills and Asha 2006). Similar results were also found for acute liver injury and the prevention of hepatic fibrosis from carbon tetrachloride. Methanol extracts exhibit impressive activity against herpes simplex virus, Sindbis virus, and poliovirus (Taylor et al. 1996).

Japanese climbing fern (*Lygodium japonicum*) is considered a noxious weed in some parts of the world and has naturalized in the Southern United States. However, it is time to reconsider this prejudice.

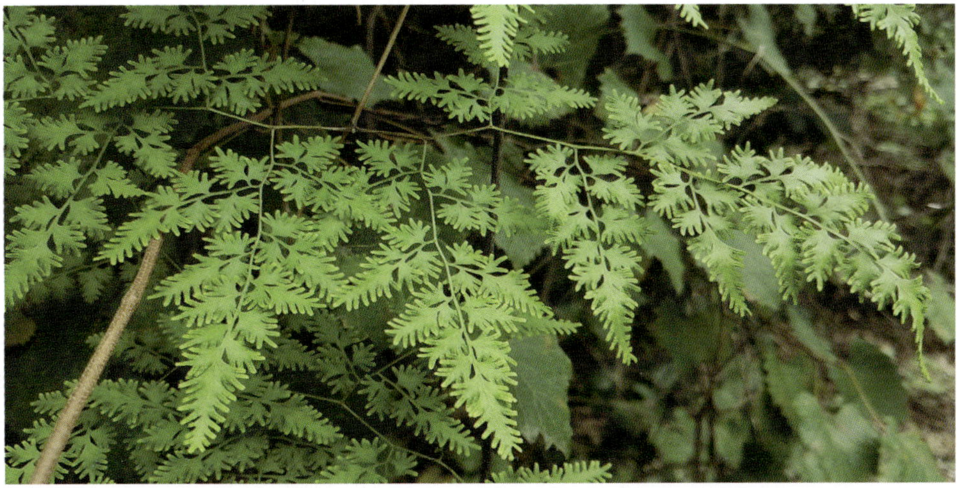

Lygodium japonicum (Japanese Climbing Fern)
Photo by Alan Rockefeller

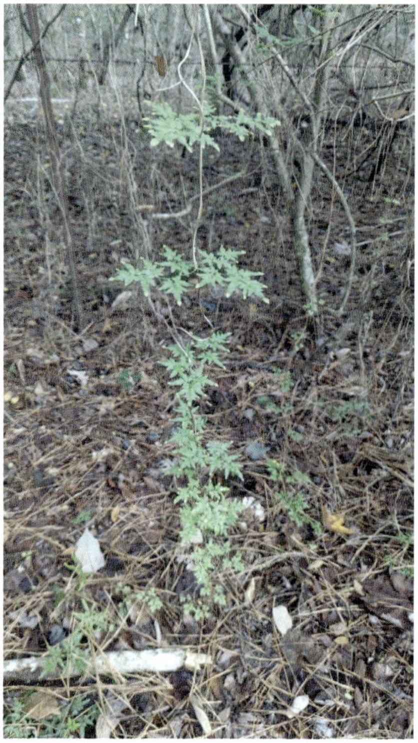

Lygodium japonicum
(Japanese Climbing Fern)
Photo by Alan Rockefeller

The roots contain the ecdysteroside, lygodiumsteroside A; 1,4-napthoquinone, 3,4-dihydroxybenzoic acid 4-O-(4'-O-methyl)-β-D-glucopyranoside, p-coumaric acid, buddleoside (linarin), diosmetin-7-O-β-D-glucopyranoside, apigenin, and acacetin.

Buddleoside regulates intestinal flora, improves intestinal barrier function, and reduces the production and penetration of lipopolysaccharide (LPS). By inhibiting the vascular TLR4/MyD88 pathway and improving vascular endothelial function, it ultimately lowers blood pressure in metabolically hypertensive rats (Wang et al. 2021). Buddleoside, also known as linarin, helps remediate central nervous system conditions, promotes sleep through sedative properties, and inhibits acetylcholinesterase. It also has anti-osteoblast proliferation and differentiation effects, suggesting benefits in bone formation for osteoarthritis and osteoporosis (Mottaghipisheh et al. 2021). Linarin inhibits TLR4 signaling, helping to prevent the inflammatory response in osteoarthritis, and it also prevents the catabolism of the extracellular matrix by LPS (Qi et al. 2021).

Linarin inhibits glioma, a malignant brain cancer, by inducing apoptosis, which is accompanied by an increase in p53 and a decrease in p65 (Zhen et al. 2017).

Acacetin is a flavonoid with anticancer, anti-inflammatory, antiviral, antimicrobial, and anti-obesity properties. It has been found to prevent cardiac damage caused by ischemia/reperfusion and myocardial infarction, reduce neuroinflammation, protect against sepsis-induced lung injury, alleviate rheumatoid and collagen-induced arthritis, and support liver function (Singh et al. 2020b).

Taylor et al. (1996) reported that acacetin also demonstrates antiviral activity against herpes simplex, Sindbis, and polio viruses.

A recent study by Wang and Renquan (2023) found that acacetin inhibits the JAK2/STAT3 pathway in TE-1 and TE-10 (esophageal squamous) carcinoma cells, inhibiting their malignant progression and promoting apoptosis. Esophageal cancer is the sixth most common cause of cancer deaths worldwide, with a five-year survival rate of only 20%. Smoking and drinking are of course significant associated risk factors, but gastroesophageal reflux is also a large contributing factor. Over-the-counter antacids begin the process, and then proton-pump inhibitors are suggested, when lifestyle and dietary changes would have helped as preventative regimes.

The aerial parts of the fern contain 4-O-caffeoyl-D-glucopyranose, 3-O-caffeoyl-D-glucopyranose, and other compounds that exhibit strong antioxidant activity. Other compounds found in the fronds are tilianin, kaempferol-7-O-α-L-rhamnopyranoside, kaempferol, p-coumaric acid, hexadecanoic acid 2,3-dihydroxy-propyl ester, daucosterol, β-sitosterol, 1-hentriacontanol, and lygodipenoids A and B.

The latter two compounds were tested in transfected cultured human embryonic kidney (HEK293) cells for an agonist assay, and lygodipenoid A was identified as a partial agonist for liver X receptor alpha (Han et al. 2012).

Tilianin is antiproliferative and induces apoptosis in PA-1 (ovarian) cancer cell lines (Xiong et al. 2021). Over eighty studies suggest that tilianin shows potential benefits in various cancers, cardiovascular health, cognitive function, asthma, Parkinson's disease, non-alcoholic fatty liver disease, and diabetic retinopathy.

The spores have been used in TCM for various inflammatory conditions. Work by Cho et al. (2017) produced an ethanol extract and examined the production of inflammatory mediators. It appears that the extract may suppress LPS-induced inflammatory responses in macrophages in vitro through the downregulation of p38 MAPK and NF-κB. Ethanol extracts of the fern spores also inhibit testosterone 5α-reductase, suggesting possible benefits as antiandrogenic compound and promoter of hair growth (Matsuda et al. 2002). Spore extracts may also be useful in preventing and treating formation of oxalate kidney stones, as demonstrated in an animal study by Cho et al. (2014).

Snake fern or small-leaf climbing fern (*Lygodium microphyllum*) is considered an invasive weed in Florida and other tropical climates. The fern contains isoeleutherol, isoquercetin, and quercetin. It exhibits moderate analgesic activity similar to diclofenac, anti-inflammatory activity similar to ibuprofen, and antipyretic effects (reduces fever) similar to indomethacin. It also exhibits antidiarrheal activity similar to loperamide, and anthelmintic activity comparable to albendazole (Alam et al. 2021b). In the Ivory Coast, the fronds are crushed and used to cure hiccups (Bouquet 1974).

Isoeleutherol exhibits a high degree of antiradical scavenging activity and is particularly stable (Nazifi et al. 2019). The compound has demonstrated the ability to cross the blood-brain barrier.

Water extracts of the fronds prevent carbon tetrachloride-induced liver damage and immune suppression in an animal study (Gnanaraj et al. 2017).

American climbing or Hartford fern (*Lygodium plamatum*) was traditionally and widely collected for Christmas wreaths, leading to the first plant conservation law in the United States, enacted by Connecticut in 1869.

Lygodium reticulatum decoctions of both rhizome and fronds are used in India to treat dysmenorrhea and as a contraceptive (Dhiman 1998; Ho et al. 2011).

The stems (rachis) of the willow-leaved climbing fern (*Lygodium salicifolium*) are sun-dried and dyed in Southeast Asia, including Thailand, for use as weaving material. Only the outer part is used.

Ethanol extracts of *Lygodium venustum* enhance the efficacy of gentamicin in an additive manner against several multidrug-resistant bacterial strains (Morais-Braga et al. 2016).

Earlier work found that ethyl acetate fractions from the fern were additive with aminoglycoside antibiotics against multi-resistant strains and showed a synergistic interaction with amikacin against *Escherichia coli* (Morais-Braga 2012). Methanol fractions also inhibit leishmanicidal and trypanocidal pathogens (Morais-Braga et al. 2013).

The fern demonstrated moderate activity against *Trichomonas vaginalis*, a frequent cause of gynecological infections in women (Calzada et al. 2007). This parasitic protozoan is sexually transmitted and is estimated to infect some 180 million people worldwide, exceeding the instances of gonorrhea and chlamydia combined. It can cause vaginitis, cervicitis, and urethritis. Moderate inhibition of diarrhea was also observed in a rat study (Calzada et al. 2010).

MACROTHELYPTERIS

Marsh Ferns

Geographic Range: damp woods of China, Southeast Asia
Medicinal Applications: anti-inflammatory, antiangiogenic, apoptosis induction, boils, burns, cancer, chronic nephrotic syndrome, COX-2 reduction, edema, hepatotoxicity protection, hydropsy, kidneys, leukemia, liver, neuroblastoma, non-bacterial prostatitis, oxidative stress regulation, renal protection, roundworms, traumatic bleeding

Large marsh fern (*Macrothelypteris oligophlebia*) rhizomes are used in Traditional Chinese Medicine (TCM), known as *zhen mao jue*, for edema, boils, burns, and roundworms.

An in vivo study on rats suggested that the rhizome provides protection of renal tissue against oxidative stress in acute kidney failure (Wu et al. 2012).

Methanol extracts from the rhizome have also shown protective effects against chronic non-bacterial prostatitis in animal trials, reducing levels of IL-10, TNF-*a*, COX-2, and PGE2 (Han et al. 2016).

Marsh fern (*Macrothelypteris torresiana* syn. *M. oligophlebia* var. *changshaensis* syn. *Thelypteris torresiana*) is used in TCM to treat edema related to bladder and kidney issues.

Hyperlipidemic mice were given a polyphenol fraction of the fern for nine weeks following the induction of chronic nephrotic syndrome, by puromycin aminonucleoside. The polyphenol fraction was able to modulate oxidative stress in the kidneys and regulating the vascular endothelial growth factor-nitric oxide (VEGF-NO) pathway (Chen et al. 2012a).

The fern's rhizome contains apigenin and protoapigenone, both of which possess activity against various cancer cell lines. A review of apigenin and cancer by Singh et al. (2022) identified twenty-five studies on various cancer types including liver, prostate, pancreatic, lung, nasopharyngeal, skin, colon, colorectal, colitis-associated carcinoma, head and neck squamous cell carcinoma, leukemia, renal cell carcinoma, Ehrlich ascites carcinoma, and breast cancer. Apigenin reduces tumor volume, weight, number, and load, mainly by inducing apoptosis.

Liu et al. (2019b) examined apigenin and protoapigenone at a protein level. While both compounds individually possess cytotoxicity, their structural similarity and close binding coefficients to identical targets result in poor efficacy when using the whole fern extract.

Neuroblastoma is a dreadful cancer, often affecting young children and has been studied with a novel flavonoid, DEDC, isolated from the fronds. This flavonoid was shown to induce apoptosis in SH-SY5Y cells by elevating reactive oxygen species (ROS) generation. The signal transducer and activator of transcription 3 (STAT3) played a crucial role in DEDC-triggered cell death (Liu et al. 2012). Another flavonoid, designated DICO, induces G2/M cell cycle arrest and apoptosis in HepG2 (human hepatoma) cell lines (Zhou et al. 2013).

Protoapigenone (PA), a flavonoid from the rhizome, shows significant antitumor activity against HepG2 (liver), TCA-8113 (squamous tongue), MCF-7(breast), M5 (acute monoblastic leukemia), and K562 (chronic myelogenous leukemia) cancer cell lines (Huang et al. 2010a).

Structural changes in PA have a significant influence on plasma albumin binding affinity and its effects on HepG2 (hepatoma) tumor cell lines compared to the flavone apigenin (Poór et al. 2013).

A protoapigenone analog, RY10-4, exhibits even stronger antitumor activity. It was shown to induce autophagy in MCF-7 (breast) cancer cells, promoting cell death (Zhang et al. 2013). When combined with a γ-secretase inhibitor (DAPT) or Notch1 small interfering RNA, the cytotoxicity of RY10-4 increases, enhancing efficacy on HER2, and SKBR3 breast cancer cell lines (Su et al. 2016a).

Protoapigenone, protoapigenin, apigenin, kaempferol, and quercetin are found in the fronds.

Ethanol extracts of the fronds protect against hepatoxicity induced by carbon tetrachloride (CCl_4) in an animal study, with efficacy comparable to silymarin (milk thistle seed extract) (Mondal et al. 2017).

Green marsh fern (*Macrothelypteris viridifrons*) has long been used in TCM to treat cancer, hydropsy (edema), and traumatic bleeding. Flavonoids found in this fern significantly inhibit tumor growth and the expression of vascular endothelial growth factor (VEGF), indicating antiangiogenic activity.

Some of the flavonoids identified in this fern include protoapigenone, protoapigenin, and protoapigenin-4'-O-β-D-glucopyranoside.

Protoapigenone and two other flavonoids showed strong antiproliferative activity on six tumor cell lines, including MCF-7 (breast) cells (Wei et al. 2011a).

These flavonoids inhibit the expression of CD34, a marker for human herpes simplex virus (HSV), and H22 (hepatoma) cancer cells in vivo (Wei et al. 2012).

Protoflavones derived from the fern have shown significant tumor inhibition in an H22 (hepatoma) cell transplantation model, but with only 20% efficacy compared to the control drug cyclophosphamide (Wei et al. 2019).

Additionally, a B-ring flavonoid isolated from the fern exhibits cytotoxicity to HT-29 (human colon) cancer cell lines (Wei et al. 2011b).

Work by Wei et al. (2022a) identified the activation of signal transducer and activator of transcription 3 (STAT3) and the suppression of NF-κB that plays a crucial role in apoptosis of HT-29 (colon) cancer cells.

MARATTIA

Ash Leaf Fern
Hawaii Potato Fern
Horseshoe Fern
King Fern

Marattia alata rhizomes have been traditionally steamed and eaten in Hawaii.

Hawaii potato fern (*Marattia douglasii* syn. *M. alata*) is also known as *pala* and *kapua ilio* on the islands. The tough stems have been traditionally woven into backing for flower leis. Decoctions made from this fern have been used to treat bronchitis and diarrhea (Uphof 1968; Usher 1971).

Ash leaf fern (*Marattia fraxinea*) was formerly used to treat ankylostomiasis (hookworm infection) in the Usambara Mountains of Tanzania and in South Africa (Watt and Breyer-Brandwijk, 1962). These intestinal parasites suck blood from the intestinal wall and lead to iron-deficient anemia, lethargy, edema, and progressive heart failure. The fertilized female hookworm can live for up to eight years, laying as many as 20,000 eggs daily, which mostly pass.

The fern was one of six plants identified (out of twenty-nine) for medicinal benefits by the Pare people in Northeastern Tanzania. Various water, ethyl acetate, and methanol extracts were tested on *Candida albicans*, *Aspergillus fumigatus*, *Fusarium culmorum*, *Staphylococcus aureus*, *Pseudomonas syringae*, and *Erwina amylovora* (de Boer et al. 2005). All plants showed activity against several test organisms.

King or horseshoe fern (*Marattia salicina* syn. *Ptisana salicina*) has fronds up to five meters tall. The starchy rhizome was a traditional food source for the Māori, known by names such as *para*, *tawhiti-para*, and horseshoe fern. This fern is endangered in New Zealand.

KING FERN ESSENCE

This essence of *Marattia salicina* facilitates inner healing, peace, and stillness at the soul level, particularly after physical and survival trauma or deep sorrow that have impacted the soul and locked into cellular memory. Find as First Light Flower Essences of New Zealand No. 37 King Fern.

MARSILEA

Pepperwort Water Clover Fern

Geographic Range: Bangladesh, China, India, Indonesia, Nigeria, Thailand, Western Himalayas

Habitat: aquatic, paddy fields

Practical Uses: aquarium plant, food

Medicinal Applications: anti-amnesic, antidepressant effects, anti-inflammatory, anticonvulsant, antiepileptic, antitussive, bones, cholesterol, diuretic, expectorant, hormones, insomnia, Leydig cell increase, liver, mental health, neuroinflammation, respiratory system, sedative, seizure reduction, sperm, testosterone, triglycerides

In Australia, the sporocarps of nardoo (*Marsilea drummondii*) are baked as cakes by Indigenous people after proper and extensive preparation.

The small aquatic water clover fern (*Marsilea minuta* syn. *M. crenata*) is found in China and India, often growing in paddy fields. It is shaped somewhat like a four-leaf clover and is served in Indonesia with sweet potato and spicy peanut sauce. In Javanese it is known as *semanggi*. It is used as vegetable in parts of India and Bangladesh. In Thailand, it is known as *phak waen* and eaten fresh with a chili dip. It is also widely available as a freshwater aquarium plant. In Indian traditional medicine (ayurveda), the fern is used for respiratory issues, insomnia, and mental health disorders. The active compound, marsiline, is reported to have sedative and anticonvulsant properties (Chatterjee et al., 1963).

The rhizomes, known as *paflu* in the Western Himalayas, are used as a diuretic (Khoja et al. 2022).

An interesting study was conducted on gerbils fed a high-fat diet. The animals were later fed the leaf extract of the fern and it reduced serum cholesterol by 31% and triglycerides by 63%. Liver cholesterol and triglycerides were lowered by 71% and 27%, respectively, compared to control animals. The treatment prevented accumulation of cholesterol and triglycerides in both the liver and aorta and dissolved atheromatous plaques in the thoracic and abdominal aorta (Gupta et al. 2000).

The frond extract contains benzoic acid-4-ethoxyethyl ester (43.39%) and farnesyl acetate (18.42%). The latter inhibits DNA replication in HeLa (epithelial/cervical) cancer cells and irreversibly block cells from progressing through the S phase of the cell cycle (Meigs et al. 1995).

A methanol extract was studied for its antitussive and expectorant properties in mice, showing a 59% and 55% reduction in induced coughs, and an 89% increase in mucosal secretions (Chakraborty et al. 2013). The methanol extract also exhibited moderate activity against the bacterium *Pseudomonas aeruginosa* (Arokiyaraj et al. 2018). A n-butanol fraction of the fern was found to reduce neuroinflammation in microglia HMC3 cell lines (Ma'arif et al. 2020a). Microglia are the first line of immune defense in the central nervous system. They play a key role in the regulation of brain synaptic functions and neurogenesis. Chronic inflammation of microglia is a common pathogenic mechanism in neurological issues.

A 96% ethanol extract of the fern leaves reduced neural inflammation through the induction of Arg1 and activation of ERb expression in microglia HMC3 cells, with the best dose being 250 ppm (Ma'arif et al. 2020b).

The fern contains phytoestrogens, which may benefit post-menopausal women by weakly binding to estrogen receptors in bone cells and modulating bone formation. The leaves contain six compounds believed to be phytoestrogenic and estrogen receptor β (ERb) agonists. This suggests possible benefits in increasing or maintaining bone mass in post-menopausal women (Aditama et al. 2021).

Ethanol extracts were tested on male rats for their influence on various hormonal issues. Both luteinizing hormone and testosterone levels increased significantly after administration. Higher doses also decreased malondialdehyde levels in monosodium glutamate-treated testes, increased sperm cell and Leydig cells counts, and increased seminiferous tubular diameter and germinal epithelium thickness (Rahayu et al. 2021).

The ethanol extract of the fern, standardized for marsiline (1.15%, w/w), was studied for its potential benefits in depression. In a forced swimming test and tail suspension test on rats, the extract significantly reduced immobility time. It also significantly relieved head twitches induced with 5-hydroxytryptophan (5-HTP), and significantly downregulated 5-HT2A receptors in the frontal cortex, but did not affect benzodiazepine receptors (Bhattamisra et al. 2008). This suggests the antidepressant effect may be due to the regulation of 5-HT2A density in the frontal cortex.

Acetylcholinesterase in the frontal cortex and hippocampus was significantly inhibited by a standardized ethanol extract of the fern. The binding of 3H-QNB in the frontal cortex indicates upregulation of muscarinic receptors. The authors suggest the fern extract possesses excellent anti-amnesic activity, probably mediated through the central cholinergic system (Bhattamisra et al. 2012).

Extracts of the fern were given to rodents to evaluate its anti-aggressive activity, and the results were qualitatively comparable to the sedative effects of diazepam (Tiwari et al. 2010).

Water clover fern or pepperwort (*Marsilea quadrifolia*) is an edible aquatic fern that is eaten in parts of Asia as a health food. In Nigeria, it is commonly known as water clover or pepperwort and is eaten to increase sexual desire in women (Nwosu 2002). The fern has been used in traditional medicine for its sedative and antiepileptic benefits. The aquatic fern is native to Europe and considered a weed in parts of the United States today.

The compound 1-triacontanol cerotate, isolated from the fern, has been shown to reduce reactive oxidative damage in the hippocampus and frontal cortex of pentylenetetrazol (PTZ)-kindled chronic epileptic rats. This suggests possible mechanisms of its traditional use (Snehunsu et al. 2015). Seizure activity induced in rat models was effectively reduced by both water and ethanol extracts of this fern. The severity of behavioral and EEG-measured seizures suggests a rational of traditional use for epilepsy in humans (Sahu et al. 2012). A methanol extract of the fern inhibits acetylcholinesterase and butyrylcholinesterase, suggestive of possible benefits in prevention or management of Alzheimer's disease (Bhadra et al. 2012).

The fern contains numerous polyphenols (at least twenty-one) including quercetin, which exhibits significant antioxidant activity (Zhang et al. 2016b).

The fern also demonstrates in vitro cytotoxicity against MCF-7 (breast) cancer cell lines (Uma and Pravin 2013).

This water fern exhibits high uptake capacity of six heavy metals: vanadium, arsenic, cadmium, chromium, mercury, and lead (Jiang et al. 2018). Research in India found that *Marsilea* species exhibit the highest specific arsenic uptake of all studied aquatic and terrestrial plants (Tripathi et al. 2012).

The chemistry and pharmacology of marsiline, derived from *Marsilea minuta* was first described by Chatterjee et al. (1963).

MATTEUCCIA

Ostrich Ferns

Geographic Range: Northern Canada, Northwest Territories, Northern British Columbia, Western Himalayas

Habitat: aquatic, forests, mountainous regions

Practical Uses: food, food for livestock, fragrances, scent masking

Medicinal Applications: antioxidant activity, antiviral, blood pressure, cancer, cytotoxicity, glioblastoma inhibition, hypoglycemic activity, immune system, kidneys, lupus, neuroinflammation, vermifuge, wormicidal

Warning: Ostrich fern should not be consumed by pregnant women, children, weak individuals, or those with peptic ulcers. It can also cause allergies in individuals sensitive to macadamia nuts. Caution is advised when consuming raw or undercooked fiddleheads due to food poisoning risk.

The genus is named in honor of the Italian physicist and neuro-physiologist Carlo Matteucci (1800–1868).

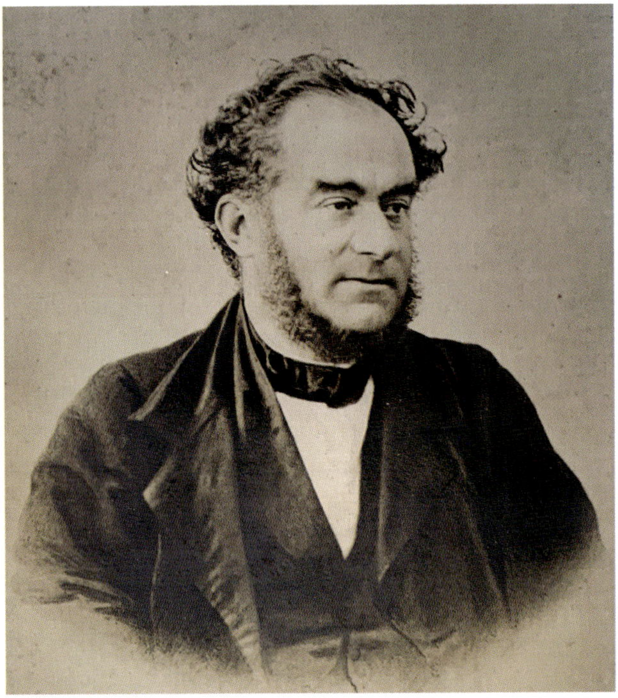

Carlo Matteucci
Photo by Nicomede Bianchi

He continued the work of Luigi Galvani on bioelectricity and proved that injured excitable biological tissue generates measurable currents.

My first introduction to the connection between humans and plants was through the book *The Secret Life of Plants* by Tompkins and Bird (1973). Although criticized by some botanists, it opened my mind to plant sentience (biocommunication).

The book noted the work of Louis Kervran, whose book *Biological Transmutations* (1972) totally shifted my awareness of transformation of molecules. How organic silica becomes calcium and how organic manganese becomes iron. These concepts later became part of my clinical herbal practice.

Many years later, I became intrigued with Music of the Plants devices designed by Silvia Buffagni Esperide Ananas. I ordered a large and later a portable machine from Italy that translates the electrical charge in plants, including ferns, into music. It has been an endless source of enjoyment.

The rhizomes of *Matteuccia intermedia* syn. *Onoclea intermedia* contain twenty-one flavanones, nine flavanone glucoside derivatives, matteflavosides H–J, and matteuinterates A–F.

A new flavanonol, demethylmatteucinol, was recently identified by Li et al. (2019c). Six flavanones in the fern show potent inhibition of α-glucosidase, suggesting hypoglycemic or blood sugar lowering activity. Matteuinterins A through C (glycosides) have also been identified, with several compounds exhibiting antioxidant activity.

Oriental ostrich fern (*Matteuccia orientalis*) contains matteucens I and J, matteuorienin and matteuorienates A through C, matteucinol, demethoxymatteucinol, and 2'-hydroxymatteucinol.

Matteurienates A through C exhibit very strong aldose reductase inhibition, suggestive of benefits in reducing eye and retinal issues associated with diabetes (Basnet et al. 1995).

The compound 2'-hydroxymatteucinol shows potent hypoglycemic activity, effectively lowering blood sugar levels in STZ-induced diabetic rats (Basnet et al. 1993).

The root extract of the fern shows moderate cytotoxicity against HaCaT (keratinocyte) cells. The extract also reduced the interleukin-8 (IL-8) and tumor necrosis factor-alpha (TNF-α) in *Propionibacterium acnes* and *Staphylococcus epidermidis*-induced THP-1 cells, indicating an anti-inflammatory effect on pus-forming acne. This suggests that the rhizome extract may have benefits in topical medications (Kim et al. 2008). The frond extract exhibits antioxidant and anti-inflammatory activity (Dion et al. 2015).

Ostrich fern spores' (*Matteuccia struthiopteris*) constituents include legumin and vicilin-like proteins.

Fronds contain L-homoserine, polyisoprenoid alcohols, ascorbic acid, γ-tocopherol, β-carotene, xanthohyll pigments (such as violaxanthin, zeaxanthin and lutein, methoxymatteucin, and thumberginol C) fatty acids (including EPA and arachidonic acid). The fronds also contain palmitic acid, astragalin, various phenolic acids (including chlorogenic acid, p-hydroxybenzoic acid, p-coumaric acid, ferulic acid, vanillic acid, and protocatechuic acid), phytosterols (including β-sitosterol, campesterol, and stigmasterol), pinosylvin (stilbene), ponasterone A, ecdysterones, pterosterone, and filicin. Betaine levels and glyco- and phospholipids are high in spring fronds and decrease as the fronds mature.

Eighty-two grams of fiddleheads contain 0.7 mg iron, 13 mg vitamin C, and small amounts of vitamins B1, B2, and B3. The fern contains various C-methyl flavanones, methoxymatteucin, and thunberginol C in both the frond base and rhizomes. L-O-caffeoylhomoserine is a major free radical scavenger.

The content of the betaine lipid diacylglyceryl-N,N,N-trimethylhomoserine (DGTS) is highest in the crosier form. Fiddleheads contain 5% protein, α- and beta-carotene, and are rich in potassium, and low in sodium.

Rhizomes of the ostrich fern contain woodwardic acid, apigenin, 3-(4-[β-D-glycophyranosyloxy]phenyl)-2-propenoic acid, 4-O-β-D-glucosyl-trans-caffeic acid, ergosta-6,22-diene-3β,5α,8 α-triol, riboflavin, D-mannitol, succinic acid, demethoxymatteucinol, matteucinol, pinosylvin, pinosylvin 3-O-β-D-glucopyranoside, matteuorienate A, glucose, galactose, xylose, various C-methyl flavanones, furfural, 2-furancarboxaldehyde, trophophyll, and sporophyll. The rhizomes also contain, apigenin, riboflavin, 4-O-β-D-glucopyranosyl-p-coumaric acid, and D-mannitol. Phenol content is particularly high.

The ostrich fern is popular as a cooked vegetable, especially in North America. The common name derives from its huge size, often up to 1.8 meters tall, and its feathery fronds that resemble plumage on the flightless avian. The species name, *struthiopteris*, derives from the Greek words *struthokamelos*, meaning "ostrich," and *pteris*, meaning "fern."

The fiddleheads are technically called crosiers due to their resemblance to a bishop's staff. The term fiddle derives from the Anglo-Saxon *fithele*, which in turn derives from the Italian *vitula*, meaning "violin." Various expressions such as "fiddlesticks," "fiddling around," "playing second fiddle," "drunk as a fiddle,"

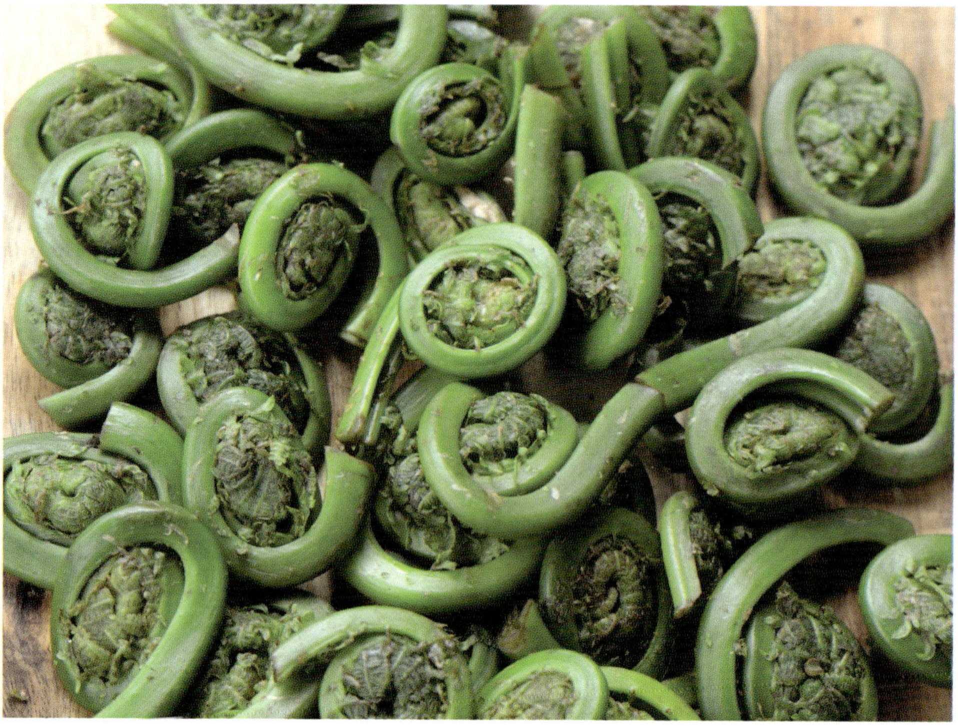

Fiddleheads of *Matteuccia struthiopteris* (Ostrich Fern)
Photo by Robert Dale Rogers

and "fiddle faddle" derive from the English puritanical scorn of having fun and pleasure instead of working hard. Ironically, "fiddle-dee-dee" is a corruption of the Italian *fedido*, meaning "by the faith of God."

Norwegians fed ostrich fern to the goats and included it in early gruit ales. Veterinarians have used the root extract to remove livestock parasites.

The fern's edible fiddleheads were used by Indigenous peoples of Northern Canada to remove placenta after giving birth and the sterile leaf stalk base was decocted and taken as needed as a tea is used to treat stomach or back pain (Leighton 1985).

The Chipewyan of Northern Alberta know the fern as *nitéli ts' uchoghé*, meaning "dry muskeg white spruce." The base of the stalk was boiled with other plants and drunk four times daily or chewed with other plants every two hours to treat a racing heartbeat. One herb I am familiar with, that is used by the Cree of Northern Alberta for bradycardia, is the tiny root of harebell (*Campanula rotundifolia* and *C. alaskana*).

The Slave or Slavey (Dene) of the Northwest Territories call this fern *eya ha dala*. The base of the green frond is decocted with other herbs to make a tea to slow a pounding heart. The stipe buds sitting on top of the rhizome are used to treat cancer and help patients gain weight (Marles et al. 2000). This is also based on information I was gifted by Russell Willier, a noted Cree medicine man.

Various Indigenous groups roasted the rhizome. The hairy exterior was peeled off, and the core ingested. Some groups ground up and dried the rhizome for winter food.

The Gitxsan of Northern British Columbia boiled or baked the fern that they refer to as *damtx* or consumed the raw fronds with grease in early spring. Various Indigenous hunters ate the fiddleheads in the belief it would mask their scent.

"If the urine is whitish, the root of Ostrich fern can be steeped, for a drink that assists urinary problems" (Rogers 2014b).

As mentioned in the introduction, the ostrich fern is a choice edible, though caution is advised. One report dating back to 1994 found that an outbreak of food poisoning in New York and Western Canada was associated with eating raw or undercooked fiddleheads. It is fortunate that my fiddlehead ice cream recipe did not become popular.

The fiddlehead is best consumed after cooking as it contains thiaminase, an enzyme that destroys vitamin B1 (thiamine). The taste of cooked fiddleheads can be described as a unique blend of asparagus, broccoli, and artichoke, with a very sweet, green flavor, and hint of bitterness.

When young, the fiddleheads contain high levels of ecdysterones and antioxidants, which are double those found in wild blueberries. They store well at just above freezing with 100% humidity and provide 95% marketable product after sixteen days, and 76% after thirty-two days. Storage in water yields similar results but requires additional labor and costs.

Thunberginol C reduced stress-induced anxiety in a mouse study. It also prevented corticosterone-induced neural cell death, reduced plasma TNF-α levels, neuroinflammation, and oxidative stress (Lee et al. 2022a). Thunberginol C also exhibits anti-allergic activity, inhibiting histamine release from rat mast cells and histamine-induced contractions in isolated guinea pig tracheal chains. The compound also shows antimicrobial activity against oral bacteria (Yoshikawa et al. 1996). Thunberginol C acts as a selective dual inhibitor of acetylcholinesterase and butyrylcholinesterase. Both enzymes interact with amyloid-beta peptide, which promotes senile plaque formation leading to Alzheimer's disease (Hwang et al. 2021).

The rhizome has been found to lower blood sugar levels and possess activity against the polio virus (Farnsworth 1999). Both frond and rhizome extracts exhibit higher α glucosidase inhibition than acarbose (Li et al. 2019c).

Pinosylvin has antifungal and antibacterial properties. The compound inhibits the migration and invasion of nasopharyngeal carcinoma (Chuang et al. 2021).

The compound matteflavoside G, isolated from the rhizome, exhibits significant inhibition against the H1N1 influenza virus, with two additional flavonoids showing moderate antiviral activity (Li et al. 2015a).

Mattecuinol induces apoptosis in human glioblastoma cell lines. The compound inhibits angiogenesis and tumor growth in vivo and may be a useful adjuvant to existing chemotherapy treatments (Silva et al. 2020a).

In fact, recent research by Netto et al. (2022) suggests that matteucinol, when combined with temozolomide, inhibits glioblastoma proliferation, invasion, and progression.

Mattecuinol is also present in Oriental ostrich fern (*Matteuccia orientalis*) (see page 188) and *Dryopteris sublaeta* (see page 156), as well as the root of kava kava, a well-known medicinal herb.

In TCM, the root is used as a substitute for thick-stemmed wood fern (*Dryopteris crassirhizoma*) and is known as guan zhong. It is considered a superior vermifuge compared to male fern because it is considerably less toxic yet effective against pinworms, roundworms, hookworms, tapeworms, giardia (beaver fever), and trichomonas infections. It is, of course, contraindicated for pregnant women, children, frail individuals, as well as those with peptic ulcers.

Guan zhong is used as a broad-spectrum antiviral and in veterinary medicine for swine ascariasis, earthworms, leeches, and various flukes, including bovine liver, flat, and broad sucker flukes. The fronds are known as *jia gou ju* and have been traditionally eaten to lower blood pressure.

Fern polysaccharides have been tested in a mouse model of systemic lupus erythematosus-like syndrome induced by *Campylobacter jejuni*. Treatment with the polysaccharides reduced weight loss, spleen swelling, and production of auto-antibodies and total immunoglobulin G compared to controls. The polysaccharides also protected against glomerular injury in the kidneys, reduced immunoglobulin deposition, and lowered proteinuria (Wang et al. 2010b). The fern exhibits antioxidant activity, while the underground parts inhibit acetylcholinesterase, suggestive of benefits in neurological disorders (Wang et al. 2024). Some of the volatile compounds in the fern's adventitious roots, trophophyll, and sporophyll are important for food, cosmetic, and pharmaceutical applications.

The fern is best eaten steamed or cooked. Rats fed fresh ferns for up to 120 days did not exhibit any carcinogenic activity, but caution is still advised (Hirono et al. 1978).

An interesting steam-distilled essential oil contains over one hundred volatile compounds, including (E)-phytol (24.8%), nonanal (15.1%), and decanal (7.6%). The oil contains two aldehydes with seaweed-like odor, suggesting possible use in ocean or beach-themed perfumes (Miyazawa et al. 2007).

Oils of ostrich fern are usually fresh, green, aromatic, and combine well with the dry notes of usnea and other tree moss absolutes. Fougère perfumes are deep-noted and typically appreciated by masculine tastes, especially in aftershaves and colognes. Coumarin notes, such as sweet clover, are complementary.

The spores of this fern contain vicilin and legumin and can cause allergies in individuals sensitive to macadamia nuts.

METAXYA

Silk Tree Fern

Silk tree fern (*Metaxya rostrata*) is common in the rainforests of Central and South America. The dried rootlets are used by Indigenous peoples to treat intestinal diseases.

The fern contains two polyphenols, cinnamtannin B2, and aesculitannin B, common sterols such as sitosterol, stigmasterol, and campesterol, as well as chlorogenic and caffeic acid. The rhizomes contain two unusual methylidenecyclopropane glucosides: (E)-4-O-β-D-glucopyranosyl coumaric acid, 2-deprenylrheediaxantone B (XB), 2-deprenyl-7-hydroxy-reediaxanthone B (OH-XB) and methyl a-fructofuranoside.

Cinnamtannin B2 exhibits moderate selective cytotoxicity against PRMI-7951 (melanoma) cell lines (Kashiwada et al. 1992). Aesculitannin B exhibits anti-corona virus (SARS-CoV-2) activity (Hirose et al. 2023). The compound is commercially available to researchers.

Two compounds, 2-deprenyl-rheediaxantone B (XB) and 2-deprenyl-7-hydroxy-reediaxanthone B (OH-XB) exhibit cytotoxicity against SW480 and CRC (colorectal) cancer cell lines (Kainz et al. 2013). Topoisomerase I inhibition is dependent on the presence of an unmethylated 7-OH group. Both XB and OH-XB are equally cytotoxic. XB arrested cells in the G2/M phase, and OH-XB induced S-phase cell cycle arrest (Mittermair et al. 2019; 2020).

MICROGRAMMA

Clubmoss Snake Fern Snake Fern Vine Fern

Clubmoss snake fern (*Microgramma lycopodioides*) is a traditional medicine in the Greater Mpigi region of Uganda (Schultz et al. 2020).

Of sixteen plants examined, fifteen displayed significant selective COX-2 inhibition, suggestive of anti-inflammatory activity (Schultz et al. 2021). COX-2 inhibitor drugs are not without controversy. The drug Vioxx was removed from the global market in 2004 due to increased risk of heart attacks and stroke. Celebrex, which was scrutinized for the same reasons, was never removed from the market. However, it now includes a warning advising not to exceed 200 mg daily and to limit use to for no more than five days. Despite these warnings, patients often ignore the advice in managing their pain. Natural COX-2 inhibiting plants do not exhibit these contraindications.

Fishscale fern (*Microgramma squamulosa*) is used to treat gastrointestinal ulcers in parts of Brazil. Work by Suffredini et al. (1999) used an acute ulcer induction test and found the crude extract comparable against reference drugs cimetidine and misoprostol.

Microgramma vacciniifolia rhizome has long been used in folk medicine. In Argentina the fern is known as *suela consuela*. Animal toxicity studies found a lectin-rich fraction caused hydropic degeneration at 5,000 mg/kg. However, neither a saline extract nor the fractions induced oxidative stress in the liver, showed genotoxicity, or were lethal, though some signs of toxicity were observed (da Silva et al. 2020). A later study confirmed that the fraction did not show genotoxicity or acute toxicity in mice. It did show antibacterial activity against *Acinetobacter baumannii*, *Escherichia coli*, *Klebsiella pneumoniae*, *Pseudomonas aeruginosa*, and *Staphylococcus aureus*. The fraction also showed the reduction of tumors on Ehrlich carcinoma-bearing mice (da Silva et al. 2022).

Other studies by the same researchers found that the saline extract and lectin-rich fraction inhibited the development of granulomatous tissue, suggesting novel therapeutic potential for pain and inflammatory conditions.

Work by Bolson et al. (2015) researched the ethno-medicinal plants of forests around Parana, Brazil. Traditional uses of this fern were reported. The rhizome lectin inhibits *Fusarium oxysporum*, a destructive fungus on tomato and other commercial crops.

The lectin from the fern was cytotoxic to NCI-H292 (lung mucoepidermoid) carcinoma cells (de Albuquerque et al. 2014) and a lectin derived from the fronds, incubated with human peripheral blood mononuclear cells (PBMCs), significantly increased TNF-α, IFN-γ, IL-6, IL-10, and nitric oxide production. The lectin stimulated T lymphocytes from PBMCs to differentiate into CD8+ cells and enhanced the activation of these cells, as indicated by CD28 expression. This activity suggests that the lectin induces a Th1 immune response, as well as activation and differentiation of T lymphocytes, suggesting immune modulation (de Siqueira Patriota et al. 2017).

The frond lectin also inhibited carrageenan-induced acute inflammation in the paws of mice, effectively reducing both edema and pro-inflammatory cytokines (de Siqueira Patriota et al. 2022).

MICROLEPIA

Hay-scented Fern
Limpleaf Fern
Rigid Lace Fern
Small Fishscale Fern

Extracts of the dry fronds of *Microlepia pilosissima* contain isopimarane diterpenoid glycosides, which exhibit activity against three pathogenic fungi and two oral pathogens, as well as moderate cytotoxicity against tested tumor cell lines (Hu et al. 2015).

Various phenylpropanoid glycosides derived from 70% ethanol extracts of the dry fronds exhibit antioxidant activity comparable to that of α-tocopherol, with several compounds displaying moderate antioxidant effects (Hu et al. 2012).

In Vanuatu, the young fronds of limpleaf fern (*Microlepia speluncae*) are lightly boiled and added to the diet of new mothers to ensure adequate breast milk production (Bourdy and Walter 1992).

Work by Kalpana et al. (2020) found extracts produced moderate activity against the sheep nematode *Gastrothylax crumenifer*.

The hay-scented or rigid lace fern (*Microlepia strigosa*) is Indigenous to Hawaii, India, and Malaysia. In Hawaii, it is also known as *palapaiai*. In ancient times, Indigenous people of the islands decorated altars with frond wreaths in honor of Laka, the goddess of hula. The fern pinnae were used as head, neck, and wrist leis, known for soothing the skin. Young fronds were reportedly fed to babies and used in baths. Some early reports suggest that the fern was used ceremonially to cure insanity, though the specific methods were not detailed.

MICROSORUM

Breadfruit Fern	Maile-scented Fern
Climbing Bird's Nest Fern	Monarch Fern
Dwarf Elkhorn Fern	Musk Fern
Fishtail Fern	Scented Oak Leaf Fern
Fishtail Strap Fern	Terrestrial Fern
Java Fern	Wart Fern

Geographic Range: Australia, Fiji, Hawaii, Ivory Coast, New Caledonia, Polynesia, Rapa Nui, Western Pacific Rim
Habitat: freshwater, rocks, tropical regions
Practical Uses: aquarium plant, fabric scent, phytoremediation (cadmium), potential sunscreen
Medicinal Applications: anti-inflammatory, antiproliferative, biofilm inhibition, cancer, cholestasis, type 2 diabetes, dermal fibroblast protection, diuretic, dysmenorrhea, gonorrhea, insulin, leucorrhea, skin, UV protection, wounds

The *Microsorum* genus presently contains 44 tropical species including several that live in fast moving water (one to two meters per second), and on rocks (lithophytic).

Scented oak leaf fern (*Microsorum commutatums* syn. *Polypodium polynesicum* syn. *Phymatosorus commutatus*) is known as *Maire Kakara* on the Cook Islands. *Kakara* means "fragrant," and the fronds are sometimes used in head garlands.

Musk fern (*Microsorum grossum*) is frequently used in Polynesian traditional medicine. Known locally as *metuapua'a*, the fern fronds and rhizome are included in formulas for a variety of ailments, including cancer (Petard and Raau 1972).

Musk fern contains phytoecdysteroids such as 20-hydroxyecdysone which are used as a safe alternative to anabolic steroid drugs.

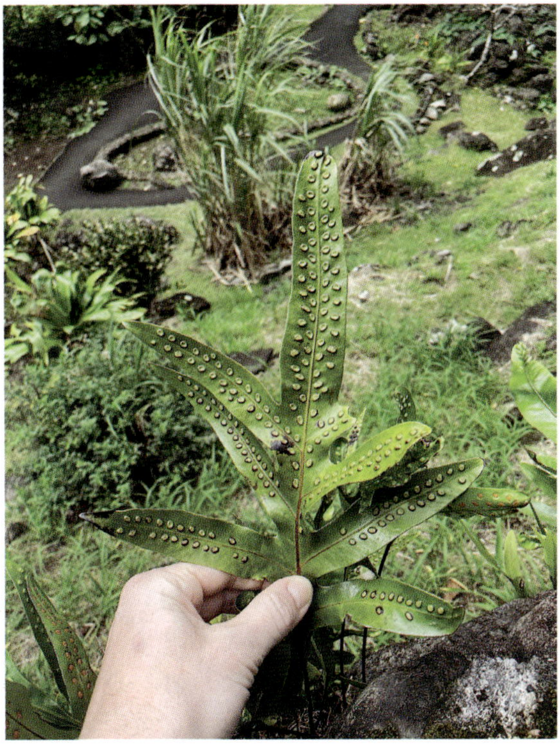

Microsorum grossum
(Musk Fern)
Photo by Drew T. Henderson

Extracts of this fern have been studied for their effects on human dermal fibroblasts. The extract upregulates *Heme Oxygenase* I, which protects skin cells from oxidative stress and provides immune protection. Additionally, when combined with repeated UV irradiation, an ecdysteroid fraction of the fern prevented premature skin aging. This suggests its potential as a novel ingredient in sunscreen products (Ho et al. 2015).

The juice of pimple fern (*Microsorum membranifolium*) has been traditionally used in dysmenorrhea, gonorrhea, and leucorrhea (Ho et al. 2011).

The fern contains various phytoecdysteroids, including ecdysone, 20-hydroxyecdysone, 2-deoxy-20-hydroxyecdysone, 2-deoxyecdysone, (E)-2-deoxy-20-hydroxyecdysone 3-[4-(1-β-D-glucopyranosyl)] caffeate, (E)-2-deoxy-20-hydroxyecdysone 3-[4-(1-β-D-glucopyranosyl)] ferulate, and (E)-2-deoxyecdysone 3-[4-(1-β-D-glucopyranosyl)] ferulate.

Cambie and Ash (1994) suggest that this fern was used in traditional Fijian medicine for antiviral activity.

The Java fern (*Microsorum pteropus*) is a popular addition to freshwater aquariums. A silver nanoparticle composite made with a methanol extract of the fern exhibits antioxidant activity (Chick et al. 2020). The fern is also a hyperaccumulator of cadmium, suggesting its potential use in phytoremediation.

Fishtail fern (*Microsorum punctatum* syn. *M. polycarpon* syn. *Polypodium punctatum*) fronds are juiced and used as a diuretic, purgative, or wound healer in the Ivory Coast (Bouquet 1974). The fern goes by other names, including terrestrial fern, dwarf elkhorn fern, crested fern, fishtail strap fern, and climbing bird's nest fern. The common names refer to the branched crest at the end of its fronds resembling a fishtail.

Monarch fern, musk fern, wart fern, breadfruit fern, or maile-scented fern (*Microsorum scolopendria* syn. *Phymatosorus scolopendria*) is found across the Western Pacific rim, from Australia to New Caledonia to Fiji. The fern is also found on the island of Rapa Nui, off the coast of Chile. The fern was introduced to Hawaii in the 1910s, where it has become naturalized and is referred to as *laua'e*, a name also given to the endemic and rare fern *Microsorum spectrum*.

When crushed, the fern releases a scent similar to maile, a Hawaiian vine (*Alyxia olivaeformis*) with small fragrant yellow flower with a sweet odor resembling vanilla, due to its coumarin content. Pieces of the fronds are woven into leis or used to scent kapa fabric made from the bast fiber of indigenous plants. In Samoa, the fronds are used for headaches, catarrh of the stomach, and as a lotion for skin sores (Uhe 1974).

The fronds of maile-scented fern contain ecdysone (0.16% dry weight) and 20-hydroxyecdysone (0.20%), along with significant amounts of makisterones A and C, inokosterone, amarasterone A, and small amounts of poststerone (Snogan et al. 2007). Later work also identified a C29 phytoecdysteroid, amarasterone A.

Makisterone A may be useful in clinical treatment of cholestasis (Kang and Li 2022).

Leaf and rhizome extracts of this fern contain up to 57% phenolic acids, as well as flavonoids such as protocatechuic acid, 4-O-glucoside, cirsimaritin, isoxanthohumol, and others.

The extracts inhibit and disaggregate biofilm formation by *Staphylococcus aureus* and *S. epidermis* cultured on human dermal fibroblast cells. They also show anti-inflammatory activity against COX-2 enzymes (Balada et al. 2022).

Cirsimaritin is a potent dimethoxy flavone also found in holy basil (*Ocimum tenuiflorum*) and several thistle species. Its antiproliferative activity has been confirmed in breast and gallbladder cancer cell lines. Work by Pathak et al. (2021) found that cirsimaritin also inhibited the proliferation of lung squamous (NCIH-520) cancer cell lines by inducing apoptosis. It also inhibited the activity of ODC and CATD responsible, enzymes responsible for the progression phase in cancer cells.

Cirsimaritin is protective of pancreatic β cells and shows significant benefits in improving insulin resistance in diabetic rats. The compound was shown to effectively suppress apoptosis in pancreatic β cells by decreasing the activation of caspase-8 and caspase-3 while increasing antiapoptotic BCL-2 protein expression (Lee et al. 2017).

When given to high-fat diet rats, cirsimaritin reduced elevated levels of serum glucose abrogated increased serum insulin in the treated group, and improved insulin resistance. This suggests possible application and therapeutic potential for treating type 2 diabetes in humans (Alqudah et al. 2023). Cirsimaritin also inhibits influenza virus A replication by downregulating the NF-κB signal transduction pathway (Yan et al. 2018).

Cirsimaritin is one of ten flavonoids isolated from birch (*Betula* sp.) tree leaf buds. The preparation of leaf buds is the basis of gemmotherapy, a modality I used extensively in my clinical practice, as a drainage remedy. The fresh buds are chopped and left to macerate in a blend of glycerin and alcohol for three weeks. Readers interested in the medicinal benefits of gemmotherapy will find several of my favorite book titles listed in the Resources section.

Work by Szoka et al. (2021) found that silver birch (*Betula pendula*) and downy birch or white birch (*Betula pubescens*) bud extracts containing cirsimaritin significantly reduced viability, proliferation, and clonogenicity of gastric (AGS), colon (DLD-1), and liver (HepG2) cancer cell lines via apoptosis. Upregulation of p53 was detected only in wild type p53 harboring cells.

The fern contains isoxanthohumol, a unique prenylflavonoid also found in craft-brewed IPA beers. The compound is a competitive ABCB1-inhibitor that reverses ABCB1-mediated doxorubicin resistance in MCF-7 (breast) cancer cells. In other words, a synergistic combination of this compound with chemotherapy resistance can increase the inhibition of proliferation and the stimulation of apoptosis in chemotherapy-resistant breast cancer cells (Liu et al. 2017b).

MOHRIA

Carrot Fern   Scented Fern

Carrot or scented fern (*Mohria caffrorum* syn. *Anemia caffrorum*) is endemic to South Africa and is currently listed as endangered. The genus is named in honor of David Mohr, a German botanist who lived from 1780 to 1808.

The species name means "from the land of the kaffirs," referring to the Cape. Traditionally, the dried, aromatic, balsamic-like fronds of the fern were smoked to relieve head colds or powdered and mixed into a cooling ointment for burns (Watt and Breyer-Brandwijk 1962).

MYRIOPTERIS

Lip Ferns

Hairy lip fern (*Myriopteris lanosa* syn. *Cheilanthes lanosa*) is native to the Eastern and Midwestern United States. It is widely grown in rock gardens due to its hardiness and tolerance for sun and hot, dry conditions.

Myriopteris notholaenoides syn. *Hemionitis notholaenoides* hyperaccumulates arsenic, making it a good candidate for phytoremediation.

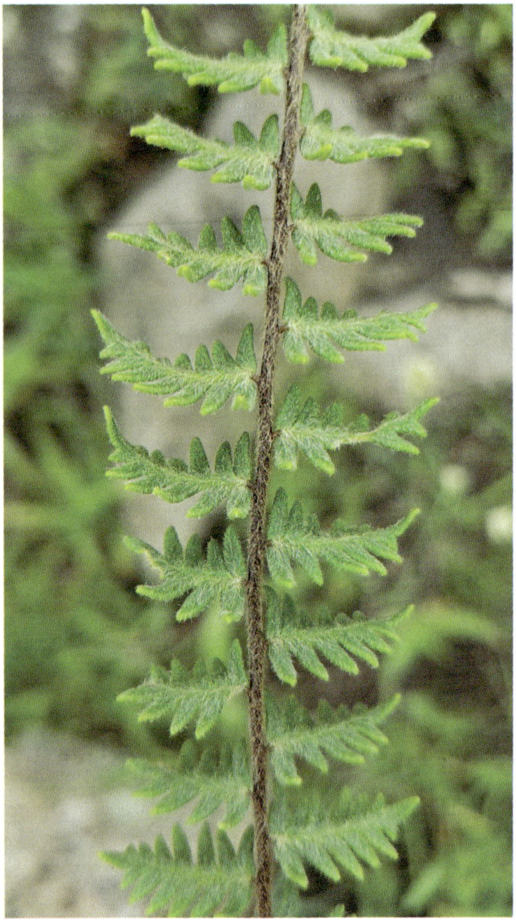

Myriopteris aurea (Golden Lip Fern)

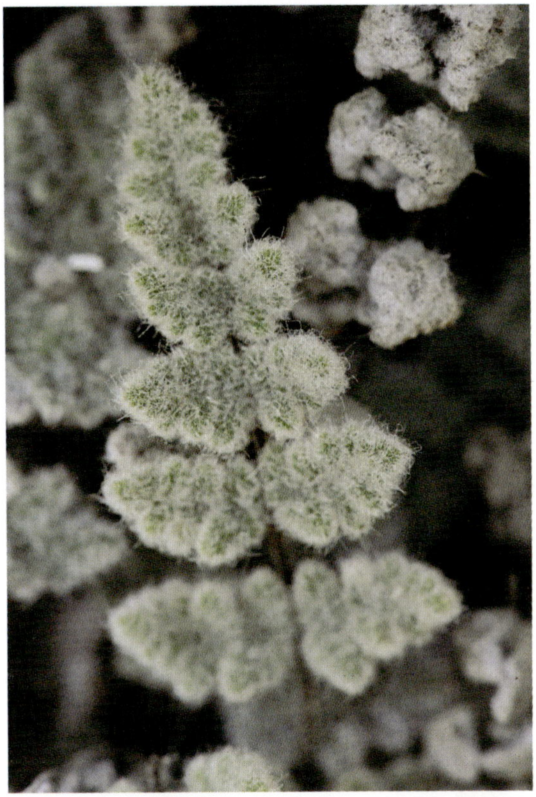

Myriopteris parryi
(Parry's Lip Fern)

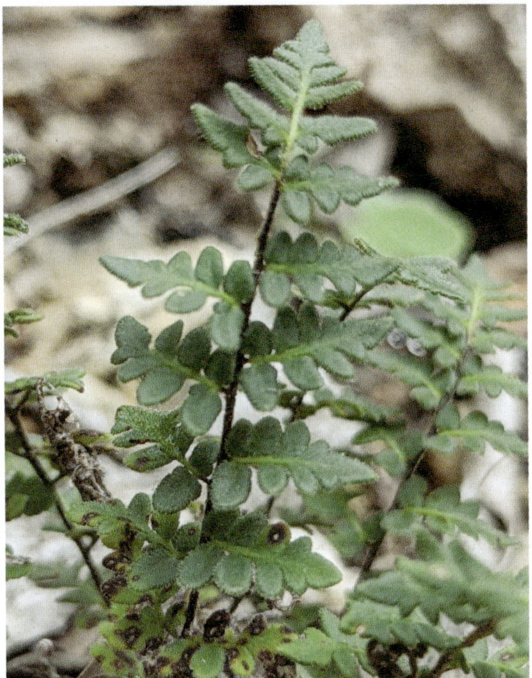

Myriopteris scabra
(Rough Lip Fern)

NEOCHEIROPTERIS

The root of *Neocheiropteris palmatopedata* contains various kaempferol glycosides, including palmatosides A through C and multiflorins A and B, as well as afzelin.

Multiflorin B inhibits aromatase enzyme activity and nitric oxide production, and afzelin shows 68.3% inhibition against quinone reductase 2. Palmatoside A inhibits COX-1 enzyme activity and palmatosides B and C inhibit tumor necrosis factor α (TNF-α). These multiple factors suggest cancer chemoprotective potential (Yang et al. 2010).

NEPHROLEPIS

Boston Fern
Fishbone Fern
Kimberly Queen Fern
Ladder Fern
Macho Fern
Sword Ferns

Geographic Range: Asia, French Polynesia, India, Ivory Coast, Malaysia, Southern Florida, Southeast Asia, West Africa

Habitat: tropical regions, wetlands

Practical Uses: air purifier, basket production, floral industry, hats production, essential oils, mats production, ornamental plant, phytoremediation (heavy metals), vase life extension

Medicinal Applications: antibacterial, antifungal, antiparasitic, antiplatelet, childbirth, blood coagulation, cancer, coughs, cytotoxic, diuretic, dysmenorrhea, liver, menstruation, neuropathic pain, sterility inducer, ulcers

Warning: The fern's sterility-inducing properties, if consumed, can lead to permanent infertility.

The meaning of the genus is somewhat obscure. *Nephro* refers to "kidney," and *lepis* derives from the Greek *lepó*, meaning "to peel or scale," referring to the kidney-shaped indusia (sori covering). The genus of around thirty species is referred to as sword ferns.

Nephrolepis acuta syn. *N. biserrata* fern has been traditionally used in India to treat dysmenorrhea (Singh and Upadhyay 2012).

The giant sword fern (*Nephrolepis biserrata* syn. *Aspidium biserratum* syn. *Hyoioektus biserrata*), locally known in tropical Malaysia as *paku pedang*, has been used in folk medicine for a variety of health conditions. The species name *biserrata* means "double-toothed" and refers to the leaf margin. The tropical giant sword fern is the largest of the sword ferns, growing up to eight meters in length in tropical regions. You can purchase it for your garden, and it is often labeled "macho fern" due to its robust size. In West Africa, the iron-rich fronds are consumed as a wild green and are used as a hemostat for wounds in Ivory Coast (Bouquet 1974).

Nephrolepis biserrata contains terpenoids such as ivalin, isovelleral, brassinolide, eschscholtzxanthin; flavonoids such as alnustin, kaempferol 7,4-dimethyl ether, pachypodol; and phenolics like piscidic acid, chlorogenic acid, and ankorine, and the aromatic 3-hydroxycoumarin. Other compounds include cinnamaldehyde, cinnamic acid, apigenin, quercetin, cymaroside, luteolin, maringenin, wogonin, 6-gingerol, nicotinamide, abscisic acid, daidzein, and salvianolic acid B.

A methanol extract of the fronds exhibits strong antioxidant activity and provides significant protection against carbon tetrachloride-induced hepatoxicity in rats (Shah et al. 2015). Carbon tetrachloride is a human carcinogen, formerly used as a dry-cleaning solvent, refrigerant, and as an additive to increase the weight of wax in old lava lamps. It was also used as a medication under the name Necatorina and Seretin. However, it is now banned due to its severe health risks.

Research by Shah et al. (2020a) found that methanol extracts of the fern possess antiparasitic activity against the marine leech (*Zeylanicobdella arugamensis*). This leech is responsible for infestations of cultured grouper fish, and the fern extract showed 100% mortality, suggesting a natural alternative to toxic chemicals used in Southeast Asia fish farms (Maran et al. 2023; Shah et al. 2020b).

Piscidic acid is found in the stem pads of prickly pear (*Opuntia ficus-indica*) cacti, a functional food with proven health benefits.

Ivalin induces apoptosis in SMMC-7721 (human hepatocellular) cancer cells. The compound induces microtubule depolymerization, blocks cells in mitotic phase, and eventually caused programmed cell death (Liu et al. 2019a).

Ivalin significantly inhibits cell proliferation, migration and invasion in breast cancer cells, by suppressing epithelial mesenchymal transition (Ma et al. 2018).

Isovelleral has been studied for relief of neuropathic pain in vitro, and pachypodol inhibits the growth of CaCo-2 colon cancer cell lines (Ali et al. 2008).

Many of the terpenoids and flavonoids mentioned above may be responsible for the antiparasitic activity of methanol extracts.

Both *Nephrolepis biserrata* and fishbone fern (*Nephrolepis cordifolia*) water and ethanol extracts were tested against nine bacterial and three fungal strains. The water extracts inhibited *Proteus mirabilis, Enterobacter aerogenes, Pseudomonas aeruginosa, Salmonella typhimurium, Escherichia coli, Klebsiella pneumoniae, Bacillus subtilis,* and *Streptococcus faecalis,* equally effective or superior to the control erythromycin (Rani et al. 2010).

Fishbone fern, also called tuber sword and ladder fern, (*Nephrolepis cordifolia*) is known in eastern Asia as *nechii*. The rhizome extract was used as a traditional medicine in Asia and French Polynesia. Approximately 10–15 ml of the rhizome extract was administered once during the menstrual period to induce permanent sterility (Dhiman 1998; Nicole 2006).

Nephrolepis cordifolia is also known as a phytostabilizer of heavy metals like copper, lead, zinc, and nickel. The fronds, when hydro-distilled, yield an essential oil found to contain β-ionone (8%), eugenol (7.2%), and anethol (4.6%) as main compounds (El-Tantawy et al. 2016). A paste made from the fronds is applied to bleeding wounds and used internally to help blood coagulation. The ferns contain antibacterial and antifungal compounds.

The fresh rhizomes are used to treat ulcers, and a tea made by simmering the rhizomes in brine water is consumed to soothe indigestion. In the Philippines, a decoction of the fronds is used for coughs (Quisumbing 1951). The fronds are also harvested by the floral industry for use as foliage in vases. Putrescine delays the senescence significantly, giving a long vase life. I often joke that the difference between a vase and a váse is about two hundred dollars.

This fern has become somewhat invasive in Southern Florida, crowding out native plants. As the name suggests, the presence of tubers is one of the main differences compared to the Boston fern.

The Boston fern (*Nephrolepis exaltata*) is a popular houseplant. It can remove toluene, xylene, and formaldehyde from the air and also acts as a natural humidifier to combat winter dryness. This beautiful fern is perfectly safe to have around children and companion animals.

It is hard to believe that toluene has not yet been classified as a carcinogen. especially since long-term exposure has been found to cause central nervous system depression, tiredness, difficulty sleeping, numbness in hands and feet, female reproductive disruption, and pregnancy loss. There is no antidote.

Xylene has also not yet been classified as carcinogenic by the International Agency for Research on Cancer (IARC) or the EPA. It is, however, neurotoxic and has been replaced in many solvent and industrial products by biodegradable PolyChem 36. Exposure to xylene can lead to symptoms such as headache, dizziness, fatigue, tremors, as well as cardiovascular, respiratory, and kidney complications. What does it take for the EPA to recognize neurotoxins as carcinogens?

Formaldehyde released from adhesives, wall coverings, rubber, water-based paints, cosmetics, and glued wood-based products like new home flooring and cupboards are absorbed by Boston ferns.

A double-blind study compared the use of a fern mask versus a regular mask in a control group. Thirty workers in a textile factory were divided into groups and observed for eight weeks. Pulmonary tests conducted before and after found that sinonasal IgA levels and pulmonary function were significantly improved in the fern mask group (Prasetyo et al. 2019).

Cytotoxicity against two prostate cancer cell lines was noted in work by Bobach et al. (2014) and water extracts combined with zinc oxide nanoparticles exhibited cytotoxicity against A549 (lung) cancer cell lines and as well as antiplatelet activity (Aboul-Soud et al. 2023).

Boston fern is known in India as fish bone fern, and its rhizome extract is used in menstrual disorders and as a birth aid during parturition (Panda et al. 2011).

The fronds, when hydro-distilled, yield an essential oil containing 2,4-hexadien-1-ol (16.1%), nonanal (14.4%), β-ionone (6.7%), and thymol (2.7%) as main constituents. The oil exhibited antimicrobial activity and cytotoxicity in MCF-7 (breast), HCT-116 (colon), and A549 (lung) cancer cell lines (El-Tantawy et al. 2016).

Fishtail fern (*Nephrolepis falcata*) is tropical, growing fronds up to two meters in length. Its common name refers to its beastly and invasive nature, escaping cultivation in Hawaii and Southern Florida.

In the horticultural trades, it is often mistaken for *Nephrolepis biserrata*.

The stems of the scaly sword fern (*Nephrolepis hirsutula*) are subjected to retting, and although originally white, they turn light brown and are then used to produce hats, mats, and baskets.

Pterosin A is found in scurfy, or Asian, sword fern (*Nephrolepis multiflora*). The compound protects pancreatic β cells, enhances glucose uptake efficiency, prevents cell death, and reduces ROS production (Chen et al. 2015). This compound also exhibits antidiabetic activity in a mouse model by significantly reversing increased blood serum insulin and insulin resistance in mice, while enhancing glucose uptake in cultured human muscle cells (Hsu et al. 2013).

Kimberly queen fern (*Nephrolepis obliterata*) also effectively removes formaldehyde as an indoor air pollutant. A study by Teiri et al. (2018) found that the fern efficiently removed formaldehyde levels by 90–100% over long-term exposure.

NOTHOLAENA

Cloak Fern   Ecklon's Lip Fern   Parry's Lip Fern

Notholaena, commonly referred to as cloak ferns, derives from the Greek νόθο(ς) and χλαῖνα, meaning "cloak." The genus contains between forty and one hundred and eight species, suggesting further taxonomic work.

Notholaena affinis is known for its ability to hyperaccumulate arsenic in its fronds.

Ecklon's lip fern (*Notholaena eckloniana* syn. *Hemionitis eckloniana* syn. *Cheilanthes eckloniana*) is on the Red List of Threatened Species in South Africa. In former times, the dried fronds were smoked to treat head colds (Watt and Breyer-Brandwijk 1962). The species name is in honor of Christian Friedrich Ecklon (1795–1868), a Danish pharmacist and collector of botanical species. Over his lifetime he named nearly two thousand different genera or species.

Fendler's false cloak fern (*Notholaena fendleri* syn. *Argyrochosma fendleri* syn. *Pellaea fendleri*) is found from Southern Wyoming to Sonora, Mexico. The Tewa people made a paste of the fern and applied it to cold sores (herpes simplex 1) on the lips (Moerman 1986).

This fern produces a white farinose exudate on the underside of its fronds, composed of waxy compounds and novel flavanones, including isosakuranetin (17%) monomethyl ether, hesperetin, sakuranetin, acacetin, velutin, pillion, quercetin 3,7-dimethyl ether of eriodictyol, and pachypodol.

Isosakuranetin, eriodictyol, and hesperetin are flavanones usually found in citrus fruit. Isosakuranetin exhibits inhibition of neuropathic pain in a rat model (Jia et al. 2017). Velutin protects against cartilage degradation and subchondral bone loss in a mouse model by inhibiting p38 signaling pathways, suggesting potential benefits in the treatment of osteoarthritis (Wang et al. 2022a). Both velutin and sakuranetin exhibit inhibition of drug-resistant hepatitis B virus (Ahmed et al. 2023). Pachypodol has been shown to inhibit the growth of CaCo2 colon cancer cell lines (Ali et al. 2008).

In Peru, the fern *cuti cuti* (*Notholaena nivea*) is widely used in traditional medicine. Early references suggest it was known as *doradilla* (Tryon 1959). The fronds contain bibenzyl derivatives that exhibit antioxidant activity and inhibit xanthine oxidase activity, suggestive of benefits in treating gout (Cioffi et al. 2011).

Most ferns require a moist environment, but Parry's lip fern (*Notholaena parryi*) found in the desert of Western Colorado, is an exception. Its adaptation to climate, light, and moisture was recorded by Nobel (1978).

Star cloak fern (*Notholaena standleyi*) thrives in the deserts of Mexico and in the Southwestern United States. The species is named after Paul C. Standley, the assistant curator of the U.S. National Herbarium, who was a student of plants in the Southwestern states.

The Seri or Comcacc people of the Sonoran Desert made a tea of the fronds to promote fertility and would carry a small bag of the fern to promote good luck.

Notholaenic acid found in this fern exhibits activity against herpes simplex 1 virus (Rinehart et al. 1990).

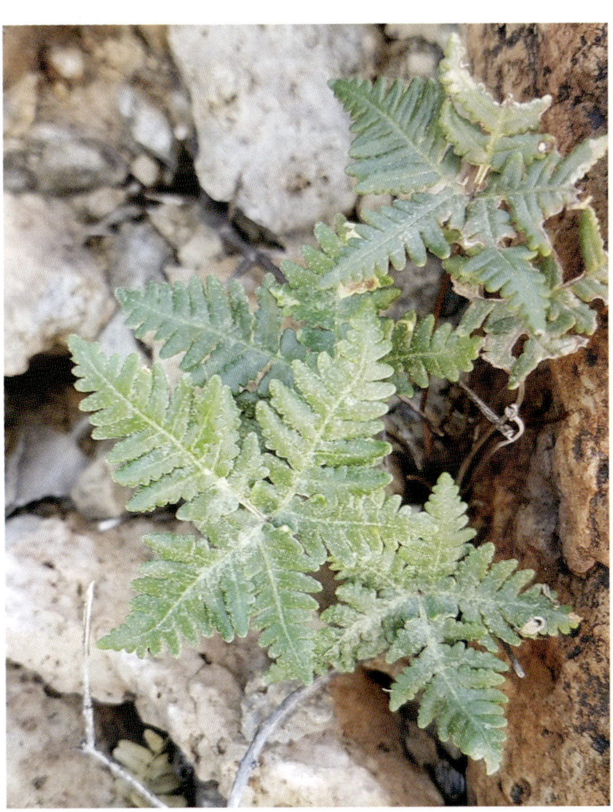

Notholaena standleyi
(Star Cloak Fern)
Photo by Alan Rockefeller

A flavonoid, 2,3-trans-5, 2'-dihydroxy-7,8-dimethoxy-dihydroflavonol-3-O-acetate, and its 2,3-cis diastereoisomer were isolated from the farinose coating on the lower surface of sulphur cloak fern (*Notholaena sulphurea*) fronds. It exhibits a yellow frond exudate, suggesting the origin of the species' name.

NOTHOPERANEMA

Lace Fern

Nothoperanema hendersonii syn. *Dryopteris hendersonii* exhibits significant antioxidant potential (Ding et al. 2008).

OLEANDRA

Strap Ferns

The *Oleandra* genus contains about fifteen species. The stipes of the snake strap fern (*Oleandra colubrina* var. *nitida* syn. *O. neriiformis*) were traditionally used as emmenagogues (May 1978). The rhizomes were used for bites (Brown 1951; Quisumbing 1951).

ONOCLEA

Sensitive Fern

The genus name is from the Greek *onos*, meaning "vessel," and *kleio*, meaning "to close," referring to the in-rolled pinnule margins.

In some parts of the world, the sensitive fern (*Onoclea sensibilis*) is considered a noxious weed. Unlike other "sensitive" plants, this fern does not contract when touched. The common name refers to the deciduous fern reacting quickly to the least amount of frost, turning it instantly from green to brown. It is usually found in marshes, swamps, and wet woodlands.

Sensitive fern (*Onoclea sensibilis*) was used by Iroquois and Ojibwa healers to treat infections, blood disorders involving cold, and to restore normal menstruation and reduce pain after childbirth. It was poulticed or decocted and applied to skin sores, mastitis, and arthritic pain. A tea was prepared for intestinal issues, and a fermented decoction was taken before meals and at bedtime to "make blood" (Moerman 1986). The Iroquois cooked the fern as a vegetable and the fronds were crushed and applied to deep wounds (Moerman 2010).

The fern extract disturbs proliferation and migration of smooth muscle cells (SMC) instigated by inflammatory macrophages in close proximity. This suggests potential in preventing atherosclerosis, which involves SMC proliferation, migration, and fibrogenic activation within blood vessels (Kang et al. 2011).

ONYCHIUM

Carrot Fern

Onychium contiguum syn. *O. lucidum* is a common fern in the Himalayas and other regions. It is often found in pastures where grazing cattle are susceptible to bovine urinary bladder cancer.

Long-term exposure to this fern in animal experiments has been linked to ileum, bladder, and mammary gland tumors. The fern's toxins increase oxidative stress and harmful lipid peroxidation in the bladders of guinea pigs.

However, the Indigenous people in the Philippines rubbed the frond juice into their hair to prevent hair loss (Quisumbing 1951).

On the other hand, three phenolic compounds isolated from Japanese claw or carrot fern (*Onychium japonicum*) fronds exhibit significant multidrug resistance reversal effects on human breast (MCF-7/ADR) and hepatic (Bel-7402/5-Fu) cancer cell lines (Li et al. 2011b). The fern extracts show more than 50% inhibition against liver toxicity induced by carbon tetrachloride and D-galactosamine (Yang et al. 1987).

The compound onychin, found in this fern, inhibits proliferation of vascular smooth muscle cells by blocking the G1 phase cell cycle. This occurs by decreasing the tyrosine phosphorylation of ERK1/2, and through the expression of cyclin D1 and cyclin E, subsequently inhibiting Rb phosphorylation (Yang et al. 2005). Excessive proliferation of vascular smooth muscle, which leads to remodeling, plays a role in vascular disorders such as restenosis, atherosclerosis, and pulmonary hypertension. After injury to arteries, platelets release platelet-derived growth factor, which can penetrate the vascular wall. Multisystem smooth muscle dysfunction syndrome is a serious genetic disease.

Onychin treatment exhibits a protective effect on ECV304 endothelial cells, shielding them from hydrogen peroxide-induced apoptosis. It also attenuates hydrogen peroxide-induced phosphorylation of P38MAPK, increases phosphorylation of ERK1/2, and decreases the activation of caspase-3 (Tuo et al. 2004).

Onitin, a compound in *Onychium siliculosum* syn. *Lomaria aurea*, also acts as a smooth muscle relaxant (Ho et al. 1985). The compound exhibits hepatoprotective activity against tacrine-induced cytotoxicity in human liver-derived HepG2 cells, similar to the compound silybin derived from milk thistle seeds. Onitin also shows free radical scavenging/antioxidant activity (Oh et al. 2004).

OPHIOGLOSSUM

Adder's-tongue Ferns Ribbon Fern

Geographic Range: China, Eastern United States, Europe, India, Madagascar, Malaysia, Philippines, South Africa, Western Himalayas

Habitat: epiphytic, forests, grasslands, tropical regions

Practical Uses: antifungal against crop diseases

Medicinal Applications: anti-inflammatory, antibacterial, antiviral, blood tonic, burns, cancer, heart conditions, diuretic, emetic, hiccups, internal bleeding, ulcers, scrofula, snakebites, sore throat, wounds

Warning: Southern adder's-tongue fern is considered emetic and should be used with caution. It may cause vomiting when consumed in certain doses, particularly in sensitive individuals.

The genus *Ophioglossum* is composed of around fifty species. The name derives from the Greek *ophios*, meaning "serpent," and *glossa*, meaning "tongue," hence "snake tongue." They are also called adder's-tongue, referring to the spore-bearing stipe, which resembles a bifurcated tongue.

Grieve (1931) notes that in England, a vulnerary preparation known as Green Oil of Charity was a remedy for wounds. He writes, "The older herbalists called it 'a fine cooling herb.' The expressed juice of the leaves drunk either alone, or with distilled water of Horse Tail, used much to be employed by country people for internal wounds and bruises, vomiting or bleeding at the mouth or nose. The distilled water was also considered good for sore eyes."

Slender adder's-tongue fern (*Ophioglossum capense* syn. *O. polyphyllum*) rhizomes were decocted and applied to boils by the Sotho people of South Africa (Watt and Breyer-Brandwijk 1962).

Adder's-tongue fern (*Ophioglossum peduncolosum* syn. *O. costatum*) contains homoflavonoid glucosides including pedunculosumosides A–G.

Homoflavonoids are distinctly different from other flavonoids and warrant further research.

ADDERS TONGUE FERN ESSENCE

This essence of *Ophioglossum petiolatum* facilitates inner healing, peace, and stillness at the soul level and calls in one's personal guardian and protector spirits from the upper heavens—the place of true wishes, hopes, possibilities, and dreams. It anchors stellar light from the upper heavens into the seventh layer of the aura. Find as First Light Flower Essence of New Zealand No. 135 Adders Tongue.

Pedunculosumosides A and C exhibit modest activity in blocking HBsAg secretion, with IC_{50} values of 238 and 70.5 μM, respectively (Wan et al. 2011). This suggests potential benefits in human hepatitis B virus liver infections. The presence of HBsAg in blood suggests that a person is infectious. This infection is a serious health issue that can lead to chronic infection, cirrhosis, and liver cancer.

A lectin from the root extract shows antifungal activity against southern blight (*Sclerotium rolfsii*), which affects hundreds of vegetables, and fusarium head blight (*Fusarium graminearum*), which causes serious damage to cereal crops (He et al. 2011).

The fern possesses the highest number of chromosomes of any known organism in the biological world (Patel and Reddy 2018).

Ribbon fern (*Ophioglossum pendulum* syn. *Ophioderma pendulum*) is epiphytic with long pendant fronds up to 4.5 meters in length. In Malaysia, it is called *daun rambu*. Hawaiian newborns were given the spores at birth to help with the first bowel movement, known as meconium, which is generally passed within the first few hours or days and is usually dark green, thick, and sticky (Fosberg 1942).

The fern contains the insecticidal protein IPDO79Ea, which is active against the corn rootworm *Dibrotica virgifera virgifera*, a serious economic pest recently introduced to Europe. It is estimated to cause over $1 billion in corn yield losses and control costs annually in the United States. IPD079Ea will soon likely find its way into GMO corn (Carlson et al. 2022).

Longstem adder's-tongue fern (*Ophioglossum petiolatum*) contains several homoflavonoids, including ophioglonin, quercetin, luteolin, kaempferol, and quercetin 3-O-methyl ether. Ophioglonin and 3-O-methyl ether exhibit slight activity against herpes B virus surface antigen at 25 μM (Lin et al. 2005).

Ophioglonin also exhibits estrogenic activity. However, the compound was unable to stimulate the proliferation of breast and endometrial cancer cells. Instead, it exhibited substantial estrogen receptor α-mediated activation of gene expression. This suggests ophioglonin's potential as a cancer chemopreventive agent (Polasek et al. 2013).

Netted adder's-tongue fern (*Ophioglossum reticulatum* syn. *O. ovatum*) rhizomes were traditionally decocted and taken for lung and heart conditions. When dried and powdered, it was applied to sores, burns, and wounds. In the Philippines, the fern is considered anti-inflammatory, and the fronds are decocted and applied to wounds. In India, the fronds are made into a paste and applied to the forehead for headaches (Singh et al. 1989).

After bracken fern (*Pteridium aquilinum*), the most common edible fern in sub-Saharan Africa is *Ophioglossum reticulatum* (Maroyi 2014). Commonly known as *Brahmi* fern or *Van palak* in India, the fresh fronds are boiled with rice and taken for up to three weeks for menstrual issues (Rout et al. 2009). The whole fern has been juiced and used for uterine hemorrhage or leucorrhea (Singh and Upadhyay 2012), and it has been given as a tonic to women after childbirth to help them recover their strength (Singh 1999).

Chan-choor (*Ophioglossum reticulatum* syn. *O. reticulatum*) rhizomes, from the Western Himalayas, are used to treat wounds (Khoja et al. 2022). The frond juice was used as a skin emollient in Madagascar (Uphof 1968).

Thermal adder's-tongue fern (*Ophioglossum thermale*) is one of the original species in the TCM formula *yizhi jian*. Also known as *Ophioglossum vulgatum* var. *thermale*, the fern itself is known in TCM as *xia ye ping er xiao cao*.

Thermalic acids A and B, found in this fern, exhibit antibacterial activity against *Staphylococcus aureus*, *Bacillus subtilis*, and *Escherichia coli* (Dong et al. 2016).

Various extracts exhibit both antioxidant and anti-inflammatory activity, with the antioxidant activity proving more potent than green tea extract (Zhang et al. 2012b).

Southern adder's-tongue (*Ophioglossum vulgatum*) is rare in Europe but found throughout most of Eastern United States towards Texas and in isolated in parts of Arizona.

A tea made from the fronds was given in traditional medicine for internal bleeding, as well as vomiting with blood. In temperate Asia, the fronds were poulticed and applied to scrofulous ulcers, with infusions taken internally at the same time.

Ophioglossum vulgatum has been traditionally used as an ointment for wounds and burns.

John Gerard wrote, "Ophioglosson, or Lingua serpentis (called in English Adder's-Tongue of some, Adder's-Grass, though unproperly) riseth forth of the ground, having one leaf and no more, fat or oleous in substance, of a finger long, and very like the young and tender leaves of Marigolds . . ." and later notes "on the end whereth doth grow a long small tongue not unlike the tongue of a serpent, whereof it took the name." When made into a green oil, this fern was considered comparable to oil of Saint John's wort.

William Coles (1657) wrote in *Adam in Eden*, "This plant is called adder's tongue because out of every leaf it sendith forth a kind of pestal like an adder's tongue, it cureth the biting of serpents."

Culpeper, the renowned herbalist, placed the fern under the dominion of the moon and cancer,

> Therefore if the weakness of the retentive faculty be caused by an evil influence of Saturn in any part of the body governed by the Moon, or under the dominion of Cancer, this herb cures it by sympathy. . . . It is temperate in respect of heat, but dry in the second degree. The juice of the leaves, drank with distilled water of horse tail, is a singular remedy for all manner of wounds in the breasts, bowels, or other parts of the body. . . . The said juice given in the distilled water of oaken buds, is very good for women who have their usual courses, or the whites flowing down too abundantly.

The Irish herbalist John K'Eogh suggested an oil or unguent prepared from adder's-tongue be used for hot tumors and St. Anthony's fire, a condition associated with consumption of ergot-contaminated rye.

Maud Grieve, in her herbal writings, notes that the Green Oil of Charity wound remedy was used in the popular adder's spear ointment for curing snakebites.

A paste of the rhizomes has been used externally for wounds, and an infusion taken internally as a vulnerary or to treat bleeding from the nose and mouth. A decoction has also been used to treat heart problems (Islam 1983).

In Oxfordshire, a tea made from the fronds was taken as a spring tonic. In India, the rhizomes were boiled in fat for wounds and to reduce inflammation.

In China, the whole fern is considered a general tonic (Roi 1955). The fern is emetic and used for scrofula, dropsy, vomiting, and hiccups. The fresh fronds are poulticed for obstinate ulcers (Uphof 1968).

American Eclectic physicians boiled the whole fern in milk, and it was taken internally for scrofulous affections, as well as a poultice of the fern applied to same region. They deemed the fern to possess astringent, tonic, and diuretic properties, and relieving dropsy, diarrhea, and sore throat.

An extract from the frond was assessed in vitro on keratinocytes, and showed increased wound closure, comparable to the platelet lysate used in clinical settings. This effect appears to work through a Ca(2+)-dependent, nongenomic pathway by activating ERK1/2 MAP kinase, suggesting a novel ointment for skin tissue repair and regeneration (Clericuzio et al. 2014).

OREOPTERIS

Lemon-scented Mountain Fern

The lemon-scented mountain fern (*Oreopteris limbosperma*) contains a variety of volatile compounds, including (E)-nerolidol, α-terpineol, beta-caryophyllene, and minor amounts of linalool, pinenes, limonene, and γ-terpinen-7-al. The fern also contains a large number of carotenoid-type derivatives (Fons et al. 2010).

OSMUNDA

Buckhorn Brake
Cinnamon Fern
Interrupted Fern
Royal Ferns

Geographic Range: Eastern Asia, Eastern United States, Europe, Florida, Galicia, India, North America, Northern Spain

Habitat: damp woods, temperate regions, tropical regions

Practical Uses: orchid potting material, horticultural use, wine

Medicinal Applications: abortifacient, antioxidant, arthritis, birth control, bones, respiratory system, diarrhea, dysentery treatment, emollient, galactagogue, infertility treatment, jaundice, joint pain, kidney conditions, lumbago, menstrual problems, musculoskeletal issues, osteoporosis, rheumatism, sciatica, skin, snakebites, splenetic disease, childbirth, wounds

Warning: The fern should not be consumed by women of childbearing age or during pregnancy as it is considered an

abortifacient. It may cause the fetus to stick to the womb or prevent the womb from distending during birth.

The genus name may refer to Osmunder the Waterman, the Anglo-Saxon equivalent of the Norse god Thor. This alludes to the large size and strength of the fern. Some authors suggest that Osmunda is a southern version of the Celtic goddess who was Thor's queen. The fern was believed to inspire prophetic dreams and symbolized reverie (Powell 1979).

A legend tells of a ferryman known as Osmunder who worked on Loch Tyne. One evening after work, he and his family were startled by an invasion of Danes. Osmunder ferried his wife and daughter to a small island in the loch and hid them among the royal fern fronds. He then returned to his ferry landing and was spared his life by the Danes by transporting them across the loch. After they moved on, he went back and returned his family to their cottage. Henceforth, the royal ferns were known as *Osmunda*. It was believed that biting the first frond of the year would prevent toothache for the entire year.

Grieve (1931) suggests that *osmund* is derived from the Saxon word for "domestic peace," from *os* for "house," and *mund* for "peace." Other authors suggest it derives from *os*, meaning "bone," and *mundare*, meaning "to cleanse." To me, this makes the most sense. Frans Vermeulen noted that a conserve of the root was once used to treat rickets.

Both cinnamon fern and royal fern have root fibers used in horticulture. The fiddleheads of cinnamon fern are eaten as a cooked vegetable. The Abnaki tribe ate the white base raw, while the Menominee simmered the frond tips to remove ants before adding them to soup stock thickened with flour (Moerman 2010).

The name *cinnamon fern* refers to the rust-colored, spore-bearing fertile fronds, not the scent.

Cinnamon fern (*Osmunda cinnamomea* syn. *Osmundastrum cinnamomeum*) was a traditional remedy used by the Iroquois and other Indigenous tribes. It was externally applied for rheumatism, and internally used for arthritic joint pain. The Iroquois also used root decoctions for treating colds in the kidneys. The Seminole of Florida used the fern for chronically ill babies and used the hot steam to bathe the body for treating "insanity." Other uses include treating infertility in women, as a galactagogue to increase breast milk, and for caked breasts, which are hardened nodules caused by stagnation of dilated veins and lactation ducts. The fern was also used for snakebite.

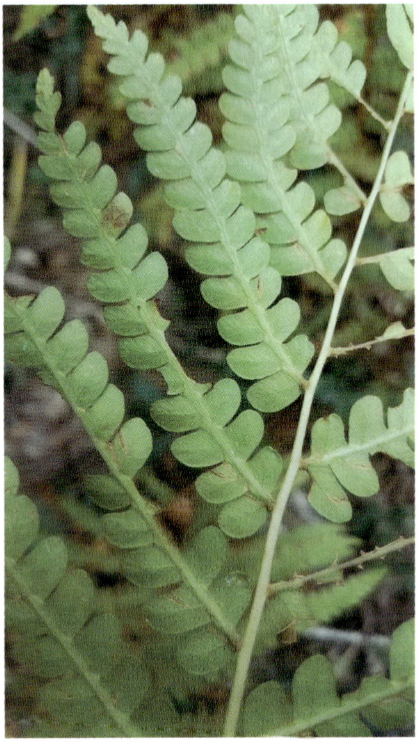

Osmunda cinnamomea
(Cinnamon Fern)
Photo by Alan Rockefeller

Infusions of the fronds were given to children suffering from convulsions due to intestinal parasites. The Cherokee cooked the young fronds as a spring tonic and chewed the rhizome to create a spit poultice for wounds. The Iroquois also decocted the rhizomes for colds, headaches, malaise, rheumatism, and painful joints (Moerman 1986).

The fiddlehead of the fern is crisp and tender and is eaten like asparagus in the Southeastern United States (Angier 1972; Core 1967; Fernald and Kinsey 1974). At one time, the old roots of the fern were harvested for use in orchid potting mixtures.

The related interrupted fern (*Osmunda claytoniana* syn. *Claytosmunda claytoniana*) was traditionally used by the Iroquois to treat weak blood and gonorrhea (Moerman 1986).

The species is named in honor of John Clayton (1694–1773), an early American botanist. He was an Anglican minister in the colony of Virginia. The flower spring beauty (*Claytonia virginica*) was also named in his honor, reflecting his contributions to botanical collections and writings. The fern is found in East to East-Central North America, as well as in Eastern Asia, along with other ferns like the ostrich, cinnamon, and sensitive ferns.

What exactly is the common name about? It describes the gap in the middle of the frond blade, left by the fertile parts as they fall off.

William Cullina (2008), in his beautiful book on ferns, moss, and grasses, notes the similarity of today's ferns and a 230-million-year-old fossil. No changes in all those years suggests a very successful lifestyle.

Recent research found that an extract from the fern acts as an active efflux pump inhibitor against *Staphylococcus aureus*, with an IC_{50} value for efflux inhibition of 19 ppm (Brown et al. 2021).

The Japanese or Asian royal fern (*Osmunda japonica*) is believed to be the original herb used in TCM under the name guan zhong (cyrtomium rhizome) (Wang et al. 2012). In Japan, it is known as *zenmai*.

Methanol extracts of the aerial parts of TCM's *osmundae rhizoma* (*Osmunda japonica*) exhibit activity against herpes simplex viruses 1 and 2 (Woo et al. 1997).

Thirty-three compounds were isolated from the rhizomes by Bowen et al. (2020).

One *ent*-kaurene terpenoid exhibited potent cytotoxicity against HeLa (human epithelial/cervical), and HepG2 (liver) cancer cell lines. A flavonoid from the rhizome showed strong antioxidant activity. The rhizome extract also exhibits antioxidant and anti-inflammatory activity (Dion et al. 2015).

Several phenolic compounds in the rhizome possess immunomodulatory activity (Zhu et al. 2013b).

An extract of the fern decreased pro-inflammatory cytokines IL-6 and IL-8 in periodontal disease. Activated NF-κB was modulated with the fern extract in both *Fusobacterium nucleatum* and *Porphyromonas gingivalis*, which are known to cause gingival inflammation (Seong et al. 2020).

Ferns growing within a 30-kilometer radius of the now disabled Fukushima Daiichi Nuclear Power Plant contain high levels of radiocesium, and residents nearby are advised to avoid eating the popular vegetable. The destroyed nuclear plant has contaminated vast regions of the Pacific Ocean, with regulatory bodies allowing the release of more stored radioactive water.

Royal fern or buckhorn brake (*Osmunda regalis*) has been traditionally used for menstrual problems, intestinal parasites, and as an anticancer remedy. This fern is widespread in temperate, damp woods. There are two varieties: the European and Asian variety *Osmunda regalis* var. *regalis*; and the (North) American gray royal fern (*Osmunda regalis* var. *spectabilis*). The species name *regalis* means "regal" or "royal." In Europe, the fern is also known

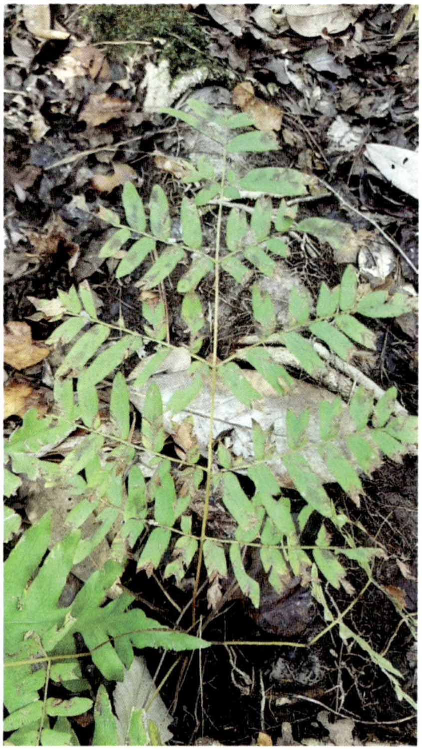

Osmunda regalis var. *spectabilis*
(North American Gray Royal Fern)
Photo by Alan Rockefeller

as bog onion. The name "buckhorn" reflects the horn shape of the main root, which is about two inches long. The roots were once used as a growing medium for orchids.

The English herbalist Gerard referred to it as water fern.

> It is called in Latin *Osmunda*: it is more truly named *Filix palustris*, or *aquatilis*: some term it by the name of *Filicastrum*: most of the alchemists call it *Lunaria maior: Valerius Cordus* nameth it *Filix latifolia*: it is named in High Dutch, *Grosz Farn*: in Low Dutch, *Groot Varen*, *Wilt Varen*: in English, Water-Fern, Osmund the Waterman: of some Saint Christopher's Herb, and Osmund.

Gerard described the rhizome as hot and dry and is used to "dissolve cluttered blood remaining in any inward part of the body, and that it also can expel or drive it out by the wound." Gerard probably derived his insights from earlier works by Dodonaeus and other herbalists of the time.

Culpeper wrote, "This has all the virtues mentioned in the former Ferns, and is much more effectual than they, both for inward and outward griefs, and is singularly good in wounds, bruises or the like: the decoction to be drunk or boiled into an ointment of oil, as a balsam or balm, and so it is singularly good against bruises and bones broken or out of joint, and gives much ease to the cholic and splenetic diseases: as also for ruptures and burstings" (Grieve (1931), quoted from the original text of Culpeper).

Grieve (1931) noted a decoction of the root is good for jaundice, and a conserve of the root was used for rickets, a bone disease in children that is associated with prolonged vitamin D deficiency. A conserve of the rhizome was also used to treat this bone condition. In Galway, Ireland, the fern was used for rheumatism and sciatica.

The rhizome contains mucilage and is a mildly bitter tonic, useful for dysentery, diarrhea, and intestinal complaints. It was often made into syrups, with caraway seeds, Dutch gin, and sugar.

Matthew Wood (2021), noted American herbalist, has also shared his insights on this medicinal fern, noting no appreciable difference between new-world and old-world royal ferns.

> Osmunda has an earthen, mucilaginous, and astringent taste. Culpeper called it an herb of Saturn because it is drying and hardening. Its constituents correlate with its properties: as an astringent it checks excess fluid losses, as an astringent with earthen salts, it hardens the bones and reinforces the mineral content of the tissues, while the mucilage soothes, nourishes, and softens the mucosa.

Grieve (1931) remarks that "the actual curative virtues of this fern have been said to be due to the salts of lime, potash and other earths which it derives in solution from the bog soil and from the water in which it grows."

Osmunda is an old remedy for the defective bone growth in infancy and the spinal deterioration in old age. "It passes with some almost for a specific in rickets," writes John Quincy (1736). Beal P. Downing (1851), writing from the wild American frontier a hundred years later, calls it the "only and absolute cure for rickets." Finley Ellingwood (1919) recommends it for osteoporosis and subluxations of the spine. Grieve (1931) mentions its common name lumbago brake. I have personally found it excellent for lumbago, and lower back pain, in clinical practice.

As a mucilaginous emollient and astringent, *Osmunda* is beneficial for the skin and mucosa. "Its soothing influence upon mucous surfaces seems to be remarkable," writes Ellingwood (1919)." It is most in esteem for restraining the whites in women, and strengthening the womb," notes Quincy.

His contemporary, Sir John Hill (1740) writes, "a decoction of the fresh roots promotes urine, and opens obstructions of the liver and spleen; it is not much used, but I have known a jaundice cured by it, taken in the beginning." The mucilage makes it of some value in acute and chronic bronchial irritation.

Note: The mucilage can be extracted after several hours in cold water, but I prefer a short extraction to take off the minerals. It tastes like Ent juice from *The Lord of the Rings*. The sweet minerally flavor is incredible.

The fern is known as *antojil* in Spain and is traditionally used to set bones and treat musculoskeletal issues, including bone fractures, osteoporosis, rheumatic, and arthritic pain. The middle part of the rhizome is soaked in white wine before use.

Antojil wine is commercially available in Northern Spain and is consumed daily before breakfast by some men. It is contraindicated for women of childbearing age and during pregnancy, as it is considered an abortifacient. Women who drink the wine report it may cause the fetus to stick to the womb or prevent the womb from distending during birth (Molina et al. 2009). This wine is recommended by biomedical doctors, osteopaths, physical therapists, and traditional healers in Spain for promoting bone regeneration, healing broken bones, and treating unspecified bone disorders.

In Slavic mythology, the sporangia of the fern, known as Perun's flowers, were believed to give the holder magical powers. Early traditions suggested it must be picked on Kupala Night, and later, following the arrival of Christianity, on Easter Eve. Collectors had to stand in a circle drawn around the fern, ignoring the threats and taunts of demons while harvesting the sporangia.

In India, a decoction of the rhizome was traditionally used as an abortifacient. A paste of the leaves mixed with milk curd was used as a method of birth control (Jain 1991).

Indigenous healers in North America used gray royal fern for various medicinal purposes.

Moerman (2004) writes, "Decoction taken by Iroquois women for watery blood. Decoction used when 'girls leak rotten; affected women can't raise children.'" Other uses included decoctions for cold kidneys and infusions in steam baths for treating insanity.

In *King's American Dispensatory* (Felter and Lloyd 1898), the accomplished Eclectic physician Dr. John King notes the fern's abundant mucilage and also the ash derived from the fern with about 50% silica. The mucilage was often mixed with brandy as an external rub for subluxations and back muscle debility. Or the rhizomes were infused and taken internally in a tea sweetened with sugar and herbs such as ginger and cinnamon.

The organic silica content of the fern is noteworthy, as it provides the scaffolding for bone health. I liken it to a modern tower construction, where the silica is the basic structure and calcium fills the gaps. Many post-menopausal women exhibit a deficiency in silica, which can lead to osteoporosis. I want to highlight again the important work by professor Kervran (1972) on biological transmutations.

An ethanol extract of the root was found to inhibit the growth of head and neck carcinoma cell lines HLac78 and FaDu. The extract significantly inhibited the invasion of these cell lines on various extracellular matrix substrates, with a particularly strong effect on laminin. The fern root extract also induced apoptosis in the two cell lines and inhibited tube formation of endothelial cells (Schmidt et al. 2017).

Osmundacetone, a compound found in the fern, protects against neurological (HT22) hippocampal cell death caused by oxidative glutamate toxicity (Trinh et al. 2021). This water-soluble compound is a 5-lipoxygenase inhibitor, with potential anti-dementia effects (Liu et al. 2022b). Osmundacetone also reduces the proliferation of A549 and H460 (non-small cell lung) cancer cell lines (Yang et al. 2022) and strongly binds to xanthine oxidase, a key enzyme in uric acid production, and provides relief for gout (Song et al. 2023). In a rat study, osmundacetone was shown to have a half-life of 5.2 hours, demonstrating its antioxidant activity (Wu et al. 2022). The compound is also found in medicinal mushrooms such as *Phellinus igniarius* and chaga (*Inonotus obliquus*).

Osmunda × ruggii is a sterile hybrid between interrupted fern (*Osmunda claytoniana*) and American royal fern (*Osmunda spectabilis*), found as only one natural population in Craig County, Virginia. A previous report of population in Fairfield County, Conneticut, has not been relocated and likely extirpated.

PARAHEMIONITIS

Rabbit Ear Fern

Rabbit ear fern (*Parahemionitis cordata*) is known in India as *chakuliya*. Juice of the whole fern was consumed as a tea to treat dysmenorrhea (Benjamin and Manickam 2007).

PARATHELYPTERIS

Ladder-shape Gland Fern   Tall Marsh Fern

A novel endophyte isolated from the rhizome of Korean maiden fern (*Parathelypteris beddomei*) possesses antifungal properties (Zhao et al. 2017a).

Parathelypterside, a stibenoid compound extracted from ladder-shape gland fern (*Parathelypteris glanduligera* syn. *Thelypteris glanduligera*), possesses antioxidant and anti-inflammatory properties.

This compound significantly alleviated neurotoxicity in the hippocampus of mice, induced by d-galactose, potentially due to the activation of cAMP-response element-binding protein. This suggests the compound may have potential in treating neurodegenerative diseases (Fu et al. 2010b).

Tall marsh fern (*Parathelypteris nipponica*) exhibits antioxidant, anti-inflammatory, and hepatic protective activities against liver injury in a mouse model (Fu et al. 2010a).

PELLAEA

Bird Rock Brake Fern
Button Fern
Cliff Brakes (Cliffbrakes)
Coffee Fern
Hard Fern
Resurrection Fern
Sickle Fern

Geographic Range: Alberta (Canada), Australia, California (U.S.), Guatemala, Limpopo (South Africa), New Zealand, Northern Quebec, South Africa, United States

Habitat: dry limestone rocks, arid environments

Practical Uses: desiccation protection, house plant, phytoremediation (arsenic)

Medicinal Applications: blood, diarrhea, fever, internal injuries, kidneys, lungs, snakebites, sunstroke

The genus name derives from the Greek *pellos*, meaning "dark," in reference to the dark brown stipes characteristic of this genus. Members of this genus are commonly known as cliff brakes.

Coffee or cliff brake fern (*Pellaea andromedifolia*) is a good example of a desiccation-tolerant organism, allowing it to survive when nearly completely dehydrated in a dormant state. When hydrated, sucrose levels in the rhizome

Pellaea andromedifolia (Coffee Fern)
Photo by Alan Rockefeller

and stele (the core of stem) drop as starch levels rise, suggesting that accumulated sucrose acts as a desiccation protectant (Holmlund et al. 2020).

Purple cliff brake fern (*Pellaea atropurpurea*) is found across most of Eastern and South-central United States, and from Northern Quebec south to Guatemala.

The Indigenous Mahuna infused the fern to flush the kidneys or to tone and thin the blood. Infusions were also taken to prevent or treat sunstroke (Jacobs and Burlage 1958; Romero 1954).

Hard fern (*Pellaea calomelanos*) grows in arid environments and has a history of use as a traditional medicine in Limpopo province, South Africa. Unlike many other medicinal plants, this fern is used for treating lung infections through the smoke inhalation of smoldering dry fronds (Braithwaite et al. 2008).

An endophyte, *Pantoea ananatis*, isolated from this fern, was genetically engineered with *Escherichia coli* as an insecticidal toxin complex, offering an alternative to *Bacillus thuringiensis* (Bt), widely used in commercial agriculture (Malomane et al. 2023).

Sickle fern (*Pellaea falcata*) is a popular tropical evergreen house plant.

Gaston's cliff brake fern (*Pellaea gastonyi*) is found in the foothills and dry limestone rocks around Banff, Alberta. The fern is an apogamous tetraploid

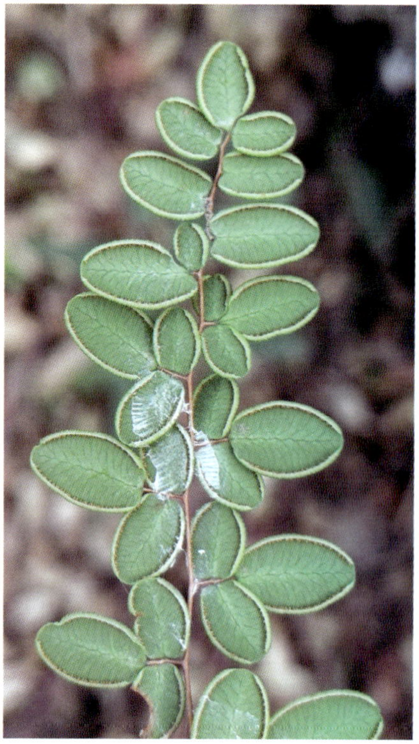

Close-up of *Pellaea andromedifolia* (Coffee Fern)
Photo by Alan Rockefeller

species with purplish black stipes and is considered a hybrid between purple cliff brake and smooth cliff brake. However, the former is an eastern species, so how did it hybridize?

Smooth cliff brake fern (*Pellaea glabella*) is found on dry limestone rock faces. The species name *glabella* means "smooth."

The rhizomes of curled brake fern (*Pellaea involuta*) were a remedy for snakebites and diarrhea in South Africa (Watt and Breyer-Brandwijk 1962).

Bird foot cliff brake fern (*Pellaea mucronata*) was used as a beverage by Diegueño, Liuseño, and Kawaiisu Indigenous people (Lloyd 1964; Moerman 2010). The Costanoan decocted the fern for internal injuries and to cough up "bad blood." They used an infusion of the new sprouts to reduce fevers (Moerman 1986).

California cliff brake fern (*Pellaea mucronata* ssp. *californica*) leaves and stalks were used by the Tubatulabal people for food (Moerman 2010).

Bird rock brake fern (*Pellaea ornithopus*) frond decoctions were used by the Liuseño for medicinal purposes (Moerman 1986).

Button fern (*Pellaea rotundifolia*) hyperaccumulates arsenic, suggesting its potential for phytoremediation. This fern is easily grown indoors, and its species name refers to the distinct, almost round leaves. The fern is native to New Zealand, Australia, and adjacent islands.

Green cliff brake fern (*Pellaea viridis* syn. *Cheilanthes viridis*) grows worldwide on limestone rocks. The species name *viridis* refers to its bright green fronds.

Wright's cliff brake fern (*Pellaea wrightiana*) was first described by Sir Joseph Dalton Hooker in 1858. This fertile allotetraploid fern is the result of hybridization between the diploid species spiny cliff brake (*Pellaea truncata*) and Trans-Pecos cliff brake (*Pellaea ternifolia*).

Research by Windham et al. (2022) suggests that this fern, common across Arizona and New Mexico, represents three polyploids originating from repeated hybridization.

PHEGOPTERIS

Beech Ferns

The genus name *Phegopteris* derives from the Greek words *phegos*, meaning "oak" or "beech," and *pteris* meaning "fern." The species name *connectilis* means "connected," and refers to the upper pinnae, which fuse to the rachis.

Akolea (*Phegopteris* sp. syn. *Athryium microphyllum*) root was cooked by Indigenous Hawaiians for food (Moerman 2010).

Narrow or long beech fern (*Phegopteris connectilis* syn. *Thelypteris phegopteris*) is native to the northern parts of North America, Europe, and Asia. It grows best on moist, acidic soil and is super hardy, surviving winter temperatures down to -46°C/-50.8°F. The fresh-cut fern contains 7.4% of coumarin, and the volatiles (E)-2-hexenal and (Z)-3-hexenol, which contribute a green odor to absolutes used in perfumes.

Japanese beech fern (*Phegopteris decursive-pinnata* syn. *Thelypteris decursive-pinnata*) is a hardy fern prized by fern gardeners for its ability to tolerate both heat and cold, enduring temperatures as low as -34°C/-29.2°F. The fern along with the perennial plant horsetail (*Equisetum fluviatile*) was screened for bioactive compounds. Protoflavonoids isolated from fern include protoapigenone, protogenkwanone, protoapigenin, 4'-O-β-D-glucopyranosyl protoapigenin, 2'3'-dihydroprotogenkwanone, and 2'3'-dihydro-2'-hydroxyprotoapigenone.

Protoapigenone is present in several ferns, including *Macrothelypteris torresiana*. The compound has demonstrated anti-cancer activity by inducing

DNA damage, apoptosis, and G2/M arrest in H1299 (human lung) cancer cell lines (Chiu et al. 2009).

Research by Pouny et al. (2011) found cytotoxicity against HeLa (cervical) cancer cells for all known compounds, leading to previously unobserved phenotypic changes characterized by the loss of centrosomal γ-tubulin labeling in both interphasic and mitotic cells.

PHLEBODIUM

Bear Paw Fern
Bear's Foot Fern
Blue Star Fern
Cabbage Palm Fern
Golden Polypody
Golden Serpent Fern
Gold Foot Fern
Hare's Foot Fern

Geographic Range: North and South America
Habitat: warmer climates, tropical and subtropical regions
Practical Uses: aquarium plant, ornamental plant, exercise performance enhancer
Medicinal Applications: anti-inflammatory, arthritis, bruises, cancer, coughs, fevers, muscles, neuritis, phototherapy for vitiligo, psoriatic lesions, oxidative stress, reducing pro-inflammatory cytokines, rheumatism

Gold foot or blue star fern (*Phlebodium aureum*) goes by a number of common names including hare's foot fern, cabbage palm fern, golden serpent fern, bear's foot fern, golden polypody fern, and gold foot fern. It was recently reclassified and separated from the *Polypodium* genus. It is common in warmer climates throughout North and South America. I was initially introduced to *Phlebodium aureum* as *calaguala* fern while living in Peru in the early 1980s.

The species name *phlebodium* derives from the Greek *phlebodes*, meaning "full of veins," referring to the internal structure of the rhizome.

The fern has been traditionally used orally (in an unspecified manner) for phototherapy in the treatment of vitiligo (Castillo et al. 2023). Indigenous groups in Mexico used the rhizome to treat coughs and fevers (Uphof 1968; Usher 1971).

Water extracts of the gold foot fern (*Phlebodium aureum*) have been combined with silver nanoparticles to produce a more cost-effective, environmentally friendly, and easily scalable medicine. Colloidal silver and silver topical ointments are known for their infection-preventive properties. Marimuthu et al. (2021) evaluated and confirmed the cytotoxic effects of the synthesized extract.

The fern has been traditionally decocted, cooled, and used as a wash for various skin conditions including atopic dermatitis and psoriasis. Indigenous groups of South America use the fern in various ways. In the Amazon rainforest, the rhizome is boiled for fever and grated fresh for tea to treat whooping cough and kidney problems. The Indigenous Bora of Peru prepare the fronds as a tea for cough, while the Witotos of the Northwestern Amazon rainforest prepare the rhizome for the same condition. Several Indigenous tribes in Peru use the fern for pancreatic concerns in unspecified manners. The Indigenous Creole of Guyana decoct the rhizome and add it to ritual baths of newborns.

Skin cancer accounts for at least 40% of all human malignancies, and fern extracts may be useful adjuncts (Parrado et al. 2016).

The fern is rich in various phenolic compounds, including benzoates, cinnamates, quinic acid, shikimic acid, caffeic acid, ferulic acid, p-coumaric acid, glucuronic acid, malic acid, vanillic acid, and 3 caffeoliquinic acid (chlorogenic acid).

Caffeic acid inhibits ultraviolet-induced peroxide and nitric oxide formation, and ferulic acid absorbs UV photons. There are several commercial products available in Europe and the United States, including Heliocare (Fernblock XP).

An excellent literature review by Segars et al. (2021) covers the fern's benefits in vitiligo, melasma, post-inflammatory hyperpigmentation, polymorphic light eruption, actinic keratosis, malignant melanoma, idiopathic photodermatoses, cutaneous lupus erythematosus, and cutaneous porphyria. Over 120 citations are available on PubMed.

The fern may also benefit other autoimmune conditions, including multiple sclerosis and lupus erythematosus (Breithaupt and Jacob 2012). One study found a reduction of inflammation in difficult-to-treat psoriatic arthritis. It should be noted that numerous human double-blind, placebo-controlled trials for the above conditions involve both oral ingestion and topical application. The authors note that as a dietary supplement, Heliocare has the strongest evidence-based recommendations.

One case report of interest highlighted the attenuation of actinic prurigo eruptions in an eleven-year-old female following supplementation (Stump et al. 2022).

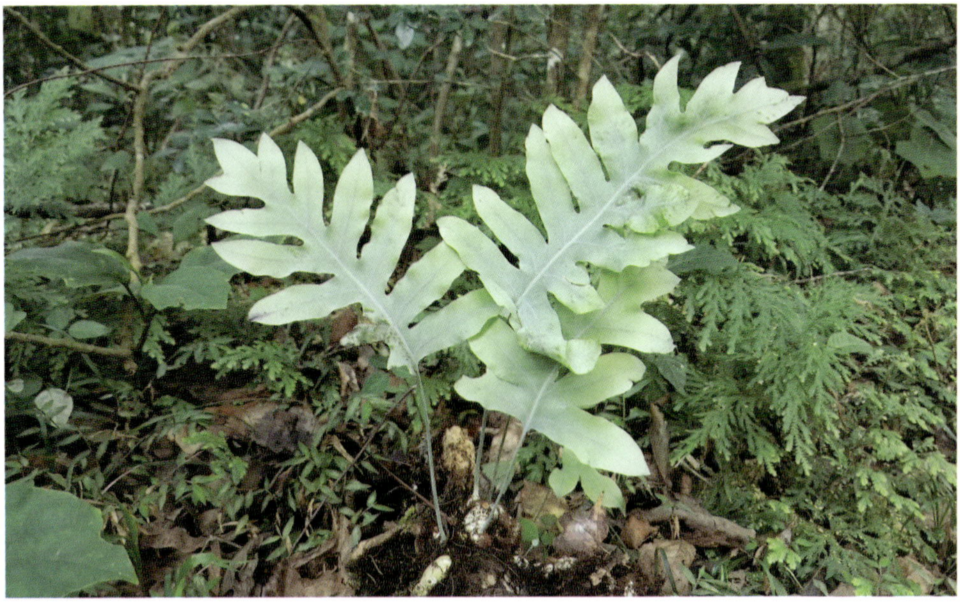

Phlebodium pseudoaureum (False Golden Polypody)
Photo by Alan Rockefeller

Vitiligo, a challenging-to-treat skin depigmentation, was also studied. Forty-four patients enrolled in a randomized, prospective, placebo-controlled trial, with half receiving an oral extract of the fern combined with NB-UVB therapy, and the control group being treated with light therapy and a placebo. Both treatments were given twice weekly for six months. The combined therapy group had a response rate of nearly 48%, compared to 22% in the control group (Pacifico et al. 2021).

A combination of Fernblock XP and sulforaphane (a sulfur-isothiocyanate found in broccoli) was shown to prevent skin aging and serves as a useful adjuvant in treating advanced melanoma (Serini et al. 2020).

A study in 2017 found that an oral extract of the fern reduced the side effects of acute phytotoxicity induced by psoralen-UVA treatment for psoriasis, vitiligo, and fungal skin infections. The study only involved twenty-two patients but all showed a significant numeric reduction of sunburn cells and a decrease in vasodilation (Kohli et al. 2017).

A multi-center, randomized, open-label study with three arms evaluated the efficacy of oral and topical applications for the treatment actinic keratosis. One hundred and thirty-one patients were involved, and the most significant improvement was noted in groups using both oral and topical applications combined (Pellacani et al. 2023).

Concentrated extracts on the market include Difur, Exply-37, Kalawalla, Leucostat, Immunotrax, and Anapsos, and are often more cost-effective than Heliocare.

The fern contains a novel (R)-mandelonitrile lyase. Unlike the compound isolated from members of the rose family, it is not a flavoprotein. Vicianin was identified as the cyanogenic compound in fern. Vicianin hydrolase catalyzes the hydrolysis of vicianin into mandelonitrile (Wajant et al. 1995).

Water extracts of creeping golden polypody (*Phlebodium decumanum*) exhibit two anti-inflammatory pathways in vitro: it decreases TNF production and increases IL-1Ra and sTNFR2, which may neutralize IL-1 and TNF activity, respectively (Punzón et al. 2003). This study validates the traditional use by the Maya of Guatemala and Belize for severe inflammatory issues such as neuritis, rheumatism, arthritis, as well as for coughs, bruises, and tumors. In vitro tests against HL-60 (acute leukemia) and MCF-7 (breast) cancer cells show only moderate cytotoxicity (Gridling et al. 2009).

A double-blind, placebo-controlled trial conducted on thirty-one sedentary males revealed that those receiving the fern extract (as compared to the control) showed significant improvement in performance parameters such as strength and interval training after one month of treatment. The extract modulated the immune system, reducing proinflammatory cytokines and increasing anti-inflammatory cytokines (Gonzalez-Jurado et al. 2011).

A follow-up study on thirty male volleyball players (aged 22–32 years) examined the benefits of the fern extract in one group and the fern extract plus coenzyme Q10 in another. The results showed significantly decreased levels of cortisol, interleukin-6 (IL-6), lactic acid, and ammonium in the group receiving the combination treatment compared to the group receiving the fern extract alone. The authors suggested that the combination of fern extract with coenzyme Q10 not only delayed fatigue and improved athletic performance but also reduced the risk of injuries associated with high-intensity exercise (Verazaluce et al. 2014).

Oral supplementation of the water-soluble fern extract during high-intensity exercise reduces oxidative stress and the inflammatory response, according to a clinical trial on adult humans. This suggests both professional and amateur athletes may be able to avoid muscle damage and other undesirable outcomes through fern extract supplementation (Díaz-Castro et al. 2012).

In a double-blind, multigroup randomized trial, sedentary students took nine doses of 400 mg fern extract capsules every eight hours for three days.

Significant differences were observed in muscle damage variables in the fern extract group compared to the placebo group (Corzo et al. 2014). Intense exercise in sedentary people can increase cardiovascular risk, making such interventions potentially valuable.

Frond water extracts of this fern reduce redness, erythema, and severity of psoriatic lesions, especially when combined with water extracts of *Calendula officinalis* leaves (Das et al. 2019b).

PHYLLITIS

See mentions of *Asplenium scolopendrium* on pages 54, 59–61.

PHYMATOPTERIS

The fern *Phymatopteris hastata* syn. *Selliguea hastata* contains constituents with remarkable antioxidant activity, including juglanin, naringenin, ethyl chlorogenate, and protocatechuic acid.

Juglanin exhibits antioxidant, anti-inflammatory, and anticancer activity, including skin, breast, and lung cancers. It also ameliorates neuroinflammation in an animal model of Parkinson's disease (Zhang and Xu 2018).

Naringenin has been widely studied for numerous health conditions, including Parkinson's disease. This compound has been shown to suppress the proliferation and migration of A2780 and ES-2 (epithelial ovarian) cancer cells lines by inhibiting the PI3K pathway and ameliorating gut microbiota, significantly increasing levels of *Alistipes* and *Lactobacillus* bacteria (Lin et al. 2022).

Ethyl chlorogenate inhibits melanogenesis in α-MSH-stimulated B16 melanoma cells (Akihisa et al. 2013). A flavanol glycoside and its naringin derivative improved glucose consumption in insulin-resistant HepG2 cells and enhanced GLUT4myc translocation in L6myc skeletal muscle cells. This suggests potential antidiabetic benefits from this fern (Ma et al. 2013).

Phymatopteris triloba fronds from the highlands of Malaysia contain flavonoids, hydroxycinnamic acids, and proanthocyanidins. Both frond and rhizome inhibit the growth of gram-positive and gram-negative bacteria. In TCM the fern is known as *san zhi jia liu jue*.

The frond extract tested against *Pseudomonas aeruginosa* showed 2.5-fold higher activity than the control drug ampicillin. It also exhibits significant antioxidant and anti-glucosidase activity (Chai et al. 2013).

The cytotoxic activity against select cancer cell lines was previously reported. Work by Tan et al. (2018) identified six differentially expressed proteins isolated from cancer cells following exposure to the cytotoxic fern extracts. The cancer-related proteins identified include elongation factor1-γ, glyceraldehyde-3-phosphate dehydrogenase, heat shock protein 90-beta, heterogeneous nuclear ribonucleoprotein-A2/B1, truncated nuclear phosphoprotein B23, and tubulin-beta chain. This suggests several possible new avenues of anticancer protein targets.

PITYROGRAMMA

Goldenback Fern Silverback Fern

Silverback fern (*Pityrogramma calomelanos*) has a long history of use due to its astringent, analgesic, antihemorrhagic, antihypertensive, antipyretic, and anthelminthic properties.

I found myself spending time in Trinidad and Tobago back in the early 1970s, where the fern was widely available at herbal markets, but I, as a newbie botanist, had no idea of its medicinal use. The fronds have been a traditional medicine in Trinidad and Tobago for flu, fever, coughs, and hypertension (Wong 1976).

Lans (2006) interviewed thirty people on the traditional uses of plants in the country and found that the fern was also used for kidney problems. Mannan and colleagues (2008) reported that the fern has also been traditionally used for amenorrhea. In the Philippines, the ferns are decocted and used to treat kidney problems (Quisumbing 1951).

Both the ethanol extract and ethyl acetate fraction of the fern are cytotoxic and inhibit the parasite *Leishmania brasiliensis* (Souza et al. 2013a). Extracts also display good activity against *Staphylococcus aureus* when combined with gentamicin, though they did not exhibit increased antifungal activity against three *Candida* species.

Luciano-Montalvo et al. (2013) found that decoctions of the fern inhibit several bacteria, confirming its traditional use in the Caribbean for the treatment of kidney infections associated with stones.

Eleven ferns, in particular silverback fern, were screened for cytotoxic and antitumor potential (Sukumaran and Kuttan 1991). A dihydrochalcone compound isolated from the fern showed activity against Dalton's lymphoma ascites and Ehrlich ascites tumor cells.

Notably, this fern is one of the few known to hyperaccumulate arsenic, with numerous published studies on this characteristic (Remigio et al. 2023).

The goldenback fern (*Pityrogramma triangularis*) stems were used by Indigenous groups of the Pacific Northwest for creating black basket designs. The fronds were chewed by Karok and Minok (Miwok) of California to relieve toothaches or the pain associated with childbirth (Lloyd 1964; May 1978).

PLATYCERIUM

Elkhorn Fern   Staghorn Ferns

Staghorn fern (*Platycerium* spp.) is a popular houseplant that can live for several decades if kept in consistent, shaded light. The common name derives from its antler-like, green, and leathery leaves.

Methanol extracts of elkhorn fern or staghorn fern (*Platycerium bifurcatum*) exhibit antibacterial activity against *Escherichia coli*, *Staphylococcus aureus*, *Klebsiella* spp., and *Salmonella typhi* (Ojo et al. 2007).

Triangle staghorn (*Platycerium stemaria*) extracts possess antioxidant and antimicrobial activity (Ngouana et al. 2021).

STAGHORN FERN ESSENCE

This essence of *Platycerium* spp. grounds, stabilizes, and strengthens the heart, making the essence beneficial before and after open-heart surgery. It helps us to let go of old, long-standing grudges that weaken the heart. It supports the liver and kidneys, and releases sadness, anger, and fear. It also promotes laughter as a healing tool, especially for those who have led an overly serious or arduous spiritual life. Find at Delta Gardens Flower Essences.

PLEOPELTIS

Scaly Polypodies   Weeping Fern

Geographic Range: Argentina, Colombia, Mesoamerica, Mexico, northern South America, Eastern and Southern United States

Habitat: tropical regions, temperate zones, growing on branches

Practical Uses: indoor plant

Medicinal Applications: abortifacient, anti-inflammatory, bleeding, chest pain, coughs, fever, gastrointestinal issues, headaches, kidneys, livers, mouth ulcers, parasites, pertussis (whooping cough), skin ulcers, snakebites, typhoid fever

Warning: Women trying to conceive should avoid consuming *Pleopeltis macrocarpa* due to its potential for causing miscarriage.

The *Pleopeltis* genus is often referred to as the resurrection fern, particularly in Mexico. There are an estimated fifty species worldwide, mostly found in tropical regions and temperate zones of the United States. The genus name derives from the Greek *pleo*, meaning "more," and *peltis*, meaning "a small crescent-shaped shield."

Pleopeltis crassinervata fronds are used in rural Mexico to treat mouth ulcers, gastrointestinal issues, and parasites.

A hexane fraction isolated from the frond by Anacleto-Santos et al. (2020) was tested against the parasite *Toxoplasma gondii* and exhibited activity with an IC_{50} value of 16.9 µg/mL. Cytotoxicity was noted against Hep-2

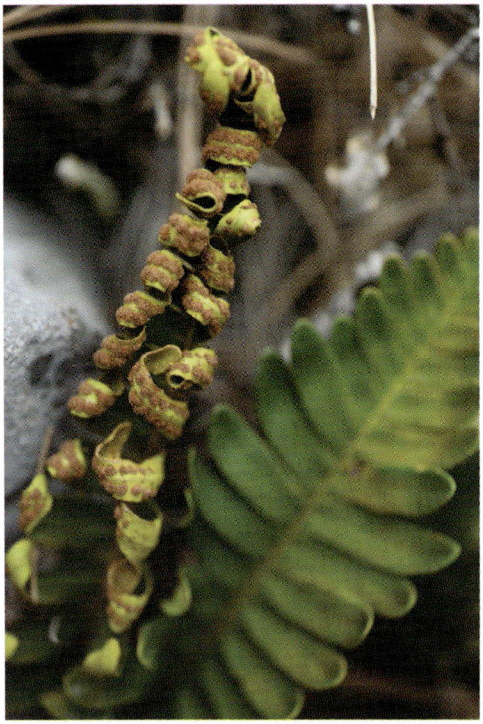

Pleopeltis guttata
(Drop Scaly Polypody)
Photo by Alan Rockefeller

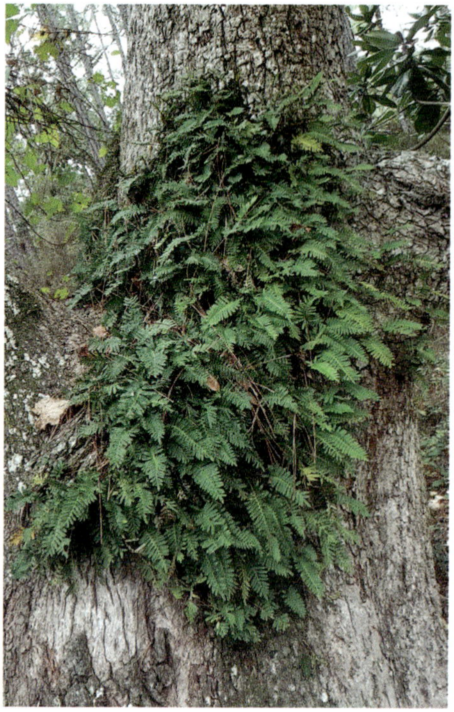

Pleopeltis michauxiana
(Resurrection Polypody)
Photo by Alan Rockefeller

(human larynx) carcinoma. Recent work on a hexane subfraction found its anti-toxoplasma activity is mainly due to effects on lipidomes and membranes (Anacleto-Santos et al. 2023).

This single-celled parasite is the leading cause of death from foodborne illness in the United States, occurs worldwide, and can persist in human bodies for long periods of time. Pregnant women can pass the infection to a fetus and is passed on from contaminated food or cat feces.

There is increasing evidence of a correlation between schizophrenia and exposure to *Toxoplasmosis gondii*, an intracellular parasite that infects one-third of humans worldwide. It is generally considered benign and asymptomatic, but a high level of behavioral and psychiatric disorders, including SSD (schizophrenia spectrum disorder) may be linked to this infection. The organism is transmitted by outdoor cats eating infected prey (rats or mice), and then spread in their feces. It is now found in raw meat including pork.

In humans, acute infection with *Toxoplasma gondii* can produce psychotic symptoms similar to SSD, and childhood exposure to cats is a risk factor. Some medications used to treat schizophrenia inhibit the replication of the organism in cell culture. A group in France looked at bipolar patients

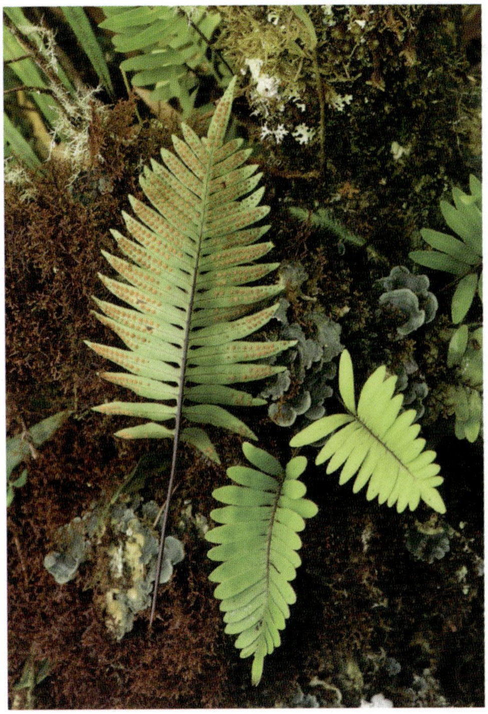

Pleopeltis plebeia
Photo by Alan Rockefeller

testing positive for *Toxoplasma gondii*, and those given valproate experienced fewer lifetime depressive episodes (Rogers 2019).

Polypodium furfuraceum syn. *Pleopeltis furfuracea* ferns have been a traditional analgesic in El Salvador (Uphof 1968; Usher 1971).

Pleopeltis macrocarpa fern decoctions were given orally at night, in Argentina to induce abortion (Zuloaga et al. 1999).

Curanderos in Columbia use the whole fern *Pleopeltis percussa* in attempts to neutralize the venom of the lethal yellow beard snake (*Bothrops asper*). This snake is responsible for the highest incidence and mortality rate among snakebites in southern North America, Central America, and northern South America.

Núñez et al. (2004) trialed twelve ethanol extracts from this fern, with ten of them showing 100% neutralization of the defibrinating effect of the venom and nine extending the coagulation time induced by the venom. Earlier studies found that the fern extract was able to inhibit the proteolytic activity of snake venom on casein.

"Yellow Beard venom contains phospholipases that show in vitro activity against *Plasmodium falciparum*, responsible for malaria. . . . Another study found a venom compound active against lymphoblastoid B cell lines, including inhibition of proliferation, apoptosis and necrosis" (Rogers 2014a).

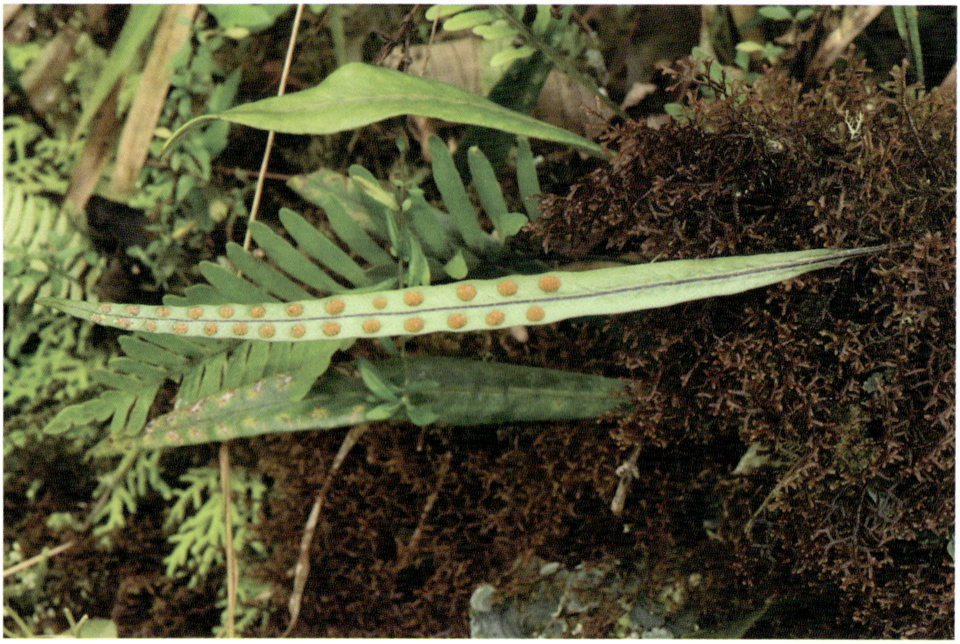

Pleopeltis macrocarpa (Big Fruit Scaly Polypody)
Photo by Alan Rockefeller

Redscale scaly polypody (*Pleopeltis polylepis* syn. *Polypodium polypodioides*) is traditionally used in Mexico to treat fever, bleeding, typhoid fever, cough, pertussis (whooping cough), chest pain, and kidney and liver diseases. The fern is sometimes referred to as resurrection fern. The Lumbee call it *tapasi moso,* meaning "a plant that grows on a rough branch." Traditionally, Indigenous healers boiled the fern down until very little water remained and combined it with tallow and rosebuds on external wounds. Other groups used ointments made from the fronds for sores and skin ulcers, as well as tea for treating headaches, dizziness, sore mouth (including thrush), and bleeding gums.

Research by Cárdenas et al. (2016) found various extracts of the fronds were active against both gram-positive and gram-negative bacteria, as well as *Candida albicans* and *Tricophyton mentagrophytes.*

Two fractions and two isolated compounds, butyl myristate and β-sitosterol, exhibited no cytotoxicity but showed anti-inflammatory activity comparable to prednisone, which was used as a control.

Weeping fern (*Pleopeltis thunbergiana*) contains pleoside, which has been shown to inhibit the proliferation of AGS (adenocarcinoma gastric) cancer cells in vitro (Jafari et al. 2018).

POLYPODIUM

Adder's Fern
Angelvein Fern
Caterpillar Fern
Common Polypody
Delicate Fern
Golden Maidenhair Fern
Lance Leaf Polypody
Licorice Fern
Oak Fern
Resurrection Fern
Rock Cap Fern
Rock Polypody Fern
Scented Oak Leaf Fern
Sweet Fern
Sweet Root Fern

Geographic Range: Americas, Baja California, Central America, Europe, Mexico, Peru, South America, Spain, United States

Habitat: epiphytic, hardwood tree trunks, rocky soil, temperate regions, tropical regions

Practical Uses: houseplant, nougat flavoring, tobacco flavoring

Medicinal Applications: antidepressant, anti-inflammatory, antimicrobial, antidiabetic, cancer, expectorant, fever, jaundice, kidney diseases, liver, melasma, nephritis, pleurisy, psoriasis, respiratory conditions, rheumatic pain, scurvy, sore throats, tuberculosis, urinary tract infections, wounds

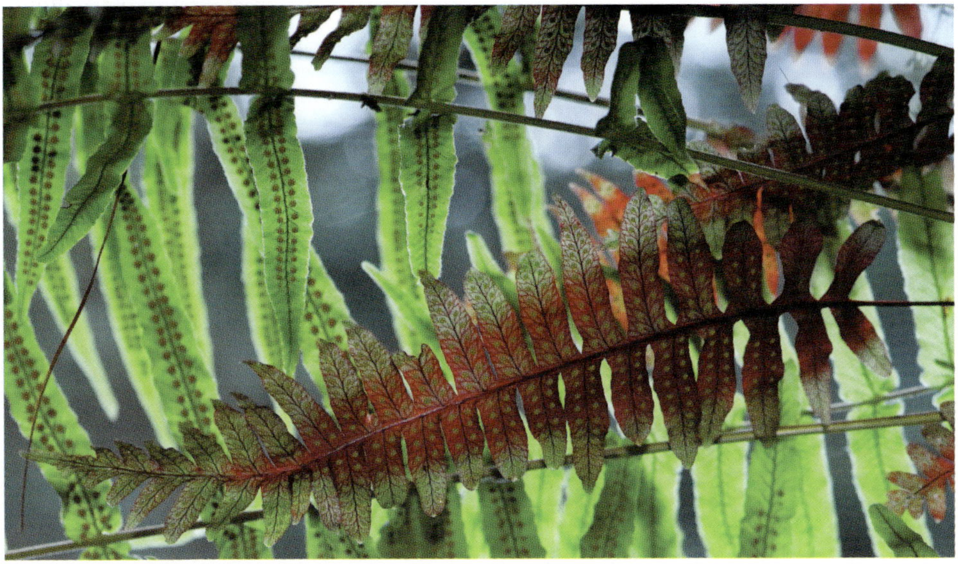

Polypodium rhodopleuron
Photo by Alan Rockefeller

The genus name *Polypodium* derives from the Greek *poly*, meaning "many," and *podion*, meaning "little foot," a reference to the foot-like appearance of the rhizome.

For blue star or gold foot fern (*Polypodium aureum*) see *Phlebodium aureum*.

California polypody or delicate fern (*Polypodium californicum*) is native to Baja California, along the coastline and mountain ranges. Indigenous groups in the area used the fern as an expectorant, diuretic, and topical application for sores and rheumatic pain. The Tolowa and Wailaki used the fern tea as an antibiotic (Stuhr 1933). The Mendocino tribe infused the rhizomes as a wash for sore eyes and the Wailaki rubbed the rhizome juice on sores and rheumatic body parts (Moerman 1986).

In South America and Spain, creeping golden polypody (*Polypodium decumanum*) is known as *calaguala* (*Polypodium leucotomos*) and used to treat psoriasis. In parts of Central and South America, the common name is

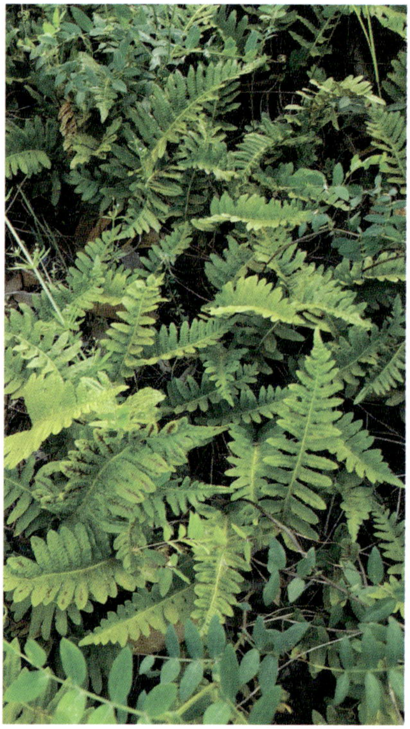

Polypodium californicum (California Polypody)
Photo by Alan Rockefeller

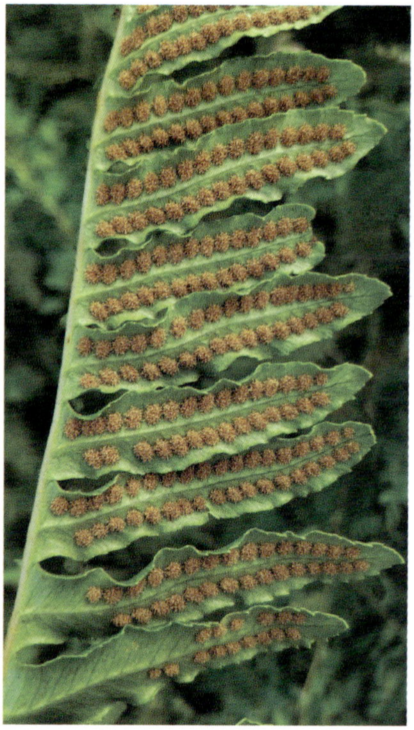

Spores of *Polypodium californicum* (California Polypody)
Photo by Alan Rockefeller

samambaia. In the early 1980s, a Spanish company created a medicine from a water extract of samambaia and marketed it as Anapsos. The prescription drug has been found to improve cognition, cerebral blood perfusion, and improve bio-electrical activity in the brain of patients with senile dementia. It is available in Spain and parts of Europe for the treatment of dementia and Alzheimer's disease (Taylor 2005).

Research by Vasänge-Tuominen et al. (1994) found that leukotriene B4, one of the inflammatory mediators, was abnormally high in psoriatic skin. The fatty acids are thought to contribute to the clinical benefits. Earlier work by Tuominen et al. (1992) suggested that the content of adenosine may contribute to the fern's therapeutic properties.

Vasänge et al. (1997) identified a sulphonoglycolipid from the fern that acts as antagonist through the platelet-activating factor receptor in human neutrophils.

Calagualine, derived from this species and *Polypodium leucotomas*, blocks tumor metastasis, proliferation, and inflammation by inhibiting the activation of NF-κB (Manna et al. 2003). Additionally, the triflavonoid selligueain is also present. In vitro, this compound was found to inhibit the proteolytic enzyme elastase. Selligueain A exhibits about thirty-five times the sweetness intensity of a 2% w/v sucrose/water solution.

Caterpillar fern (*Polypodium formosanum*) is named for its blue-green, white rhizomes that resemble a caterpillar or grub, and is also called grub fern.

The Central American fern *Polypodium friedrichsthalianum* has been traditionally used for treating syphilis and as a remedy for the bite from the *toboba* (*Porthidium ophryomegas*), a venomous snake. The snake's name may derive from the Chibchan language in Costa Rica (Portilla 2022).

The rhizome of licorice fern or sweet root fern (*Polypodium glycyrrhiza*) has a pleasant licorice-like flavor, favored by Indigenous people of the Pacific Northwest. I have tasted it raw and collected and dried the root for a pleasant tea. It goes dormant in summer, but the fall rains help it produce new fronds. The fern is epiphytic, meaning it does not need soil but can attach to vertical surfaces, including moss-covered rocks and trees, particularly big leaf maple (*Acer macrophyllum*).

The species name *glycyrrhiza* derives from the Greek *glykys*, meaning "sweet." The rhizome contains compounds sweeter than sugar. Ferns in general contain various sugars, including xylose, arabinose, glucose, galatose, mannose,

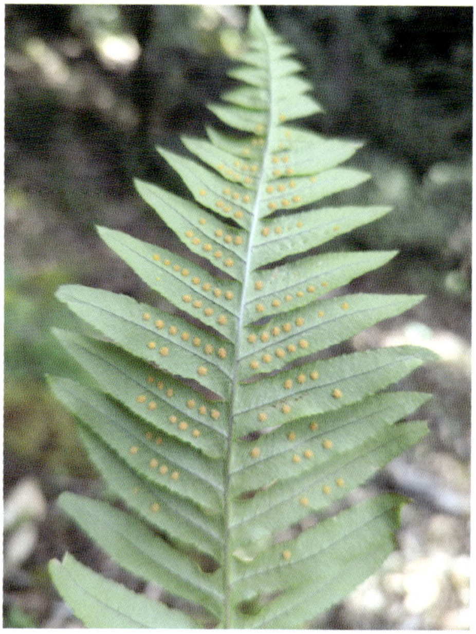

Polypodium glycyrrhiza (Licorice Fern)
Photo by Alan Rockefeller

and rhamnose, albeit mostly in small amounts. The rhizomes are alterative, carminative, hemostatic, and pectoral.

Polypodoside A, derived from the rhizomes, was rated by a human taste panel as exhibiting 600 times the sweetness intensity of a 6% w/v aqueous sucrose solution. It is so sweet that the taste lingers for over an hour.

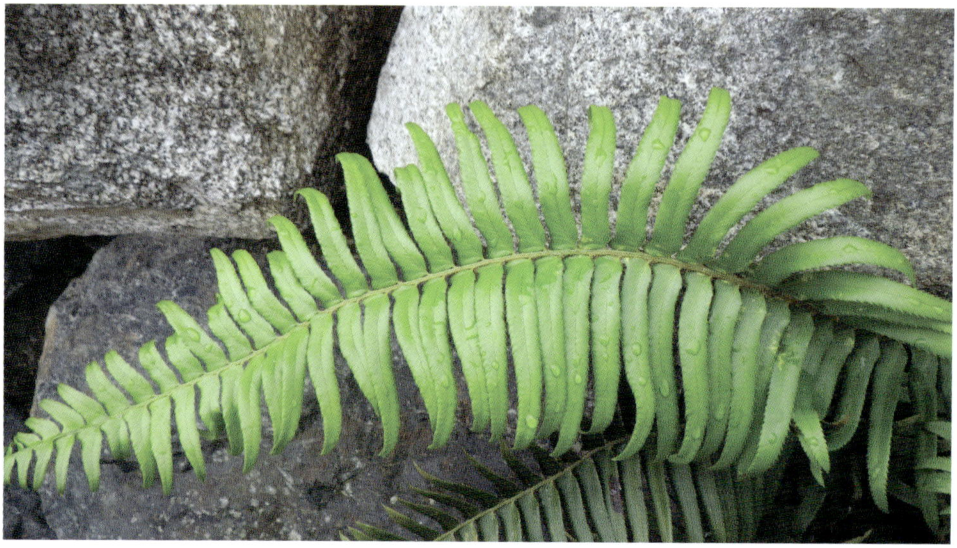

Polypodium glycyrrhiza (Licorice Fern)
Photo by Drew T. Henderson

Indigenous people of Haida Gwaii know the fern as *tsagwal* and the fronds as *dlaayéngwaal-xil*. The long green rhizomes are sweet, and elders mention that after chewing them drinking water tastes sweet. The Kaigai Haida used the rhizomes to flavor labrador tea (*Rhododendron groenlandicum*). The Haida and other Northwest Coastal Peoples used it for colds and sore throats, simply chewing the rhizome or decocting it for coughs, including whooping cough (Turner 2004).

The Tlingit call it *ssaach*, the Yupik *plzuut*, and the Nisga'a *ts'ak'a aam*. The Kitasoo name is *ts' igeʔaém*, and the Haisla refer to the rhizome as *ts'gaʔám*, and the entire plant as *k'ts' aʔam'ás*. The Hesquit ate the long, slender rhizomes raw, and the Southern Kwakiutl sucked on the root to prevent hunger and thirst. The root juice was swallowed to stop vomiting blood. The Makah chewed the peeled stalks for coughs. Their name for the rhizome is *xixiitap*, meaning "crawling root thing." The Quinault ate the baked rhizomes and chewed them raw for coughs (Moerman 1986). The dried roots were steamed as survival food, or scorched, cut into small pieces, dipped in oil, and chewed by elders (Moerman 2010).

The Heiltsuk name is *ʔháixp'axst'auxw us tl'uk'um*, meaning "it's kind of sweet when you bite it." The Lummi call it *k'esíp*, and the Quinault *tsumanáa-mats*. On Wsánec territory on Vancouver Island, licorice fern is called *tesip*

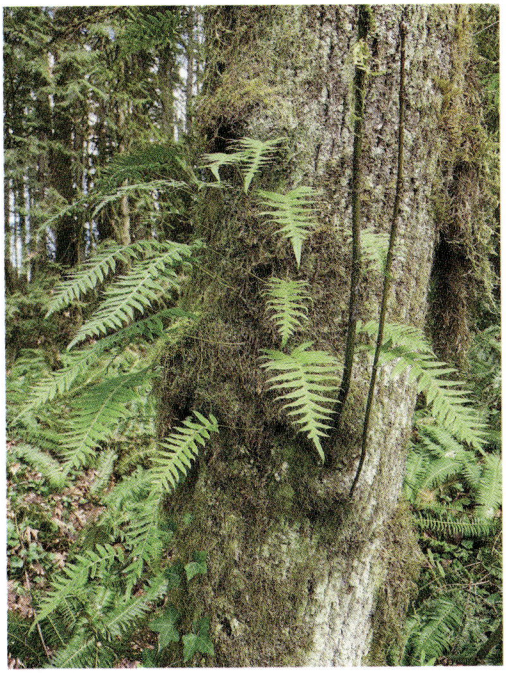

Polypodium glycyrrhiza (Licorice Fern)
Photo by Drew T. Henderson

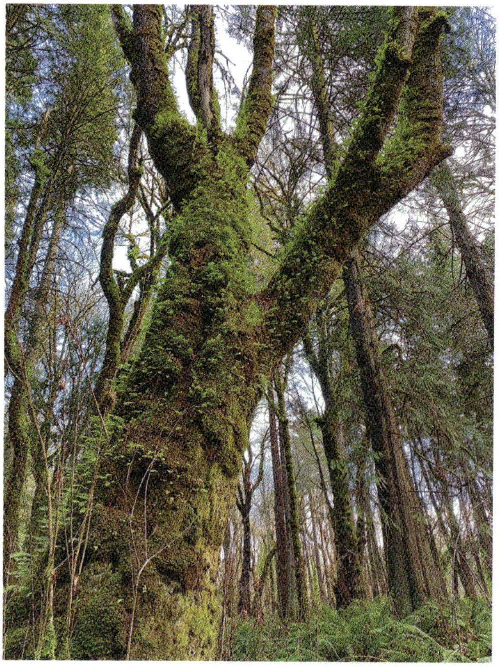

Polypodium glycyrrhiza (Licorice Fern)
Photo by Drew T. Henderson

(*tl'esip*). The Stl'atl'imx (Pemberton) use the same word for licorice fern. The fern grows on rocky soil and on big-leaf maple (*Acer macrophyllum*) trunks. The Comox name is *t'th úshen*, and the Sechelt know the fern as *lekw 'ay*. Across the ocean strait, the Squamish refer to it as *tl' esip* or *ilténtin*, meaning "appetizer." Ilténtin comes from ílen which means "to eat."

The sweet root tea was used to improve the taste of bitter medicines. Indigenous healers used it for treating colds, coughs, sore throats, and more severe respiratory conditions such as tuberculosis. A piece of root was chewed, and the juice swallowed for coughs and digestive complaints (Turner and Hebda 2012).

The Cowlitz people infused the crushed stipes for treating measles (Moerman 1986). The Lower Cowlitz refer to the fern as *tl'ewilqw*, and the Upper Cowlitz know it as *l'lwéelk*. Mixed with fir needles, the rhizome has been decocted, and the liquid consumed to treat measles. The Nlaka'pamux name is *leqieqáy'st*.

The fern exhibits antiviral activity against herpes virus type 1 (McCutcheon et al. 1995). The rhizome tea is anti-inflammatory and possesses a mild antihistamine activity.

Polypodium hastatum fern contains chlorogenic acid, ethyl chlorogenate, and polypodiside (Li et al. 2018).

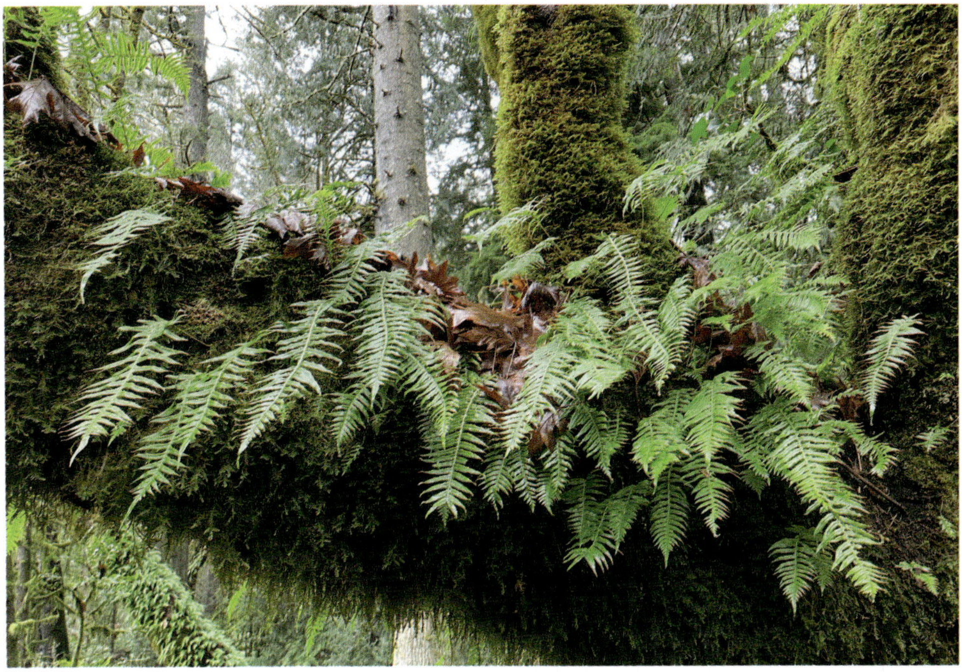

Polypodium glycyrrhiza (Licorice Fern)
Photo by Drew T. Henderson

The increasing incidence of diabetes worldwide is a most serious concern, amounting to over 540 million people worldwide. Diabetes affects over 10% of the population in the United States (32.2 million people) followed by Mexico, where nearly 17% of the population (14 million people) are diabetic.

Polypodiside is a natural Nrf2 activator found in this fern that shows in vitro potential to reduce diabetic complications. Work by Li et al. (2022b) showed that polypodiside reduces pro-inflammatory cytokines activated by high glucose levels and inhibits the MAPK/NFκB pathway, leading to reduced inflammation. Furthermore, the anti-inflammatory effects are closely related to the activation of Nrf2.

Sixty volatile compounds were identified in the whole fern, mainly composed of fatty acid esters, especially methyl and ethyl esters.

Western polypody (*Polypodium hesperium*) rhizomes were chewed by the Nlaka'pamux (Thompson) for their sweet flavor (Moerman 2010).

Lance leaf polypody (*Polypodium lanceolatum*) rhizomes have been traditionally used in Mexico and Guatemala to treat fevers and coughs (Usher 1971). Decoctions were also prepared in South Africa for colds and sore throats (Watt and Breyer-Brandwijk 1962).

Polypodium nipponica and *P. formosanum* contain triterpenoids that exhibit in vivo activity in a two-stage carcinogenesis model on mouse skin papilloma (Konoshima et al. 1996). The Japanese name is *aonekazura*, and *Nippon* (the local word for the country).

Polypodium plebeium ferns in central Mexico provide nectaries on the fronds to attract ants for protection. Studies have shown that when young fronds were examined, the damage from sawflies and caterpillars was significantly greater when ants were removed (Koptur et al. 1998). In Mexico, the rhizomes are used for coughs and as a purgative (Usher 1971).

Cultivars, such as 'Southern Cross' and 'Tahitian Fern,' are popular houseplants. In Samoa, the frond juice is used as ear medicine (Uhe 1974).

Resurrection fern or gray polypody (*Polypodium polypodioides* syn. *Pleopeltis polypodioides*) is an epiphyte, native to the Americas and Africa. It favors hardwood tree trunks in Eastern and Southeastern United States but is also found in Southern Africa. The Houma of Louisiana decocted the fronds for headaches, dizziness, bleeding gums, and used the cooled liquid as a wash for babies' sore mouths or thrush.

Leathery polypody (*Polypodium scouleri*) fern rhizomes were chewed by Hesquiat children as candy. The Makah people may have also used the fern as a food source (Moerman 2010).

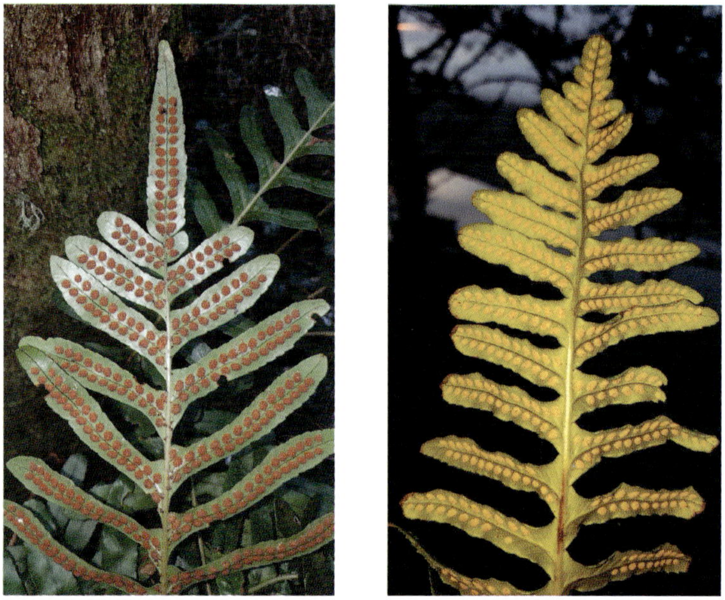

Polypodium scouleri (Leathery Polypody)
Photos by Alan Rockefeller

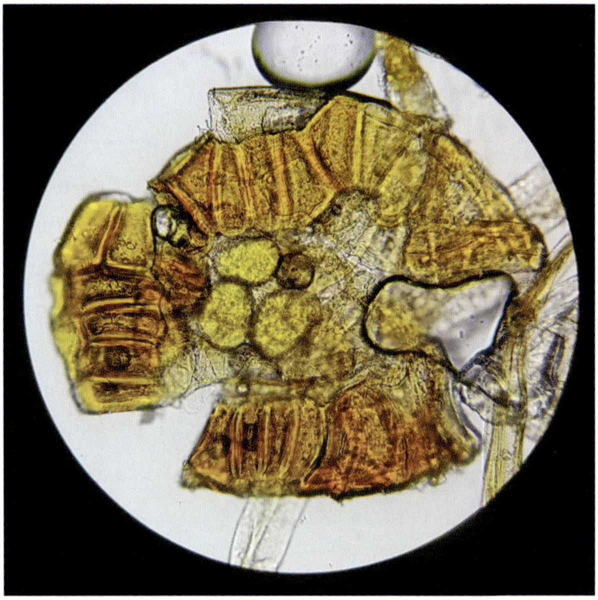

Magnified cross-section of *Polypodium scouleri* (Leathery Polypody)
Photo by Alan Rockefeller

Angelvein fern (*Polypodium triseriale*) contains selligueain and melilotoside.

Rock cap fern or rocky polypody (*Polypodium virginianum* syn. *P. vulgare* var. *virginianum*) was used by the Lenape and Iroquois for various respiratory conditions, including sore throats, colds, coughs, lung congestion, and tuberculosis. It was also taken for measles, cholera, and stomach aches. The Cherokee applied fern poultices for inflamed swellings and wounds and drank frond infusions for hives. The Mik'maq of Eastern Canada drank root decoctions for pleurisy, and the Eastern Cree of Quebec drank the tea for neuralgia and kidney problems.

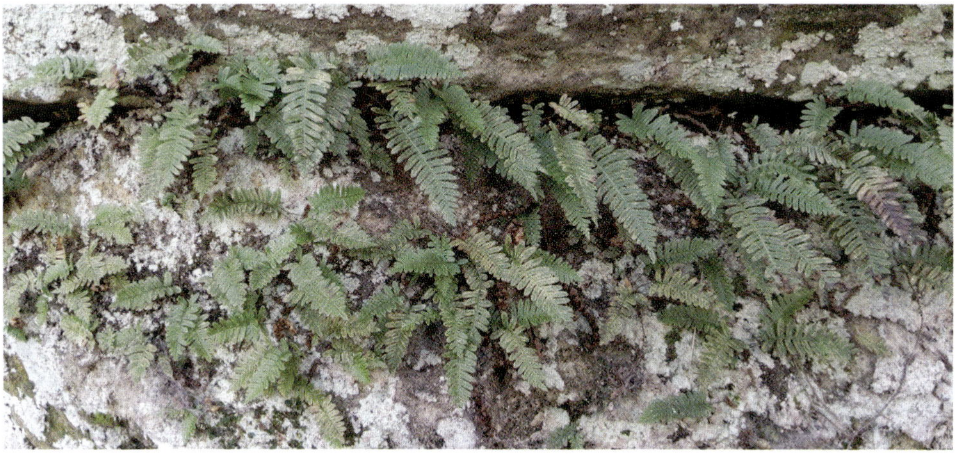

Polypodium virginianum (Rock Cap Fern)
Photo by Alan Rockefeller

Early North American settlers used the root to flavor tobacco, and decoctions were used to treat depression and "fearsome and troublesome" bad dreams. The fern also contains ecdysterone and ecdysone.

Common polypody or western polypody, also known as sweet fern, adder's fern, rock polypody fern, and golden maidenhair fern (*Polypodium vulgare* var. *columbianum* syn. *P. hesperium*) has been used in traditional medicine as an expectorant for treating coughs, including whooping cough (pertussis), and as a diuretic in various kidney diseases such as chronic nephritis and pyelonephritis. Decoctions of the root and fronds have been traditionally used to treat tuberculosis (Leighton 1985).

The Cree of Northern Canada know the fern as *kānākiwîkoc*, *kāthîthîkipakākî*, or *kinîpikōtîthaniwîpak*. The fern was known in Western Washington state to the Cowlitz as *k'lwe'lk*, Green River as *skiwëlk*, Klallam as *kla'sip*, Lummi as *k'est'p*, Makah as *xëxi't*, meaning "crawling root on trees," Quinalt as *tsumana'amats*, Skagit as *klë'tcai*, Snohomish as *k!ëtcai*, and Swinomish as *stsloqwi'lk* (Gunther 1945). The term *licorice fern* is commonly used, but the binomial name is *Polypodium vulgare*.

The rhizome was roasted by the Makah, with its juice swallowed for coughs. The Cowlitz crushed the rhizome and mixed it with young fir needles, boiled it, and drank the infusion, or possibly the decoction, for measles. The Quinault believed the best ferns grow on alder moss. They either baked the rhizome on coals or used it raw as a cough medicine (Gunther 1945). The people of Bella Coola decocted the roots for stomach pain or chewed them for colds, sore throats, gums (Moerman 1986). The Nootka rubbed the sweet roots on their hands to bring good luck while fishing. The fern was also used for designs in basket weaving, to line steam pits, and woven into rugs and sleeping mats.

The rhizomes have a bittersweet licorice-like flavor—likely due to the intensely sweet osladin, a steroid saponin that is up to 500 times sweeter than sugar—similar to the sweetness of western licorice fern. Chewing the root before drinking water made the water taste sweeter. Even the whole ferns are sweet and were chewed and their juice swallowed to ease sore throats. Sweet fern has been traditionally used to make nougat candy (discussed more on page 249).

The Eclectic physician Dr. John King noted the fern is pectoral, demulcent, purgative, and anthelmintic when used as a decoction (30 ml to 120 ml up to four times daily). Water extracts of the rhizome led to the isolation and identification of flavan-3-ol derivatives, including (+)-afzelechin, a known

α-glucosidase inhibitor, suggestive of benefits in managing elevated blood sugar levels.

Polypodium vulgare has a long history of use in Europe, and in 2008, the European Medicines Agency published a monograph on the rhizome, indicating its medicinal significance.

The fern has been known by various names throughout history. Early Greeks called it *polypodion* or *filicula*, according to the Roman Pliny the Elder. The German physician Dr. Valentino Kräuterman (1725) wrote a book suggesting oak fern (*Polypodium vulgare*) be taken after the evening meal in order to have happy dreams.

The presence of osladin in ferns gave rise to names like the Dutch engelzoet, meaning "angel sweet," and Swedish *stensöta*, meaning "stone sweetness," given to a rock fern.

The connection between fern and oak led to a need in early 18th-century Ireland to import the fern from other countries. It was believed to be more effective than ferns gathered in other locations. This belief persisted, and over a century later on the Aranislands, it led to the practice of gathering the rhizomes during a new moon and burying them in porridge overnight to ensure their medicinal potency (Allen and Hatfield 2004). In Herefordshire, fronds for treating whooping cough were only considered effective if they bore spores.

Maud Grieve (1931) describes the fern as an alterative, tonic, pectoral, and expectorant, useful in treating dry coughs and formerly used for consumption.

I've noted,

> A mucilaginous decoction of the fronds was formerly . . . used in country places as a cure for whooping cough in children. . . . The fresh root used to be employed in decoctions, or powdered, for melancholia and also for rheumatic swelling of the joints. It is efficacious in jaundice, dropsy and scurvy, and combined with mallows removes hardness of the spleen, stitches in the side and colic. The distilled water of the roots and leaves was considered by old herbalists good for ague, and the fresh or dried roots, mixed with honey and applied to the nose, were used in the cure of polypus.
>
> The dried root is used for stimulating bile secretions, as a laxative and for visceral obstructions and worms. It is also mildly expectorant and used for bronchial congestion, and asthma, combining well with marshmallow

> root. External washes are used for wounds, while poultices or sun-infused liniments are used for arthritic pains in the limbs and lumbar regions. It is an ingredient in plasters for dislocated fingers and applied to sores between the fingers (Rogers 2014b).

Hieronymus Brunschwig (1500) recommended water (hydrosol) from polypody ferns to clean the blood, soothe irritated coughs, soften the belly, and alleviate melancholia. Gerard (1597) notes that Dioscorides recommended the root for members out of joint and for chaps between the fingers.

Culpeper (1652) suggested harvesting the rhizome in October or November when the leaves have done their service. He writes,

> Then the body of the root swells, and acquires twice its former thickness; it then grows tender, and its juice, when broken, is saccharine, thick and gummous. . . . It is under Jupiter in Leo. With laxatives it gently carries off the contents of the bowels without irritation. . . . With mucilaginous herbs, such as white beet and mallow, it is excellent for cholics. The powder taken to half a drachm daily, and fasting three hours after, is good for the spleen, jaundice and dropsy. . . . Some use its distilled water in cough, asthma, diseases of the lungs, pleurisies, obstructions of the mesentery, and in whatever cases acrimony is to be subdued.

John K'Eogh recommended the fern for purging bilious substances, adding anise seeds to open obstructions of the spleen and ease fevers. A dried powder was suggested for snuff to reduce nasal polyps.

In *Potter's Cyclopedia of Botanical Drugs and Preparations*, it is mentioned that "its action is peculiar in that it occasionally produces a rash of red spots, but this disappears in a short time and causes no inconvenience."

William Salmon (1710), in his *Botanoligia. The English Herbal*, wrote, "It prevails in peculiar against Frensies, and radically cures the most profound madness whether it be raging or otherwise."

The fern was combined with digitalis (foxglove) to treat epilepsy (Barton 1877). In traditional Polish medicine, the fern was used as an expectorant, as well as chronic nephritis and pyelonephritis.

Research by Gleńsk et al. (2019) found that osladin inhibits various strains of *Escherichia coli* and its biofilm formation. *E. coli* is the most common pathogen associated with urinary tract infections (UTIs).

The rhizome contains at least eight phytoecdysteroids (PEs), composing 2%, with a molecular structure similar to insect molting hormone. PEs are found in algae, fungi, ferns, gymnosperms, and angiosperms, with more than 500 different PEs identified in over one hundred terrestrial plants. The most common PE is 20-hydroxyecsysone. In humans, PEs exhibit benefits as antidiabetics, antioxidants, antimicrobials, hepatic protectants, anticancer agents, anti-inflammatories, and antidepressants (Arif et al. 2022). Ecdysterones are also used to increase muscle mass in athletes, weightlifters, and bodybuilders.

Other compounds in the rhizome include polypodine, filicinic acid, methyl salicylate, triterpenoids, glycyrrhizin (0.6%), catechin (3.7%), and phloroglucinol (0.5%) as well as sucrose (15%) and fructose (2%). Due to its sweet nature, the rhizome was used in the past to flavor tobacco.

Water extracts of the rhizomes have demonstrated central nervous system (CNS) depressant effects and ß-adrenoceptor agonist activities. These extracts also show positive inotropic and chronotropic effects on the perfused frog heart, cause hypotension and tachycardia in dogs, and inhibit contractions in the small intestine of the rabbit (Mannan et al. 1989).

Ethanol extracts (80% maceration) have been shown to be cytotoxic to A375 (human melanoma) cancer cell lines while remaining safe for normal fibroblast cells (Tabeshpour et al. 2023). Extracts of this fern also regenerate skin epidermis and increase vascularization in a mice model (Batur et al. 2020).

The fronds were extracted with methanol and were found to contain significant amounts of shikimic acid, epicatechin, catechin, which are possibly related to the fern's wound-healing properties and lack of toxicity (Farràs et al. 2021).

Research by McCutcheon and colleagues (1995) found that the fern extract possesses activity against bovine herpes virus type 1.

Water extracts of the rhizome improve the efficacy of ciprofloxacin in inactivating uropathogenic *Escherichia coli* strains (Tichaczek-Goska et al. 2021).

Nougat candy is a chewy combination of roasted nuts, sugar, or honey, and whipped egg whites. The name derives from the Southern France Occitan *pan nogat*, and in turn from the Latin *panis nucatus*, "nut bread." It has a long history, possibly dating back to early 7th-century Spain. In parts of Europe, it is still made with traditional ingredients, but no longer contains the aromatic sweet fern rhizomes once used. In the United States, nougat is often adulterated with corn syrup, hydrolyzed soy protein, vegetable oils, and milk powder. Your local European food stores will carry the more authentic nougat versions.

No homeopathic remedy with *Polypodium vulgare* is currently available. According to Jörg Wichmann, noted homeopath, the skin problems caused by this fern are unproblematic sporadic red spots that quickly disappear. Wichman passed away on April 23, 2020, but his family continues his brilliant work at the Provings Info website.

Juliane Hesse conducted a homeopathic trituration proving in 2014 and published it in her book *Die Urweltpflanzen*.

Hesse observed an alternation between effort and resignation, indicating possible tinea miasm (ringworm), as well as skin rashes similar to pityriasis (miasm).

POLYSTICHUM

Christmas Ferns
Eastern Maidenhair Fern
Holly Ferns
Korean Rock Fern
Shield Ferns
Tassel Fern
Western Sword Fern

Geographic Range: Alaska, Asia, Central North America, Eurasia, Europe, Greenland, Iran, Pakistan

Habitat: calcareous soil, cliffs, limestone rocks, high elevations, mountains, pavements, red alder trees, western red cedar trees

Practical Uses: bedding, decoration, erosion control, houseplant, steam pit, basket, and storage box lining

Medicinal Applications: anthelmintic, antibacterial, anti-inflammatory, antipyretic, antispasmodic, arthritis, asthma, diarrhea, fever, inflammation, liver, pneumonia, pulmonary edema, rheumatism, snakebites, sore throat, stomachache, tuberculosis

Warning: Polystichum squarrosum may not be safe for consumption as it produces pathological changes in laboratory animals.

The genus name *Polystichum* derives from the Greek *poly*, meaning "many," and *stichos*, meaning "rows," referring to the multiple rows of sori. Collectively, the genera are known as holly ferns.

Hard shield fern (*Polystichum aculeatum*) is a European/Asian evergreen, usually found on limestone cliffs at higher elevations.

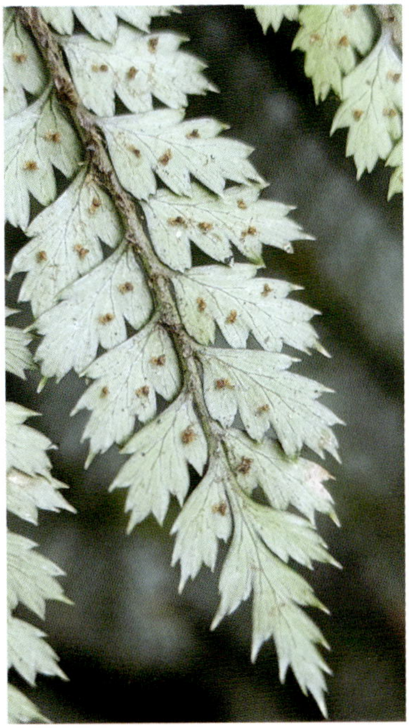

Underside of *Polystichum vestitum* (Prickly Shield Fern)
Photo by Alan Rockefeller

The fronds are decocted in Iran as an anthelmintic (Bahadori et al. 2015). Both fronds and rhizomes have been shown to exhibit significant activity against *Staphylococcus aureus* and *Escherichia coli*.

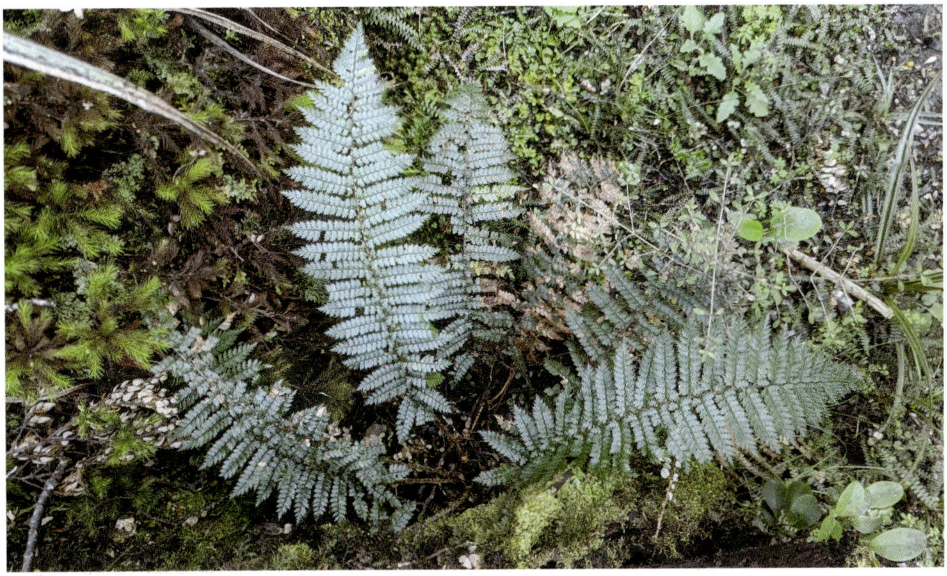

Polystichum vestitum (Prickly Shield Fern)
Photo by Alan Rockefeller

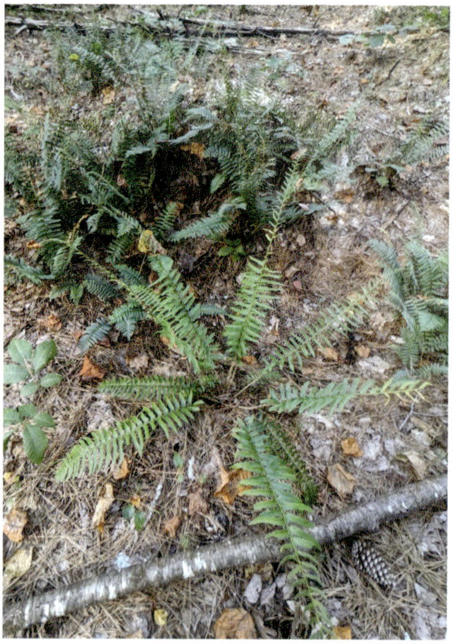

Polystichum acrostichoides (Christmas Fern)
Photo by Alan Rockefeller

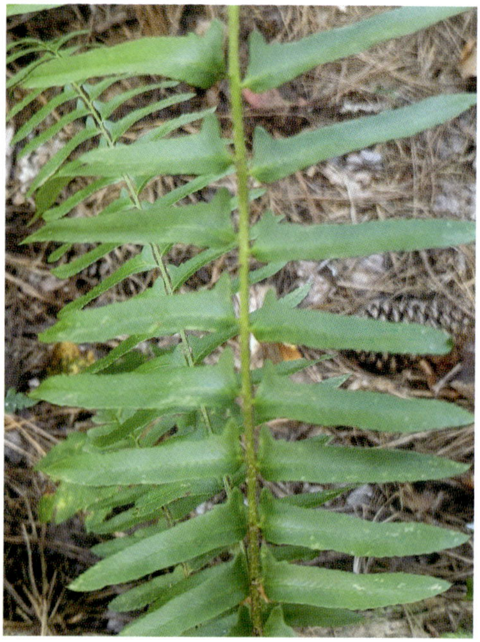

Close-up of *Polystichum* sp.
Photo by Alan Rockefeller

Christmas fern (*Polystichum acrostichoides*) has a wide range of traditional uses among Indigenous people of Eastern North America. The fresh rhizome was crushed and applied externally for rheumatism and red spots (possibly liver spots) on the skin. The rhizome was decocted and ingested for fevers, chills, hoarseness of the throat, pneumonia, and tuberculosis, or applied externally to rheumatic joints. The fern tea was ingested for stomachache, intestinal cramping, and diarrhea, and chewed on for toothache. The dried rhizome was powdered and inhaled as snuff to help restore vocal cords. The Mi'kmaq also used the rhizomes for hoarseness (Moerman 1986).

Moerman (2010) notes that the Cherokee used the fiddleheads as a food source. A cold infusion of the rhizomes was given to the elderly for stomach and bowel complaints. When planted on a shady hillside, it can help control soil erosion. For fern gardeners, it is recommended to plant it at an angle to prevent water and snowmelt from collecting inside and decaying the center.

The rhizomes of Braun's holly fern (*Polystichum braunii*) have been traditionally used in Pakistan and other countries for chronic health conditions such as arthritis. Saleem et al. (2019) found that methanol, ethyl acetate, and water extracts of the rhizome demonstrated good antiarthritic potential in orally fed

Wistar rats. The benefits may be due to the inhibition of protein denaturation and lysosomal membrane stabilization.

Both water and methanol extracts significantly reduced IL-4, IL-5, IL-6, IL-13, IL-1β, TNF-α, and NF-κB, and upregulated aquaporins (1 and 5) in a mouse trial on airway inflammation and pulmonary edema. Both extracts also restored activities of superoxide dismutase (SOD), catalase (CAT), glutathione (GSH), and reduced levels of malondialdehyde and possess significant potential in the management of allergic asthma (Saleem et al. 2022).

Northern holly fern (*Polystichum lonchitis*) is found throughout the northern hemisphere, from Eurasia to Alaska to Greenland, and in the mountains of central North America. It loves calcareous soil and the nooks and crannies of limestone rocks and pavement. The fern contains α-D-galactopyranoside, and methyl and n-hexadecanoic compounds.

Sher et al. (2023) tested its anti-inflammatory, analgesic, antipyretic, and antispasmodic activities in a mice model. The effectiveness of the methanol extract, followed by ethanol and then water extractions, suggests more study is required to test its effectiveness against various diseases.

Makino's holly fern (*Polystichum makinoi*) is an Asian evergreen fern, highly prized in the horticultural world. It is hardy to –29°C/20.2°F.

Western sword fern or giant holly fern (*Polystichum munitum*) is known to the Indigenous people of Haida Gwaii as *ts'aagul*, *ts'aagwaal*, or *ts'áagwaal*.

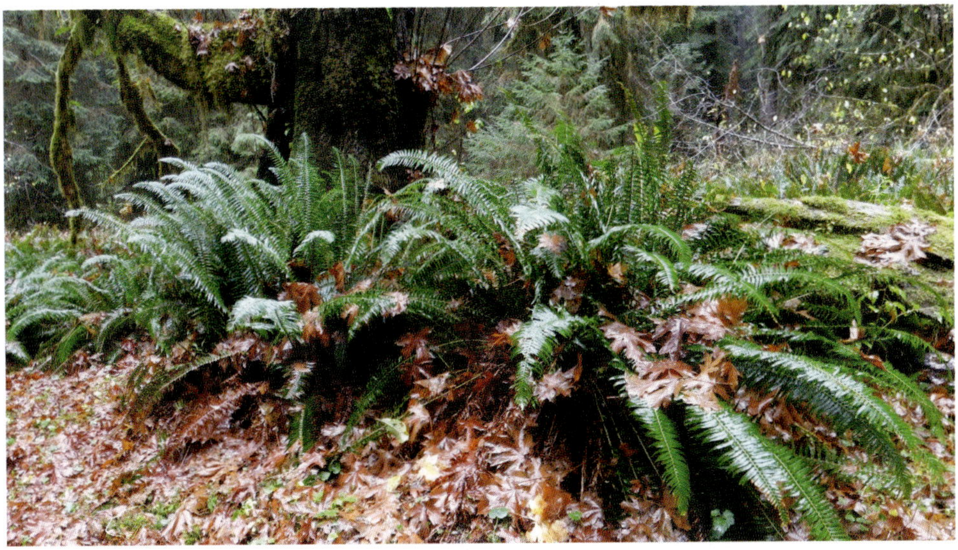

Polystichum munitum (Western Sword Fern)
Photo by Alan Rockefeller

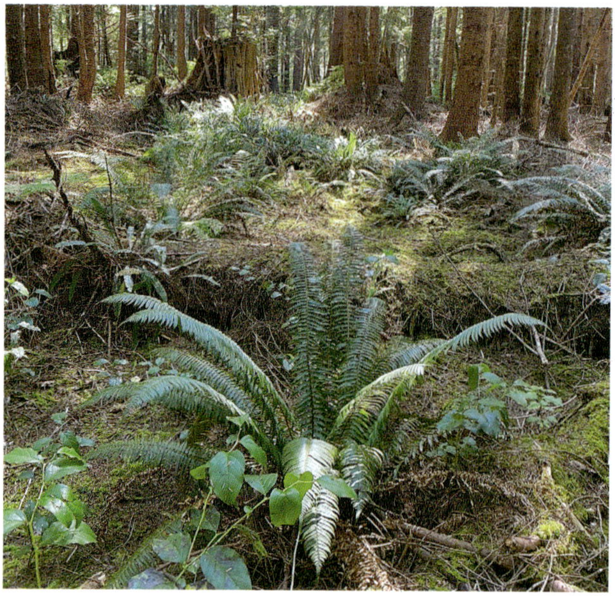

Polystichum munitum (Western Sword Fern)
Photo by Drew T. Henderson

These names were sometimes also applied to spiny wood fern (*Dryopteris* sp.) The rootstocks were called *snanjang*, or *sk'yaaw*, a term also used for wood fern, as both rhizomes are edible. The smaller rootstocks were called *snaal jaad* (scabby woman or girl), a term also reported by ethnobotanist Newcombe (1897) and also applied to *Blechnum spicant* rhizomes. Sword fern is important in Haida medicine and in their narratives.

The word for shrew (sometimes called mouse) is *Jigul ʔawga*, *Jiigwal ʔawga*, or *Kaagan Jaad* as "Mouse Woman," and *Jagul ʔaww* translates as "Fern Mother" (Swanton 1911).

Mouse Woman, in Haida tradition, lives under a clump of western sword fern. In one story, the "hero" helps a shrew cross a log, and the shrew (or mouse) disappears under a clump of ferns. When the man draws the ferns aside, he finds the painted house front of the Fern Mother, with planks sewn together in the old style. The Fern Mother calls him grandson and gives him supernatural medicine (Swanton 1905).

Fern Woman was a supernatural being (Haida), and Sword Fern was a supernatural person who controlled the weather and had a hairy face, ear-rings of dentalia, and cheeks smeared with red ochre, used in weather rituals (Swanton 1905).

The name *Mouse Woman* is interesting. My friend and colleague David Young (2014), who lived near the grandmother spirit as depicted in a petro-glyph on a large boulder oceanside on Gabriola Island, British Columbia,

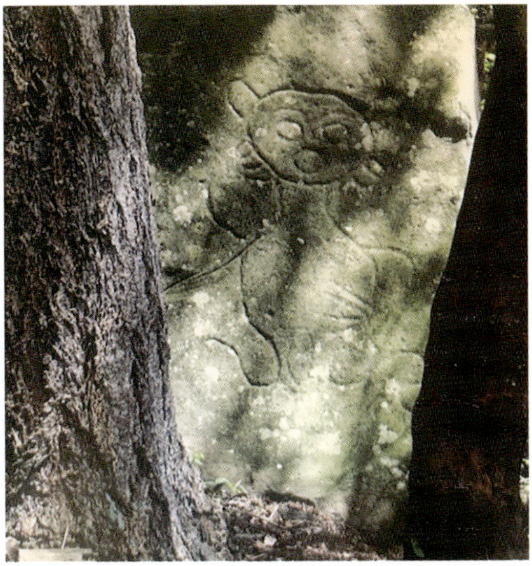

Mouse Woman
Photo by David Young

Canada, cited numerous accounts of people experiencing spontaneous healing from touching or embracing the monument.

Sword fern fronds were used to line steam pits, storage boxes, baskets, and drying racks for berries, lay fish, cover the floors of summer houses and dance houses, and for bedding. The Nlaka'pamux copied the sword fern patterns in the design of their split cedar root coiled baskets.

Children of Squamish and other Southern British Columbia tribes played a game to see who could pull off the most pinnae, saying "*pála*" with each one, in a single breath. According to Turner (1998), this tradition was more serious for the Ditidaht and some Salish Coast people. The contest was part of a young man's training, teaching him to train his breath so he could dive to the base of bull kelp forests and cut off the stipe from the ocean floor. The Klallam and Makah of Washington state also performed this endurance game.

Sword fern is mainly found under Western red cedar and red alder trees. The Makah used the fronds to steam salmonberry sprouts on hot rocks to give them flavor (Moerman 2010). Sword fern was known by different names to various tribes of Western Washington. The Lower Chelhalis know it as *sa'xalum*, the Upper Cowlitz as *tsli'mai*, the Green River tribe as *sxa xitc*, the Klallam as *pilapilaxiltc*, the Lummi as *s'xe'lem*, and the Makah as *plipla'bupt* or *totoqwa's*, meaning "roots above the ground." The Quileute call the roots *pila'pila'bupt*, and the fronds *tsato'tsa*, and the Quinault name for the rhizome is *sk'ë'ë'tckl* or *sk'okots'a*, and the Skagit call the roots *saq!* and the whole plant *stca'lasets*.

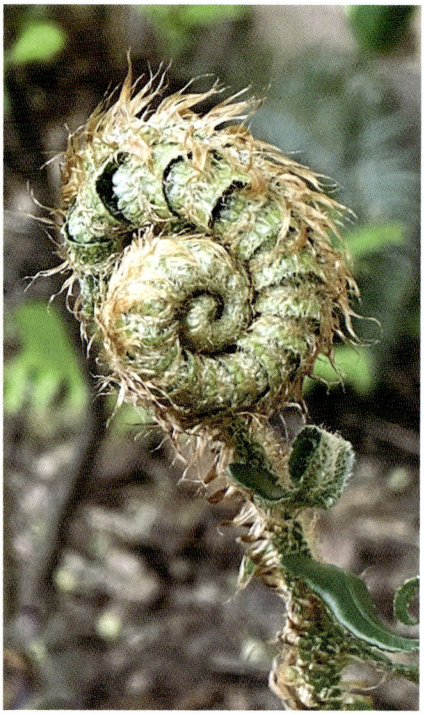

Fiddlehead of *Polystichum munitum* (Western Sword Fern)
Photo by Drew T. Henderson

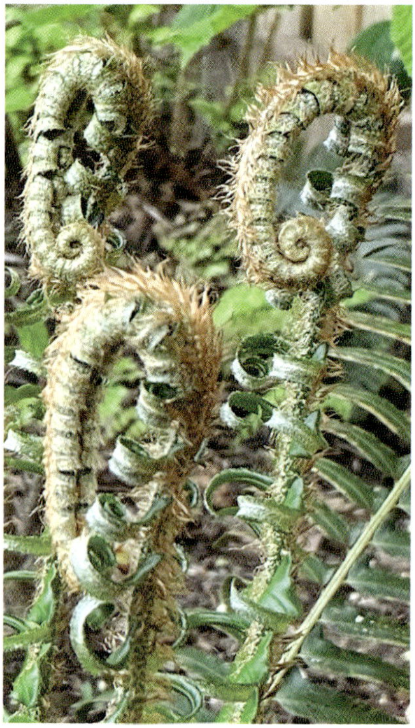

Polystichum munitum (Western Sword Fern)
Photo by Drew T. Henderson

The neighboring Snohomish and Squaxin know the fern as *sx'xaltc* and *sxa'xaltc*, respectively. The Swinomish name is similar, *sxa'xalatc*, meaning "small sprout" (Gunther 1945). They chewed the raw fern for sore throat or tonsillitis. The Hul'q'umi'num' also know sword fern by the similar *sthxelum*. According to Luschiim and Turner (2021), this is a sacred plant used in ceremony by the Coast Salish people. It was used for food all year round and in the Winter Dance.

The Quileute peel the *pilápila* rhizome and baked it in a steam pit with fresh salmon or dried salmon eggs. The Makah and Klallam boiled the rhizome. The Nitinaht steamed the large rhizomes for food in summer, while the Thompson (Nlaka'pamux) used the roots for food in an unspecified manner (Moerman 2010). They call the fern *sxáʔy' eq* or *s-xal-m*, similar to the Tillamook name for western sword fern.

The fronds were used by several tribes for bedding. The Quileute placed the chewed leaves on the inner bark of salmonberry and applied the poultice to sores and boils. The Cowlitz boiled the rhizome or infused the stems, cooled the liquid, and strained it for treating skin sores. The Quinault did the same

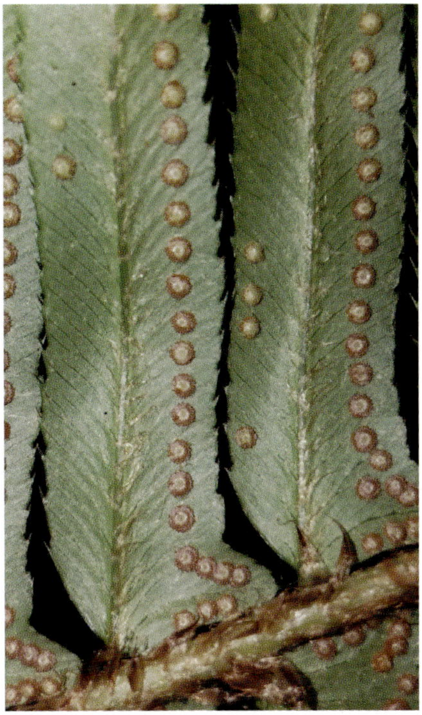

Spores of *Polystichum munitum* (Western Sword Fern)
Photo by Alan Rockefeller

and washed their hair with the water to cure dandruff. The spore sacs were scraped off the fronds and applied to burns (Moerman 1986).

Lummi women chewed the fronds to aid in childbirth (Gunther 1945). Various Indigenous groups chewed the fiddleheads and consumed the juice for uterine cancer.

Indigenous healers from Wsánec territory on the Sannich peninsula of Vancouver Island know sword fern as *stxálem* (*sthxélem*). The rhizomes were picked in spring, cooked in an open fire or steam pits, then peeled and eaten with grease or salmon eggs. The fronds were used to line the pits or baskets for picking berries or carrying food. One resident remembers clams were covered with fronds and salal (*Gaultheria shallon*) branches in steam pits.

The fronds were picked by two or four men to cover the floor for new dancers or used in initiation rites or bathing rituals (Turner and Hebda 2012). The Squamish, across the straits, call sword fern *tsxálem*, as do the Halkomelem and Strait Salish.

The Songhees are an Indigenous Salish people living on Vancouver Island. Early work by Turner and Bell (1971) reported that the Salish people used the fern spores to cure skin sores. The fern juice inhibits gram-positive and gram-negative bacteria, as well as mycobacterium species. McCutcheon et al. (1995) found moderate inhibition of both *Mycobacterium tuberculosis* and *M. avium*. The rhizomes show significant activity against strains of *Pseudomonas aeruginosa* K99.

In Japan, the fern *Polystichum ovato-palaceum* is known as *Tsuyanashiinode*. Potent 2,2-diphenyl-1-picrylhydrazyl (DPPH) radical scavenging activity was found by Masuda et al. (2012).

Tassel fern (*Polystichum polyblepharum*) gets its name from the innovative manner in which the ferns emerge in spring. After the crosiers (fiddleheads) begin growing, they bend over backwards so the unfolding tips of the fronds look like tassels. As they mature, the tassel effect disappears as they fully unfurl. The species name means "many eyelashes," referring to the numerous brown hairs on the stem.

Forest shield fern (*Polystichum pungens*) has been traditionally used in East Cape, South Africa, to treat wounds. A methanol extract exhibits significant inhibition of both gram-positive and gram-negative bacteria. An acetone extract only inhibited gram-positive species (Grierson and Afolayan 1999).

Polystichum semifertile fern exhibits significant antioxidant activity and inhibits xanthine oxidase, associated with gout (Chen et al. 2005; Ding et al. 2008).

Soft shield fern (*Polystichum setiferum* syn. *P. angulare*) is a European species. The species name *setiferum* means "with bristles," due to the soft bristly tips of the fronds. During the Victorian fern obsession, nearly 400 varieties were identified and named.

The spores of *Polystichum setiferum* have been studied for the phytoendocrine disruption posed by nonylphenol. This toxic compound is considered a high risk to human health and the environment, yet is widely used in cleaning products, adhesives, paints, varnish, food packaging, agricultural pesticides, and cosmetics.

As an endocrine disruptor, this toxin can interfere with normal estrogenic processes, potentially causing early menstruation in young girls and low sperm counts in men. Pregnant women should exercise caution when using any product containing this toxin.

Research by Esteban et al. (2016) suggest that this toxin can interfere with higher plant germination and poses a risk to riparian plants and irrigated crops. The fern also contains the volatile compounds (E)-2-hexenal and (Z)-3-hexenol, which add a green odor to absolutes used in perfumes.

Red-bearded Christmas fern (*Polystichum squarrosum*) when fed to laboratory animals, produces pathological changes and preneoplastic lesions almost comparable to those caused by bracken fern. This suggests it may not be safe for consumption.

Korean rock fern (*Polystichum tsus-simense*) is often offered as a house gift in Asian communities. The fronds are long-lived and used in the cut flower industry.

Eastern maidenhair fern (*Polystichum woronowii*) frond decoctions were used in traditional Iranian medicine, internally for hepatitis and externally for inflammation. Both the frond and rhizome contain polyphenols, anthraquinones, quinones, and cardiac glycosides. Research by Bahadori et al. (2015) found that frond extracts possess activity against *Staphylococcus aureus*, and rhizome extracts are active against *Escherichia coli*.

PRONEPHRIUM

Chinese Peng Fern Flatfork Fern Kidney Fern

The genus name may derive from the Greek *pro*, meaning "before," or "in front of," and *nephrós* meaning kidney. *Pronephros* refers to the first-formed anterior part of the human embryonic kidney. As of June 2022, there were over forty species.

Pronephrium megacuspe contains the flavonoids pronephrones A through D. The compounds are cytotoxic to ovarian cells of the tobacco cutworm (*Spodoptera litera*).

Chinese peng fern (*Pronephrium penangianum*) is used to relax muscles and tendons, promote blood circulation, reduce bleeding, and relieve pain and edema in patients with metabolic syndrome (Zhou et al. 2019).

The rhizomes of *Pronephrium penangianum* were analyzed, revealing six flavonoid glycosides (jixueqisus A through F) along with nine other known flavonoids. Jixueqisus A and B are red pigments, jixueqisus C is a dihydrochalcone glycoside, jixueqisus D a chalcone glycoside, jixueqisus E an aurone glycoside, and jixueqisus F a flavanone glycoside.

Four known flavane-4-ol glycosides, as well as abacopterin A, abacopterin C, eruberin A, eruberin B, and triphyllin A exhibit moderate anti-proliferation against MCF-7 (human breast), HepG2 (human hepatic), HCT-116 (human colon), and BGC-823 (human gastric) cancer cell lines (Shen et al. 2020). Abacopterin A and C and eruberin B are also found in *Abacopteris penangiana*, and were discussed earlier (see page 11).

Eruberin A, a 2,3-dehydroflavonoid, has been shown to be significant in the activation of pancreatic stellate cells (PSCs), the initial step in pancreatic fibrosis associated with chronic pancreatitis and adenocarcinoma.

Research by Tsang et al. (2015) found that eruberin A significantly suppressed fibrotic mediators in PSC cells, possibly by influencing the P13K/AKT/NF-κB signaling pathway. PSCs are involved in crosstalk between pancreatic cancer cells and the cancer stroma, contributing to tumor growth, metastasis, tumor hypoxia, immune evasion, and drug resistance (Bynigeri et al. 2017).

A nano drug delivery system incorporating a compound from the fern combined with Prussian blue nanoparticles exhibits strong antitumor effects in the treatment of cervical cancer. This combination suppressed B-cell lymphoma 2 (BCL2) and increased BCL2-associated X protein (BAX) levels, along with the cleaved caspase level, indicating enhanced apoptosis (Daniyal et al. 2020).

Pronephrium simplex syn. *Thelypteris simplex* hyperaccumulates yttrium (atomic number 39). This rare earth element is used in oncology radiation therapies. High-temperature super conductors of yttrium are used in magnets for MRI machines. Yttrium is also used to make synthetic diamonds and other gemstones. Yttrium-90 is widely used in radiation therapy for hepatic cancer, leukemia, and lymphoma. Yttrium is rarely found in its pure form, but often occurring in other minerals. It was first discovered by a Swedish army officer in 1787 who called it ytterbite, after the nearby village of Ytterby, meaning "outer village," located just a ferry ride away from Stockholm.

In Japan, the fern is known as single leaf bat fern, *hitotsuba-komori-shida*.

Pronephrium triphyllum contains triphyllin A, which exhibits strong anticancer activity against HepG (hepatoma) in vitro.

Triphyllin A (first mentioned on page 12) is also present in *Pronephrium penangianum* and *Abacopteris penangiana*.

PSILOTUM

Whisk Fern

The genus name *Psilotum* derives from the Greek *psilos*, meaning "smooth." In tropical climates, *Psilotum* species are epiphytic, but in more temperate climates, they may be found among rocks or even in plant pots in greenhouses.

Whisk fern (*Psilotum species*) is the only living vascular plant without leaves or roots, instead having hairlike rhizoids covered in round sporophytes that turn yellow when mature. The stem has tiny leaf-like projections called enations.

The prehistoric fern has developed a mycorrhizal relationship with its rhizoids that serves it well. In turn, of course, the fern provides the fungi with carbohydrates, produced by photosynthesis. The relationship is more parasitic than mutualistic, however. Or to be more accurate, a form of life known as mycoheterotrophy.

The underground gametophytes, containing male and female organs, rely on fungi for nutrients. When fertilized, they will grow into a new sporophyte, which then supports the fungi. It was formerly speculated that whisk ferns originated with rhyniophytes some 400 million years ago. However, recent DNA studies suggest a closer relationship with ferns, possibly related to the order adder's-tongue fern (Ophioglossales).

The common name *whisk fern* derives from the historical use of the stiff, upright stems as whisks and small brooms.

The fronds of the naked whisk fern (*Psilotum nudum*) exhibit antibacterial and antifungal activity (Rani et al. 2010). It has been traditionally used to treat constipation and respiratory complaints. The common name also references its early use, with several ferns tied into a small broom. *Nudum* from the Latin *nudus*, refers to the smooth, naked stem of the fern. Other authors suggest it means "bare naked," due to the lack of typical vascular plant organs as the fronds are minimal.

In Japan it is cultivated as a garden ornamental, with over one hundred varieties. The fern is known as *matsubaran*, meaning "pine-needle orchid."

In Hawaii, it is known as *moa*, due to the chicken foot-shaped stems. The spore powder has been traditionally gathered as a waterproof body powder to prevent or treat chafing, and it was taken internally to promote vomiting.

A traditional Hawaiian children's game, *moa nahele*, involved intertwining the branches and pulling them apart, and the winner would crow like a rooster (Pukui and Elbert 1986, 248). Today, the fern is also used in the preparation of traditional Hawaiian leis.

The fern contains the alkaloid psilotin and 3-hydroxypsilotin (glycoside). A water extract has shown to exhibit antibacterial inhibition against *Salmonella typhimurium*, *Escherichia coli*, *Proteus mirablis*, *Enterobacter aerogenes*, *Klebsiella pneumoniae*, and *Bacillus subtilis*, outperforming the control antibiotic erythromycin. Ethanol extracts inhibit *Trichophyton rubrum* (Rani et al. 2010).

The only other whisk fern is the epiphytic flatfork fern (*Psilotum complanatum*) which sometimes hybridizes with *Psilotum nudum*, forming *Psilotum* × *intermedium*.

NAKED FERN ESSENCE

This essence of *Psilotum nudum.* Guardian of the Rainbow Bridge, calls in one's personal guardian and protector spirits of the center, the place of the true soul self. It also anchors stellar light from the center into the fifth layer of the aura. Find as First Light Essence of New Zealand No.133 Naked Fern.

PTERIDIUM

Bracken Ferns   Eagle Fern   King Charles in the Oak

Geographic Range: British Columbia, Canary Islands, Colorado Desert, Eastern North America, Europe, Heilongjiang Province (China), Ireland, Japan, Liberia, Norway, Siberia, United Kingdom, Venezuela

Habitat: forests, grasslands, tropical regions, woodlands

Practical Uses: animal bedding, biofuel, bread flour, cheese packing, clover fertilizer, fire fuel, food, garden mulch, insect repellent, kitchen strainer, mulching potato mounds, dye, wreaths and flower arrangements

Medicinal Applications: arthritis, burns, chest pain, diarrhea, digestive issues, headaches, infections, insect bites, intestinal worms, mastitis, mosquito bites, nausea, rheumatism, spleen, stomach cramps, tuberculosis, uterine prolapse, weak blood

Warning: Bracken fern contains the toxin ptaquiloside, which is carcinogenic and mutagenic. Consumption of fresh bracken fern can release cyanide and cause harmful effects such as breakdown of vitamin B1 (thiamine), leading to potential poisoning in both humans and animals. Additionally, cattle that eat the fern may pass toxins into their milk. The fern should only be consumed after proper preparation, and its use as food is increasingly questioned due to associated health risks.

Bracken fern or eagle fern (*Pteridium aquilinum* syn. *Pteris aquilina*) is common worldwide. Some authors suggest it is the fifth most widely distributed weed species in the world!

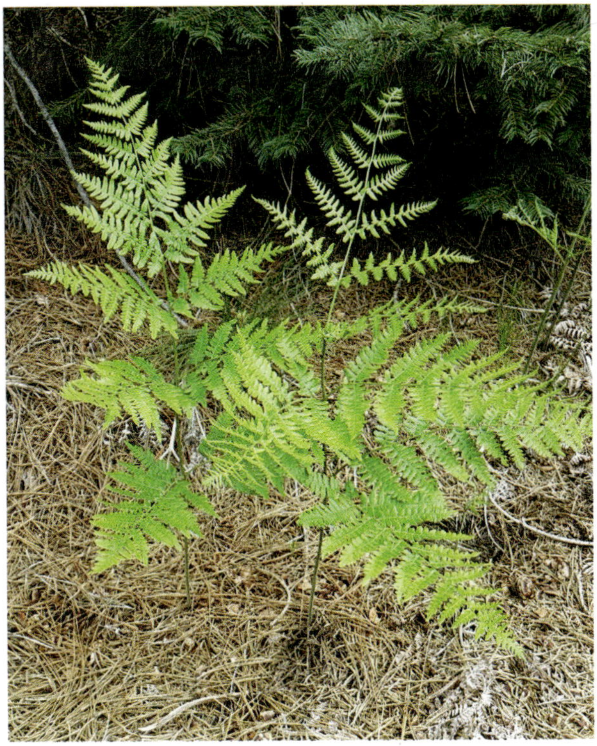

Pteridium aquilinum
(Bracken Fern)
Photo by Alan Rockefeller

It has long, underground stems with very large fronds, some up to six feet in height. Bracken may derive from the German *brache*, a term suggesting fallow or uncultivated land, or from the Swedish *bräken* or Danish *bregne* with similar meanings.

In Europe, the fern has been used for centuries as animal bedding, and garden mulch to inhibit insects and weeds. The species name *aquilinum* means "eagle-like" and was named by Linnaeus who called it eagle fern. Other names are King Charles in the oak, and in Scotland the fern is known as devil's hoof. When the bracken stem is sliced at an angle, it reveals a pattern resembling the Greek letter X, which is also the initial of Christ. Carrying the stem was said to keep one safe from evil spirits, witches, and werewolves. In Ireland, it is called the Fern of God, as the stem cut in three sections reveals the letters G, O, and D. That is a bit of a stretch, except perhaps for Christians. In Germany, the fern is known as *Christwurz* and in Norway *korsblom*. In West Sussex, the fern was cut above the root to predict the initial of a future husband or wife. It was believed that this fern was the only plant in Jesus' manger straw that did not produce beautiful flowers in celebration. And since then, it has not blossomed.

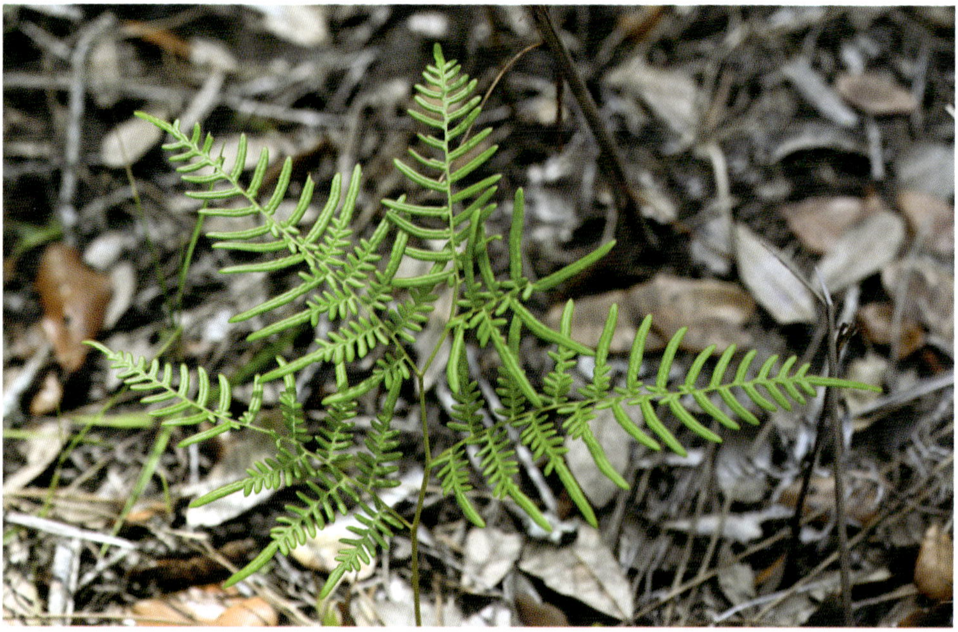

Pteridium caudatum (Southern Bracken Fern)
Photo by Alan Rockefeller

A witch could be banished by waving a frond, similar to the idea of protection from vampires by holding a cross. Shepherds in parts of Britanny and Normandy created fern crosses from the midrib to protect themselves and their flocks. In some Norman churches, such as the crypt of York Minister (built in 1171) and St. Peter's Northampton, there are carvings of unfolding fronds of this fern (Dowling 1900).

The dried root was carried by sailors as a remedy for seasickness. Culpeper (1652) recommended burning the ferns, noting that the smoke drove away serpents, gnats, and other noisome creatures. He writes, "The roots being bruised and boiled in mead and honeyed water, and drunk kills both the broad and long worms in the body and abates the swelling and hardness of the spleen. The leaves eaten, purge the belly and expel choleric and waterish humours that trouble the stomach." Ointments from the simmered roots were recommended for wounds, and the dried powder sprinkled into foul ulcers. The English herbalist Gerard (1597) notes "the root of Ferne cast into an hogshead of wine keepeth it from souring."

In Siberia and Norway, the uncoiled fronds were combined with two thirds of their weight of malt for a special ale.

The underside of frond produces a saccharine and glucose-rich nectar that provides immediate relief to mosquito and insect bites. When broken, the stems will produce sweet nectar for several days.

The author Gertrude Jekyll noted in the early 20th century that the scent of bracken fern is "like a smell of the sea as you come near if after a long absence." The root has been traditionally dried, baked, and then peeled and pounded into a powder. The powder, when kept dry, lasts for years as a source of starch (60%).

Early German settlers in Eastern North America recognized the uses of the fern. Johann Christopher Sauer wrote *Compendious Herbal* (1762–1778), translated into English by W. W. Weaver (2001). He highlighted that the bracken rhizome was noted for its placement under the tongue of a horse that has fallen. It will begin to urinate and stand up again, according to Mattioli (1500–1577), a famous Italian author and commentator on Dioscorides. If burned by fire, boiling water, or oil, the bracken rhizome is moistened and the juice pressed over the wound. Sauer recommended taking a dose of up to one quint of dry powder prior to consuming food as a vermifuge, particularly during the waning of the moon.

The phases of the moon influence intestinal parasites, such as pinworms, whipworms, roundworms, hookworms, and tapeworms. They are most active in laying eggs during a full moon, so treatment is best during the few days before and after this time.

In Eastern North America, the Lenape and Iroquois used the bracken fern externally for rheumatism, but mainly internally as a tea for weak blood, uterine prolapse, caked breast (mastitis), headaches, infections, tuberculosis, chest pain, and digestive issues including diarrhea, vomiting, nausea, and stomach cramps. The Iroquois also used the rhizome as witchcraft medicine, shaping it into a person in a coffin to cause death within ten days. They and the Delaware also prepared a tea from the rhizome to increase urine flow.

The Iroquois used the fern in a combination for treating prolapsed uterus or to make "good blood" after childbirth. The Ojibwa infused the rhizome for stomach cramps in women (Moerman 1986). The Cherokee used the fern for rheumatism, based on the signature of its emerging curled fronds, to strengthen bent muscles and limbs. The rhizome was used as a tonic and given for "cholera-morbus," meaning acute gastroenteritis with severe cramps, diarrhea, and vomiting (Moerman 1986).

The Montagnais used frond beds for comfort and relief from arthritis, and to strengthen babies' backs. Decoctions of the root were given for tuberculosis.

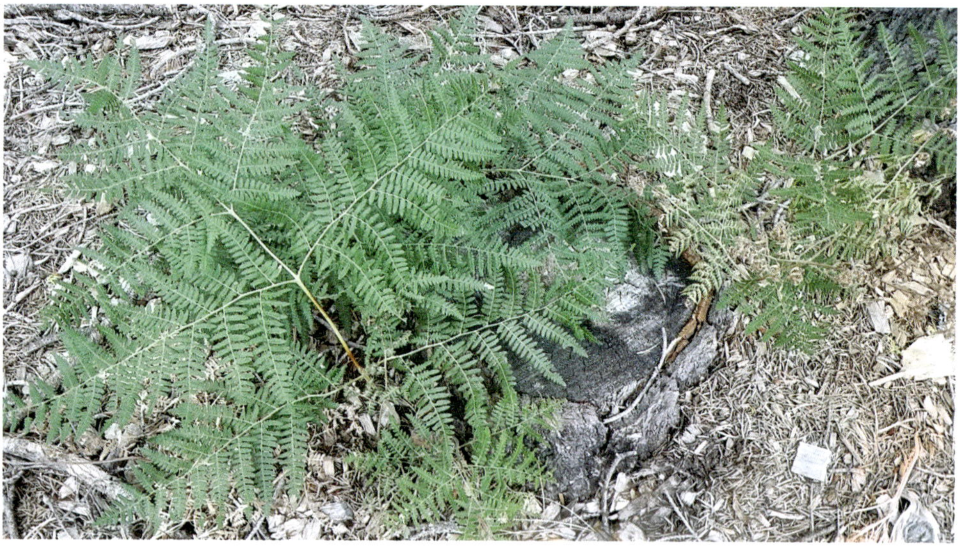

Pteridium aquilinum var. *pubescens* (Hairy Bracken Fern)
Photo by Alan Rockefeller

Hairy bracken fern (*Pteridium aquilinum* var. *pubescens*) was used in a similar manner by many Indigenous groups.

The Haida name is *hlt' anʔanda* (Newcombe 1901), while some people call it *ti tagansk'yaaw* or *ta.ansk'yaaw*. Basket weavers would use the fronds for design and the fern's rhizomes were dug in the fall, cooked in steam pits, and eaten with eulachon grease (*t'aaw*) (Turner 2014).

Indigenous people of British Columbia used the fronds to line steam pits, cover berry baskets, store dried food, wipe fish, and make bedding.

The Ktunaxa made sunshades from the fronds. In recent times, the Nuxalk use dead fronds, *qamats*, to mulch their potato mounds. This was due to the high content of potash, a valuable fertilizer for potatoes. It is estimated that fifty kilograms of dried fern ash yields one kilogram of potash.

Several groups, including the Nuu-chah-nulth, Kwakwaka'wakw, and Oweekeno, saved the fibrous leftovers from the edible rhizome and dried them as tinder for "slow matches." When contained in clam shells or tightly bound in cedar bark, the fibers would smolder for many hours, even days (Turner 1998).

The Nuu-chah-nulth and Ditidaht call the rhizomes *shitlaa* and the curled-up fronds *shitlmapt*. The Kwakwaka'wakw call the fern *sag*^{w} *m*, and the rhizome *ság*^{w} *emi*. The Oweekeno also refer to the rhizomes as *sag*^{w} *m*. The Wsánec of Vancouver Island know bracken fern as *sekán* (*seqéen*). The coarse-textured fern was used to clean fish, and then added to fire to create red-colored smoked food. The fall or winter rhizomes were cooked in pit fires or roasted over coals. The tough skin and fibers were removed, and the white starchy interior eaten with fish eggs or other fats. It was said to cause constipation when eaten alone. The fern is associated with snakes, with many taboos surrounding the digging of summer rhizomes (Turner 1973). Turner and Hebda (2012) record one version about Snake Island (a small Gulf Island in Canada). The story involves a young boy eating bracken fern without oil or fats. He became constipated and when laying down, snakes entered him. He was ultimately rescued by canoe, but Snake Island remains overrun by snakes to this day. The Nanaimo tribe, further north on Vancouver island, collected the dried central fibers as fire fuel or torches (Turner and Hebda 2012).

The fern was widely used by Indigenous people of the region now known as Western Washington. The Klallam, Snohomish, Squaxin, and Swinomish all know the fern as *tc'a'lacasats* or a close variation of the name. The rhizomes were harvested in the fall.

All tribes of the region roasted the rhizome, peeled it, and ate the starchy center. The Cowlitz ate the fronds raw, which was not advisable due to the fern's toxicity (discussed on page 268). They call the fronds *tc'a'latca*, and the rhizome *tc'a'kum*. The Skagit know the whole fern as *stca'lasets*, and the roots as *saq'* or *sqî'üx* (Gunther 1945).

The Cahuilla of the Colorado Desert boiled the young shoots for food. The flavor is said to be similar to asparagus. The Blackfoot ate the cooked stems and roasted roots. Moerman (2010) summarizes the use of the rhizome roasted or for bread flour by various Indigenous groups, including the Bella Coola, Hawknut, Hesquiat, Southern Kwakiutl, Montana, Nitinaht, Okanagan, Salish, Sierra, Upper Skagit, and Thompson (Nlaka'pamux). The Quinault call bracken fern *tsumxéxnix*, and the Nlaka'pamux *séʔaq*, similar to the Stl'atl'imx (Pemberton) name.

The fronds were consumed as a vegetable by Indigenous Alaskans, Atsugewi, Costanoan, Mahuna, and Ojibwa. The Sekani call it flat leaf, or *utoh dahbudzi*. The Northern Gitxsan refer to the fern as *demtx* (*damtx*) or *hap'ibaʔa*. The Costanoan decocted the rhizome or rubbed the raw root on the scalp for hair growth (Moerman 1986).

Moerman (1986) notes that the Costanoan threw fern tips into hot water to get rid of ants, and then added the water to soup stock, adding fern rhizome flour. It was said to taste similar to wild rice. In spring, male hunters would eat the fronds of the bracken fern, mimicking the diet of female deer to disguise

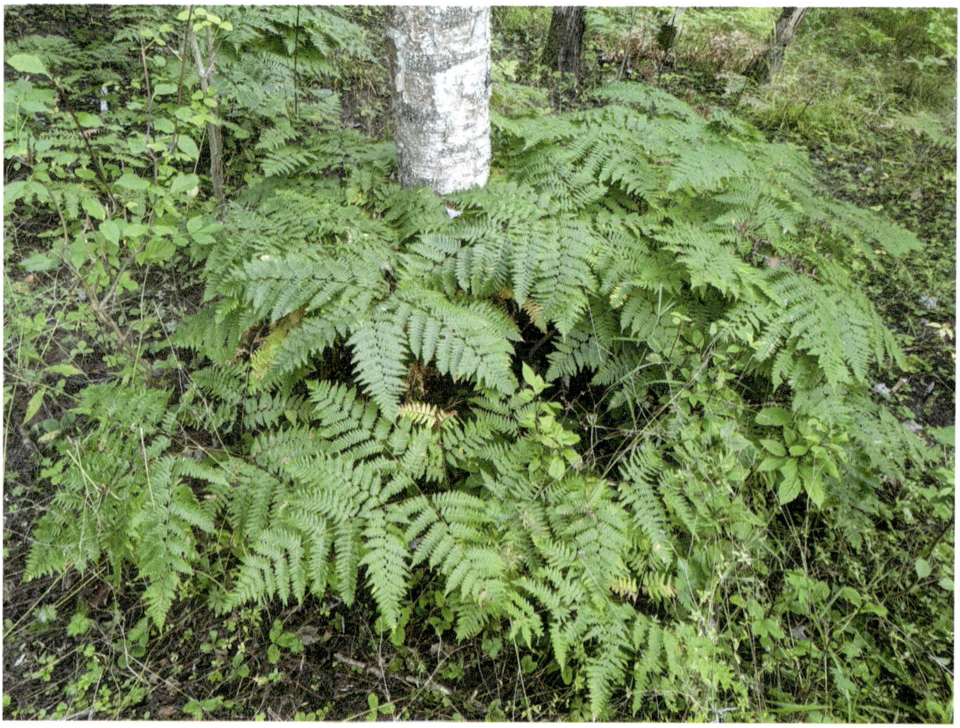

Pteridium aquilinum var. *latiusculum*
(Western Bracken Fern)
Photo by Alan Rockefeller

their scent, which allowed them to approach within six meters of the animals, making for an easy kill with bow and arrow.

In tropical Africa, fresh rhizome juice is combined with ginger root and taken orally as an aphrodisiac (Jansen 2004). However, it is important to note that fresh bracken fern is toxic. When mammals, including humans, chew the young fronds, they release cyanide and two hormones that cause insects to molt frequently until they die, and an enzyme thiaminase, which breaks down vitamin B1 (thiamine).

These ferns have been cooked and eaten for thousands of years, but the wisdom of this practice is being seriously reconsidered as the fern is believed responsible for the high rate of stomach cancer in Japan.

In the U.K., for example, a Bracken Advisory Commission is addressing the health risks for humans and livestock.

The myths surrounding fern "seed" and invisibility even led to "Operation Bracken," a secret British military operation in Iraq in 2005. No ferns were harmed in the campaign.

Bovine papilloma virus (BPV) is responsible for numerous benign and malignant diseases, including urinary bladder cancers and squamous cell carcinomas of the upper digestive tract. Ptaquiloside and other illudane glycosides inactivate cytotoxic T lymphocytes and natural killer cells, and over twenty-four genotypes of BPV are now recognized (Medeiros-Fonseca et al. 2021). This is a serious concern as cattle, sheep, and free-range pigs are susceptible to poisoning. Cows eating the fern can pass ptaquiloside through their milk. Although not proven useful in livestock, some research suggests that selenium supplementation may help prevent and fully reverse the immunotoxic effects of fern ingestion.

The fern contains the toxin ptaquiloside (PTA) but is still frequently eaten in East Asian countries. Work by Kim et al. (2023a) found that the concentration of PTA is reduced by up to 99% after boiling the fern for twenty minutes.

On the other hand, extracts of the fern have been found to induce cell cycle arrest and apoptosis in certain cancer cell lines. Work by Roudsari et al. (2012) evaluated the extracts against normal cells HDF1 (human dermal fibroblasts) and HFF3 (human foreskin fibroblasts), as well as TCC (a rare human kidney cancer), NTERA2 (human embryo cancer), and MCF-7 (breast cancer) cell lines. Ptaquiloside is cytotoxic to HGC (human lymphoma-related gastric cancer cell lines) (Yurdakok et al. 2014). A polysaccharide, also derived from the fern, exhibits immune modulation and antioxidant activity (Zhao et al. 2022c).

At high concentrations, the extract caused DNA damage and apoptosis, but induced cell cycle arrest in the G2/M phase at mild concentrations, depending on the cell type and tumor origin. This suggests that bracken fern extracts may be a potent source of anticancer compounds requiring further exploration.

A study by Rasmussen (2021) examined the presence of ptaquiloside in fern-based food products and in traditional medicine. Boiling and drying reduces the toxin content somewhat but cannot remove it completely. The author found crosiers from the United States contain no ptaquiloside nor pterosin B, suggesting potential for commercial production of toxin-free fronds.

Like many other ferns, bracken fern contains phytoecdysterones. Fresh ferns contain 0.25 to 0.53 µg/kg, compared to 0.1µg/kg in spinach. The fern also contains the volatiles (E)-3-hexenoic acid and (E)-2-hexenoic acid with herbal and fruity notes. The essential oil contains compounds with anticancer properties (Nwiloh et al. 2014).

Despite its potential risks and benefits, bracken fern is used in various industrial contexts, including soapmaking, glass, leather tanning, and other industries around the world. In Venezuela, the fronds are used for packing and wrapping heads of curing cheese. Bracken fern is considered a valuable biofuel when made into bales or briquettes. The leftover ash contains up to 50% potassium when harvested in June, with a pH of 12 or higher. Yields of 250 kilograms of potassium per hectare can be achieved. In pot trials, ash harvested and burned in September increased clover yields by 150% and the number of root nodules by 140%.

The fern has been used throughout the world as a natural dye. Early colonists at Plymouth Rock produced an olive-green dye using alum and copper as mordants.

A dark yellow dye for tartans was produced in the Scottish Highlands, while in Ireland, a light green color was obtained from the young fronds. In France, silk was dyed a gray green using ferrous sulphate and cream of tartar. American weavers used the rhizome to obtain black wool, the fiddleheads with alum for a yellow-green dye, and lime-green with chrome mordant. The Washoe, Mono, and Yokut of California boiled the rhizome for black dye, but untreated rhizomes gave a brown pattern material used for weaving.

In Liberia, the fern is known as "strainer weed," due to the layering over the top of a kettle to serve as a strainer. The stems are woven into wreathes and flower arrangements (Hartley 1962). The ferns can be decocted and sprayed on aphids attacking cultivated roses.

In Japan, the almond-flavored starch known as warabi is used in pastries. The local name is *kusasotetsu*, and the fern is boiled and then deep-fried in batter or slowly cooked in soy sauce. *Warabimochi* is a popular traditional dessert. In China, the fern is called *juecai* and is eaten in soups and stews. On a recent visit to Atlanta, Georgia, I enjoyed delicious cooked bracken fern served by robots in an upscale Korean-style restaurant.

On the Canary Islands, one of my personal favorite vacation spots, the rhizome was dried and ground into flour after roasting. With or without barley this is known as *gofio*, an easily digested flour, similar in taste to wild rice. It was considered a survival food.

Bracken fern is harvested for food in China, with an annual output of two thousand tons from Heilongjiang province alone.

However, it is important to note that bracken fern is considered carcinogenic and mutagenic. Gastric cancer rates in Japan, North Wales, and Venezuela are associated with eating this fern.

Bracken Fern (*Pteridium aquilinum*) has undergone three comprehensive modern remedy provings by Doris Drach and Franz Swoboda (2005), Marie Geary (2000), and Lisa Griffiths (1998). See the Homoeopathie-wichmann denmark website.

Symptoms associated with bracken fern include bursting headache, rash on scalp, heartburn worsened by eating or lack of appetite leading to forgetting to eat, and feelings of being overwhelmed by day-to-day life. Emotional symptoms include weeping, suicidal despair, violent aggression wishing to kill others or self, claustrophobia, and choking pressure in the throat that cannot be removed by swallowing.

> Bracken fern (*P. aquilinum*) is for a detached, distant feeling, desire to hide, disinclined to make small talk. Patient is irritable, short tempered, negative with thoughts of verbal and physical violence. Lethargy, woolly, fuzzy, inability to focus. Delusions of being a failure, haggard and old, with erratic behavior in traffic. Dreams of death of horses from starvation, being criminal, underground activities, theft and capture, or of traveling. Sensations of head constriction, sensitive sense of smell. Ovarian pain alternating sides (Drach and Swoboda 2005).

To summarize Lisa Griffiths's proving: The most striking characteristic of bracken is its capacity for rapid and invisible travel. What is particularly intriguing about the recurring theme of India in the dreams is that the spores are exceptionally good at colonizing poor and devastated land. The huge rhizome that moves outward and engulfs everything in its path is evoked in the dream of the octopus in the sea pool, which the dreamers cannot escape as it approaches with its tentacles reaching out to consume her.

Its increased vigour, aggression, and suppressive abilities when exposed to higher light intensity are echoed in several incidences of uncharacteristic behavior of some provers. There are great waves or rushes of energy and outbursts of anger and aggression towards others who threaten or obstruct in some way. There is also claustrophobia, with an overwhelming desire to be out in the open air. Attempts to control bracken involved the beating, cutting, spraying, and burning of the fronds, which are the "head" of the plant body. It seems quite extraordinary therefore to find repeated head pain, and dreams of the tops of heads being cut off or blown off. Lisa Griffiths proved with three females and one male at 30 C in 1998.

Griffths suggested there will be big issues around being overwhelmed and being overwhelming. The rage is overwhelming, the person is overwhelmed with rage, nausea is an overwhelming feeling, cancer is a disease that "takes over." Things come in waves, waves of nausea, waves of rage. Waves are overwhelming.

Marie Geary proved with five females and one male at 6C, 12C, and 30C in 2000.

Drach and Swoboda note, "Symptoms like the deep bone pains of this carcinogenic, neurotoxic plant makes us think of the syphilis miasm" (*Mosses and Ferns* 2021). Doris Drach and Franz Swoboda offer a case history in the same journal. They suggest that the core attribute of the bracken persona is adapting instead of showing oneself, remaining hidden, secret, feelings of shame, and keeping silent when the group is in charge, and showing spontaneous violence instead of open conflict.

The full version with exact proving symptoms can be found in *Documenta Homeopathica* 27: "*Adlerfarn, Pteridium aquilinum, eine arzneimittelprüfung mit hindernissen*" (in German).

BRACKEN FERN ESSENCE

This essence of *Pteridium aquilinum* is very helpful for those who fear their psychic sensitivity and feel pressured to accept and use these gifts. These imbalances are often caused by a left-brain-dominant approach to living with a need to search out and examine the artistic and creative side. It is useful to use this remedy alongside a program of artistic and creative endeavors.

Bracken essence combined with alcohol and water is recommended for feelings of frustration and defeat. It is particularly helpful for people who have difficulty expressing their true selves to the world. They often play the childlike role in life, frustrated by their inability to accept their own power. This essence has also been found useful in cases involving cancer. Find at Bailey Essences.

The related spider bracken fern (*Pteridium arachnoideum*), found in South America, contains toxic ptaquiloside and its degradation product, pterosin B, in both its mature green fronds and new sprouts.

Similar to bracken fern, it is responsible for bovine enzootic hematuria and upper alimentary squamous cell carcinoma in cattle (Ribeiro et al. 2020).

Longud (*Pteridium brownseyi*) fronds from the Western Himalayas are used as a vegetable, while the young fronds are used to treat asthma (Khoja et al. 2022).

Austral bracken (*Pteridium esculentum*) contains ptaquiloside, ptesculentoside, and caudatoside, highly unstable, and toxic norsesquiterpene glycosides. The species name *esculentum* means "edible."

In Māori mythology, this bracken was believed to originate from Tanepukkupukurangi, a son of Rangi, the Sky Father, and Papa, the Earth Mother. One of their sons, Haumia, clung to Rangi as hair on his back, but when they separated, he fell down and buried himself in the Earth Mother. Only the hair on his head (the fern fronds) remained visible, which were harvested for food and as a medium for consulting spiritual beings.

A piece of fern stalk was used when a man could not attract a desired woman, burying it in a spot near her house, so that she would walk over it daily, in hopes of attracting attention (Riley 1994).

The rhizome of this fern, known to the Māori as *aruhe*, was second only to kumara (sweet potato) as a staple food. "Fern root was the food of war, kumara that of peace" (Riley 1994). The dry rhizomes contain about 60% starch after separation from the fibers.

Hairy bracken fern (*Pteridium revolutum*) contains pterosin A and its derivatives, which help regulate blood sugar homeostasis and protect pancreatic β-cells, preventing their death, and reducing reactive oxygen species (ROS) (Chen et al. 2015). However, the fern itself is carcinogenic and should not be consumed.

PTERIS

Amakusa Fern
Blunt-lobed Fern
Brake Ferns
Huguenot Fern
Many-leaved Fern
Ribbon Ferns
Saw-leaved Bracken
Silver Lace Fern
Spider Fern
Table Fern

Geographic Range: Africa, Asia, Europe, Malaysia, Malay Peninsula, North America, Papua New Guinea, Philippines, South America, Southwestern China

Habitat: cemeteries, forests, limestone-rich ground, old shady walls, temperate zones, tropical regions

Practical Uses: cosmetics for spot and freckle reduction, decoration, houseplant, phytoremediation (copper and arsenic), traditional tea, wedding garlands

Medicinal Applications: Alzheimer's disease prevention, antibacterial, antitumor, anti-inflammatory, antioxidant, atherosclerosis, cancer, cytotoxic, diarrhea, dysmenorrhea, kidneys, menstruation, liver, melanin, neurodegeneration, neuroprotection, platelets, prostate, snakebites, toothaches, tuberculosis

Warning: The consumption of certain ferns in large quantities, such as *Pteris species* containing ptaquiloside, may lead to neoplastic lesions or other adverse effects, particularly in livestock and possibly humans.

There are about 300 species of *Pteris* worldwide. The genus name comes from the Greek word for fern, meaning "feathery."

Various extracts from *Pteris* exhibit antitumor, antifungal, and antibacterial activity, as well as inhibition of platelet aggregation and anti-inflammatory properties.

Cretan brake, also known as table fern or ribbon fern (*Pteris cretica*), is an evergreen species native to Europe, Asia, and Africa. It is widely cultivated by nurseries for either gardens or as a potted houseplant. In traditional Iranian medicine, the fronds were applied topically for their antibiotic benefits. The fern contains triterpenoids, saponins, alkaloids, polyphenols, and tannins. Bahadori et al. (2015) found rhizome extracts inhibit *Staphylococcus aureus*.

The fern exhibits antimicrobial and antioxidant activity (Saleem et al. 2016) and the aerial part of the plant contains nine identified pterosins, including creticolacton A and 13-hydroxy-2(R),3(R)-pterosin L, which both showed cytotoxicity against HCT-116 (human cancer) cell lines (Lu et al. 2019).

Research by Luo et al. (2016) identified several sesquiterpenoids and identified four with lipid-lowering effects in 3T3-L1 adipocytes, more potent than berberine in reducing triglycerides. One compound exhibited the most potent activity and probably reduces total triglycerides through the regulation of LXRa/b by activating liver X receptors (LXRs) via hydrogen bonding.

The fern contains ptercresions A–C, callisalignene D, berberiside A and D, and creoside I. Ptercresion B and C, as well as callisalignene D, show moderate protection against liver cell injury (Hu et al. 2022). Berberiside A and D exhibit antiproliferative activity against A549 (lung), HepG2 (hepatic), and

MDA-MB-231 (breast) cancer cell lines (Dong et al. 2022).

The varietal hardy ribbon fern (*Pteris cretica* var. *nervosa*) is widely used in TCM to treat hepatitis.

Work by Xiong et al. (2022) identified luteolin-7-O-rutinoside, which significantly reduces levels of alanine aminotransferase and aspartate aminotransferase levels.

The compound also significantly reduces the release of tumor necrosis factor-α, interleukin-6, and interleukin-1b and inhibits P13K/AKT/AMPK/NF-κB pathways. It also increases superoxide dismutase and glutathione levels, helping to reduce oxidative stress.

The dried fronds of the related *Pteris cretica* ssp. *laeta* is a popular traditional tea in Southwestern China. Extracts from this species were evaluated for possible benefits in the prevention of Alzheimer's disease both in vitro and in vivo on amyloid precursor protein/presenilin (APP/PSI) in mice. The extracts diminished oxidative stress damage and apoptosis of Ab-induced HT22 cells and improved cognitive deficits, while also reducing pathological injury and inflammatory response in mice.

Pterosin A (PA) and other compounds were identified in the ethanol extract of this fern. PA reduced apoptosis of APP-overexpressing neural stem cells and promotes their proliferation and neuronal differentiation. Both the extract and PA promoted hippocampal neurogenesis by activating the Wnt signaling pathway (Shi et al. 2023).

The consumption of thickleaf brake fern (*Pteris deflexa*) and striped brake fern (*P. plumula*) by cattle in Northwestern Argentina has been related to bleeding neoplastic lesions in the mucosa of urinary bladder. This is probably due to the presence of ptaquiloside and pterosin B in the ferns (Micheloud et al. 2017).

Amakusa fern (*Pteris dispar*) is an evergreen perennial native to the temperate zones of South China and Eastern Asia. Ethanol extracts (95%) of this fern revealed diterpenes, including geopyxin B and E. Both compounds exhibit moderate cytotoxicity against Bel-7402 (hepatoma) and HepG2 (hepatic) cancer cell lines (Wang et al. 2017b).

The fern compound *ent*-11α-hydroxy-15-oxo-kaur-16-en-19-oic acid exhibits inhibition of melanin synthesis by suppressing tyrosinase gene expression. This suggests potential use in cosmetics for reducing spots and freckles associated with aging (Kuroi et al. 2017).

Water extracts of the sword brake fern or silver lace fern (*Pteris ensiformis*) reduce inflammation and modulate the immune system (Wu et al. 2005a).

Caffeic acid and hispidin derivatives from the fern inhibit low-density lipoprotein (LDL) oxidation and reactive oxygen species (ROS) production, suggesting its potential for preventing atherosclerosis (Wei et al. 2007). The compound (2S,3S)-12-hydroxypterosin, isolated from the fern, exhibits activity against *Mycobacterium tuberculosis* (H37 Rv) in vitro (Chen et al. 2013). Pterisolic acid A and C, pterosin P, and dehydropterosin B were later obtained from slender brake or silver lace fern (*Pteris ensiformis*) for the first time (Zhang et al. 2016c). Various dihydrochalcones and diterpenoids from the fern exhibit anti-inflammatory activity. One compound exhibits moderate activity against HCT-116 (colon), HepG2 (liver), and BGC-823 (gastric) cancer cell lines (Shi et al. 2017). Pterosin B, and 2R,3R-pterosin L 3-O-glucopyranoside exhibit cytotoxicity against HL60 (leukemia) cancer cells (Chen et al. 2008).

Flavonoid-enriched extracts exhibit antiproliferative activity against MCF-7 (breast) and HepG-2 (hepatoma) cancer cell lines (Hou et al. 2020).

The fern has been traditionally used to treat dysmenorrhea (Mannan et al. 2008). In the Philippines, a decoction of this fern was used for dysentery (Quisumbing 1951). On the Malay Peninsula, the astringent frond juice was used to clean the unhealthy tongues of children, and the rhizome juice was applied to glandular swellings of the neck (Burkill 1966). In parts of Papua New Guinea, the fern is used to regulate menstruation (Blackwood 1935).

The fronds of *Pteris henryi* contain henrin A, an *ent*-kaurane diterpene. When trialed against a panel of dental biofilm, cancer lines, and HIV, it exhibited potential against HIV with an IC_{50} value of 9.1 μM (Li et al. 2015).

Hardy ribbon fern (*Pteris laeta* syn. *P. cretica* ssp. *laeta*) has been widely used in TCM to treat nervous system diseases. Some pterosin sesquiterpenes found in the *Pteris* species show neuroprotective activity. Work by Cheng et al. (2023) found that pterosin B, derived from the fern, exhibits significant neuroprotection against glutamate excitotoxicity, enhancing cell viability from 43.8% to 105%. Pterosin B works on the downstream signaling pathways of glutamate excitotoxicity rather than blocking activation of glutamate receptors directly. It restores mitochondria membrane potential, and alleviates intracellular calcium overload, eliminates cellular ROS, and downregulated Kelch-like ECH-associated protein expression 2.5-fold. This suggests pterosin B could be a potential candidate to treat neurodegenerative diseases.

Pteris melanocaulon is a hyperaccumulator of copper and arsenic, suggesting its potential use in the phytoremediation of abandoned mine sites.

Spider brake fern (*Pteris multifida* syn. *Pcynodoria multifida*) is native to East Asia but naturalized in parts of the United States. It is also known as spider fern, huguenot fern, and saw-leaved bracken. The fern is found on old shady walls and masonry around cemeteries.

The name Huguenot fern originated from the (false) belief that it was collected in a Huguenot cemetery in Charleston, South Carolina, in 1858. The fern has since become invasive.

Fern decoctions are used in TCM to relieve symptoms of benign prostatic hyperplasia (BPH). The fern is known in TCM as *feng wei cao* and is available as a granule preparation.

A double-blind clinical trial with 155 patients was conducted by Xue et al. (2008). One hundred and eight patients received the granules (5 grams) twice daily and 47 patients were given Proscar (5 mg) once daily for three months. Both groups showed significant improvement of symptoms associated with BPH, with the fern group experiencing fewer adverse reactions.

Pterosin C 3-O-β-D-glucopyranoside and 4,5-dicaffeoylquinic acid, isolated from the fern, show significant selective cytotoxicity against KB (epithelial carcinoma) cells (Harinantenaina et al. 2008). Their research also identified other compounds, including wallichoside, which decreases BMI1 protein (B-cell-specific Moloney murine leukemia virus insertion region 1) protein levels in HCT116 (human colon) carcinoma cells and inhibits sphere formation of Huh7 (human hepatocellular) carcinoma cells, indicating it diminishes the self-renewal capabilities of cancer stem cells (Kaneta et al. 2017). A flavonoid extract of the fern given to mice for sixty days decreased the prostate index of BPH. A ninety-day sub-chronic toxicity test showed no safety issues (Dai et al. 2017).

Rats fed a high-cholesterol diet along with lyophilized fern powder were compared with those given β-sitosterol. Results showed that the spider brake powder lowered the hyperlipidemic levels (Wang et al. 2010a). Twelve pterosin glycosides have been identified in the roots of the fern.

One of these compounds showed moderate cytotoxicity against HCT-116 (human colon) cancer cell lines and induced the upregulation of the caspase-9 and procaspase-9 levels. Multifidosides A and B, isolated from the whole plants, exhibit cytotoxicity against the Hep-G2 (human liver) cancer cell line with an IC_{50} value less than 10 μM (Gee et al. 2008). Dehydropterosin B, isolated from the fronds, shows potent cytotoxicity against PANC-1 (human pancreatic), and

NCI-H446 (human small-cell lung) cancer cell lines (Ouyang et al. 2010).

Early work by Woerdenbag et al. (1996) identified two diterpenes from the fronds that exhibited moderate cytotoxicity against Ehrlich ascites tumor cells. Two novel pterosin dimers, named bimutipterosins A and B were isolated from the whole fern by Liu et al. (2011). Both exhibit cytotoxicity against HL60 (human leukemia) cell lines.

Multikauranes A and B, as well as multifidarin A, exhibited cytotoxicity against a panel of five human tumor cell lines (Ni et al. 2015). Crotonkinins E and F, and pterisolic acid A and C show moderate activity against HCT-116 (human colon), HepG2 (human liver), and BGC-823 (human gastric) cancer cell lines. Total flavonoids inhibited the growth of transplanted H22 (hepatoma) tumors in mice (Yu et al. 2013).

Alzheimer's disease involves cellular neuroinflammation and is among others associated with activated microglia. Various *ent*-kaurane diterpenes, derived from the fern rhizome, exhibit significant nitric oxide inhibition in lipopolysaccharide (LPS)-activated BV-2 microglia cells (Kim et al. 2016).

Blunt-lobed fern (*Pteris obtusiloba*) contains various pterosins and dimers, including obtupterosins A through C. The latter three compounds exhibit cytotoxicity against HCT-116 (human colon) cancer cells but were inactive for α-glucosidase inhibition (Peng et al. 2020). The species name means "blunt-lobed," referring to the round edges of the fern's leaves.

Many-leaved fern (*Pteris polyphylla*) is used in TCM and exhibits in vitro mutagenic activity (Lee and Lin 1988).

Both crude extracts and gold nanoparticles of striped brake fern (*Pteris quadriaurita*) possess antiproliferative and apoptosis-inducing properties against MCF-7 and BT47 breast cancer cell lines (Rautray et al. 2018).

The fresh frond juice is mixed with toddy (the sap of *Phoenix sylvestris*) and taken as a drink early in the morning before food for two to three days to correct irregular menstrual cycles (Rout et al. 2009).

Half-pinnate brake fern (*Pteris semipinnata*) is known as *ban bian qi* in TCM and is widely used to treat toothaches, diarrhea, jaundice, and snakebites. In Singapore, the common name for the fern is *paku pelanduk*. Ethanol extracts of the fern exhibit cytotoxic activity against HepG2 (liver), SPC-A-1 (lung), MGC-803 (gastric), CNE-2Z (nasopharyngeal), and BEL-7402 (liver) carcinoma cell lines. The active antitumor compound appears to be an α,β-methylene cyclopentanone moiety (Li et al. 1998).

Pteisolic acid G, derived from the fern, inhibits cell viability and induces apoptosis in HCT116 (human colorectal) cancer cell lines (Qiu et al. 2017). The compound *ent*-11α-hydroxy-15-oxo-kaur-16-en-19-oic acid (also referred to as 11aOH-KA or 5F), is an important compound found in *Pteris semipinnata* and its cognate, Amakusa fern (*Pteris dispar*) (see page 275). This compound may protect mammalian cells from oxidative stress and aging (Batubara et al. 2020).

Other compounds of importance, with binding affinity to protein receptors, are β-caryophyllene and cyclobarbital. Beta-caryophyllene is a terpene, which acts as a cannabinoid and binds to CB2 receptors. It is generally regarded as safe (GRAS) and is used as a food additive. When combined with paclitaxel, beta-caryophyllene inhibits colorectal carcinoma in vitro.

A water extract of the fronds was shown to exhibit high anti-melanogenic activity. Research by Hamamoto et al. (2020) found approximately 2.5% of 11α OH-KA in the dry leaf. Treatment with the water extract suppressed pigmentation of hair in mice.

This small-scale study suggests the potential development of future products to treat patients with hyperpigmentation conditions, such as melasma.

The compound *ent*-11-α-hydroxy-15-oxo-kaur-16-en-19-oic acid, derived from the fern, inhibits the proliferation of HO-8910PM (metastatic ovarian) cancer cell lines (He et al. 2005). The compound also induced apoptosis in HT-29 (human colon) cancer cells by increasing both p38 and inducible nitric oxide synthase (iNOS) levels (Chen et al. 2004).

Ent-11α-hydroxy-15-oxo-kaur-16-en-19-oic-acid (5F) exhibits cytotoxicity and apoptosis on HepG2 (liver) carcinoma cell lines (Li et al. 2010) and induced apoptosis in SGC-7901 (human gastric) cancer cell lines by activating mitochondrial apoptotic pathways (Chen et al. 2011a).

Earlier work by Liu et al. (2005; 2009) found that the compound induced cell death in the FRO (anaplastic thyroid) cancer cell line.

Three breast cancer cell lines (MCF-7, MDA-MB-231, and SK-BR-3) were treated with *ent*-11α-hydroxy-15-oxo-kaur-16-en-19-oic-acid. The compound inhibited proliferation and induced apoptosis in all cell lines, decreasing the expression of Bcl-2 and increasing expression of Bax, Bak, and caspase-3 (Wu et al. 2017a). Semipterosins A through C were shown to exhibit minor anti-inflammatory activity.

5F significantly reduced the volume of implanted pathological scars in nude mouse models (Zhang et al. 2007).

Cisplatin is synergistic with 5F in reducing proliferation and inducing apoptosis in NCI-H23 (human non-small lung) cancer cell lines (Li et al. 2017b). 5F nanoparticles have been shown to inhibit nasopharyngeal carcinoma (CNE2) tumors transplanted into mice, with minimal side effects reported (Liu et al. 2021a).

Rhizomes of giant brake fern (*Pteris tripartita*) are used in parts of Africa and Indonesia in an unspecified manner involving childbirth.

Brake fern, or ladder brake fern (*Pteris vittata*), absorbs copper and heavy metals, such as arsenic, from contaminated soils. Numerous scientific articles highlight its role in phytoremediation, including a recent publication by Guo et al. (2023a).

The fern is native to Asia, Europe, tropical Africa, and Australia. It loves limestone-rich ground and has been introduced into regions like California, Texas, and Southeastern United States gardens.

Methanol extracts of this fern exhibit antioxidant activity and significantly inhibit 4NQO-induced mutagenicity in *Escherichia coli* PQ 37. Reduced viability of MCF-7 (breast) cancer cells was also noted (Kaur et al. 2014).

An ethyl acetate fraction of the fern contains the polyphenols epicatechin and umbelliferone.

Research by Kaur et al. (2017) found that the fraction alleviated 2-acetylaminofluorene–induced liver damage in rats by modulating the expression of p53 and restoring hepatic enzymes and normal liver architecture after treatment. Water extracts were also tested by Kaur et al. (2023) and found to modulate genotoxicity and oxidative stress, as well as induce apoptosis in human MCF-7 (breast) cancer cell lines.

Umbelliferone is widely present in numerous medicinal plants and has been cited over 4,000 times on PubMed. A recent study found that umbelliferone and *Lactobacillus acidophilus* combined in pre-treatment reduced methotrexate-induced intestinal injury. This significant adverse effect limits its clinical use (Hassanein et al. 2023).

Hexane extracts exhibited cytotoxicity against MCF-7 (breast cancer) cells through apoptosis and autophagy (Mohany et al. 2023).

The endophyte *Diaporthe ueckerae*, associated with the fern, contains ueckerchalasins C and D, which display cytotoxicity against HeLa (cervical/epithelial) and HepG2 (hepatoma) cancer cell lines. Ueckerchalasin C also exhibits activity against *Staphylococcus aureus* and MRSA (Gao et al. 2022).

Ethanol extracts of Wallich's giant table fern (*Pteris wallichiana*) alleviate induced ulcerative colitis in mice by enhancing the intestinal barrier through the upregulation of tight junction proteins, including ZO-1 (zonula occludens). The fern extract reduces intestinal inflammation by suppressing the TLR4/MyD88/NFκB signaling pathway (Tao et al. 2022).

SHAKING BRAKE FERN ESSENCE

This essence of *Pteris tremula* facilitates inner healing, peace, and stillness at the soul level after experiences of disempowerment trauma or deep sorrow that have impacted the soul and are locked into cellular memory. It helps the unconscious mind release the belief that it is not safe to relax or let one's mental guard down. Find as First Light Flower Essences of New Zealand No. 39 Shaking Brake Fern.

PYRROSIA

Dragon's Scale Fern   Felt Ferns   Tongue Ferns

Geographic Range: China, Korea, Mongolia
Habitat: temperate zones, tropical regions
Practical Uses: food source for insects
Medicinal Applications:, anti-inflammatory, antioxidant, antibacterial, asthma, bronchitis, cytotoxicity, diabetic nephropathy, diuretic, dysentery, cancer, gout, herpetic keratitis, hyperuricemia, kidneys, nephrolithiasis, pneumonia, osteoporosis, pyelonephritis, rheumatism, schistosomiasis, skin, snakebites, urinary infections, urolithiasis, vaginal bleeding

Pyrrosia and other fern genera support various insects, including butterflies and moths.

A rare, fern-spore-feeding micro-moth larvae *Stathmopoda tacita* has been rediscovered after over a century (Shen and Hsu 2023). The consumption of fronds is widespread, but consuming fern spores as a source of food is less common in the animal kingdom. The genus name derives from the Greek *pyrrhos* "red" referring to the color of the frond sporangia.

Three *Pyrrosia* species (*P. sheareri*, *P. lingua*, and *P. petiolosa*) are used in TCM for urinary infections, urolithiasis, hematuria, abnormal uterine bleeding, cough, and asthma caused by damp heat and phlegm in lungs (Xiao et al., 2017).

All three fronds, known in TCM as *shiwei*, show slightly different chemical profiles, suggesting more specificity would result in more scientific benefits. Chlorogenic acid, mangiferin, and eriodictyol-7-O-glucuronide is present in most species of this genera.

Chlorogenic acid is widely present in a number of medicinal plants. It has a wide range of benefits due to its antioxidant, anti-inflammatory, antibacterial, antiviral, hypoglycemic, lipid-lowering, cardio-protectant, antimutagenic, anticancer, and immune modulating properties (Miao and Xiang 2020).

Mangiferin benefits have been discussed under other ferns (Imran et al. 2017).

Eriodictylo-7-O-glucuronide is a potent inhibitor of the dengue virus (Dwivedi et al. 2016).

Bare tongue fern (*Pyrrosia calvata*) contains a number of compounds, including hemipholin, mangiferin, diploptene, and chlorogenic acid. In a rodent model of crystal-induced kidney injury, mangiferin reduced the deposition of calcium oxalate crystals and alleviated kidney tissue damage (Pan et al. 2021).

Felt fern (*Pyrrosia davidii* syn. *P. gralla*) contains stigmasterol, ursolic acid, sucrose, and mangiferin.

Fronds from TCM's *pyrrosiae folium* contain six compounds with binding affinity to regulate target genes affecting prostate cancer, including tumor necrosis factor and hepatitis B signaling pathways (Guo et al. 2022b).

An earlier clinical trial by Rodgers et al. (2015) involving eighteen healthy males who consumed 1,500 milligrams of the fern extract for seven days found no benefits for the treatment of calcium oxalate kidney stones. A rather short trial and why were healthy subjects used? Why not individuals with a previous renal history or those with recently diagnosed kidney stones?

The rhizome of three-finger tongue fern (*Pyrrosia hastata*) inhibits matrix metalloproteinase-9 (MMP-9) activity, with results slightly lower than epigallocatechin gallate (EGCG) from green tea. This suggests potential application in antiaging cosmetics.

Tongue fern (*Pyrrosia lingua*) is widely used in Korea and China for treating pain, vaginal bleeding, and urolithiasis (kidney stones). Ethanol extracts from the fern suppress osteoclast differentiation by acting on osteoclast precursor cells, suggesting benefits in preventing or treating postmenopausal osteoporosis (Jang et al. 2022a).

Both petroleum ether and dichloromethane fractions of the fern exhibit benefits in preventing and reducing calcium oxalate stone formation in a rat study. The fractions contained caffeine, citric acid, and tartaric acid, which may have played a role in reducing renal oxalic acid and inhibiting stone formation (Wang and Yang 2018).

The fern powder and extract, which contain quercetin and kaempferol, may play a role in reducing nephrolithiasis (Xu et al. 2022). In rat models, the fern significantly reduced levels of urine oxalic acid, urine calcium, and osteopontin. It also decreased populations of various gut bacteria, including *Oxalobacter formigenes*, *Bacteroidetes*, *Bifidobacterium*, and *Fecalibacterium*.

The leaves of this fern contain flavonoids, including mangiferin and isomucoside.

During the COVID-19 pandemic, numerous medicinal plants were tested for their potential to prevent or treat this devastating virus. In one study by Shoaib et al. (2021), this fern and three other plants (out of 200) were found to possess anti-SARS-CoV effects.

In a clinical trial involving seventy-eight cases of herpetic keratitis caused by herpes simplex virus type 1, eye drops made from this fern and *Prunella vulgaris* led to a cure in thirty-eight patients, with improvement in thirty-seven others. Only three patients did not experience benefits (Zheng et al. 1990).

A study on diabetic, high-fat diet rats showed that the fern extract significantly decreased serum creatinine, blood urea nitrogen, and total urinary protein levels. It also improved renal pathology and downregulated the inflammatory markers 1L-6, TNF-α, and IL-1β. The serum reductions in advanced glycation end products (AGEs) and RAGE ligands suggests potential benefits in diabetic nephropathy (Liu et al. 2018b).

The essential oil of this fern exhibits significant activity against *Staphylococcus aureus*. The major compounds were 2,4-pentadienal, phytol, and nonanal (Fan et al. 2020a).

Pyrrosia petiolosa is a hardy fern found in the temperate zone five of China, Korea, and Mongolia. *Xiao shi wei* is valued in TCM for treating acute pyelonephritis, chronic bronchitis, and bronchial asthma. Ethanol extracts from this fern exhibit antioxidant activity (Hsu 2008).

Petiolide A, barbatic acid, and kaempferol have been identified in a 95% ethanol extract. Its diuretic benefits are due to the presence of kaempferol, which is comparative to orally bioavailable inhibitors (Lang et al. 2021).

Barbatic acid, also present in some lichens, is cytotoxic to adult worms of *Schistosoma mansoni* (Silva et al. 2020b). Schistosomiasis affects approximately

260 million people in tropical regions. The drug praziquantel has saved millions of lives, but drug-resistance is becoming more common in recent years.

Ethanol extracts of the dried fronds exhibit significant anti-inflammatory activity but low toxicity against A549 (lung cancer) cell lines. Various solvent extracts inhibited eight out of thirteen tested microorganisms (Cheng et al. 2014).

An ethyl acetate extract of the fern shows strong inhibition of *Staphylococcus aureus* by decreasing the expression of human leukocyte antigen (HLA) and staphylococcal enterotoxin A (SEA) virulence genes. The authors suggest eugenol likely contributed to the antibacterial activity (Song et al. 2017). Another study found that an ethyl acetate extract relieved the inflammation of *Staphylococcus aureus*–induced pneumonia in mice (Cheng et al. 2021).

A rat study found that fern extracts ameliorated induced urolithiasis by inhibiting oxidative stress and inflammation, notably attenuated renal tissue injury (Zhou and Wang 2022).

The fern exhibits significant diuretic activity without any obvious toxicity in a rat study. The Na-Cl cotransporter inhibition of methyl chlorogenate was greater than hydrochlorothiazide, a standard drug known for its side effects (He et al. 2023).

The essential oil contains 2,4-pentadienal (12.5%), phytol (10.5%), and nonanal (8.6%) as main constituents. The oil possesses broad antimicrobial activity, especially against *Shigella flexneri* and *Staphylococcus aureus* (Fan et al. 2020b).

Dragon's scale fern (*Pyrrosia piloselloides*) is a facultative mild hemiparasite fern. The fronds were extracted with water and methanol, with the methanol extract exhibiting antiproliferative effects on HeLa (human cervical carcinoma) cells, but neither extract showed any significant effects on apoptosis. The methanol extract revealed the presence of 5-hydroxymethylfurfural (23.1%), allopurinol (8.66%), and 3,5-dihyroxy-6-methyl-2,3-dihydropyran-4-one (7.41%) (Sul'ain et al. 2019).

Allopurinol, an analog of hypoxanthine, has been used as a drug for over fifty years to treat gout and hyperuricemia. About 2% of patients develop a skin rash, hepatitis, or interstitial nephritis.

Five finger Taiwanese tongue fern (*Pyrrosia polydactylis*) inhibits matrix metalloproteinase-9 (MMP-9) activity in WS-1 cells after ultraviolet B irradiation. This suggests potential use in anti-aging skincare products (Lee et al. 2009).

Shearer's felt fern (*Pyrrosia sheareri*) also contains mangiferin, diplotene, and chlorogenic acid. An analysis of the beneficial therapeutic effects of the fern, based on 1,148 cases of bacillary dysentery, was conducted by Zhao (1985).

Fifty plants used in TCM for rheumatic disease, were screened for antioxidant activity. This fern rated in the top six, based on its highest antioxidant capacity and total phenolic content (Gan et al. 2010).

The fronds of narrow-leaved felt fern (*Pyrrosia tonkinensis* syn. *Pyrrosia stenophylla*) have been steam-distilled and yield twenty-eight compounds, including trans-2-hexenal (22.1%), nonanal (12.8%), limonene (9.6%), phytol (8.4%), 1-hexanol (3.8%), 2-furancarboxaldehyde (3.5%), and heptanal (3.1%). The oil showed good antibacterial activity against all tested strains (Xin et al. 2016).

RUMOHRA

Leatherleaf Fern

For leatherleaf fern see *Arachniodes adiantiformis* syn. *Rumohra adiantiformis* syn. *Polypodium adiantiforme* on page 44.

SADLERIA

Rasp Fern Red Pig Fern

Amaumau or rasp fern (*Sadleria cyatheoides*) inhabits old lava flows and wet forests in Hawaii. The young fronds and pith are eaten steamed or roasted.

When young, the fronds and stems are bright red and block UVA radiation. The stems are up to ten centimeters in diameter and were traditionally used to produce a red dye. The cortex was mashed, and the red juice was boiled down by dropping hot stones in a gourd.

Palapala'ā, or *palae*, a common lace fern (*Sphenomeris chinensis*) in Hawaii, also produces a red-brown dye (Fosberg 1942).

The fern was used for "female ailments" and its fronds were braided into leis.

The related red pig fern (*Sadleria pallida* syn. *S. hillebrandii*) is native to Hawaii, where it is also known as *'ama'u*, *'aamau'i'i*, *àma'uma'u*, and *pua'a 'ehu'ehu*. The fronds are up to a meter long, and the stems have long been used for ornamental plaiting. The stipe base and brownish "wool" around the growing tip is known as *pulu*.

A large export market for pulu existed in the late 19th century in Hawaii for pillow stuffing and packing material. Fortunately, better fibers were found elsewhere, saving the fern from being harvested to extinction. Extracts from the spores damage K562 (human premyeloid leukemia) cells (Simán et al. 2000).

SALVINIA

Butterfly Fern	Salvinias
Eared Water Moss	Water Butterfly Wings
Giant Water Fern	Water Mosses/Watermosses
Kariba Weed	Water Splangles

Geographic Range: Africa, Antarctic waters, Asia, Europe, South America

Habitat: aquatic environments, catfish ponds, coal mine runoff streams, contaminated water sources, dairy wastewater, freshwater lakes, mine sites, ponds, small lakes

Practical Uses: bee attractant, bio-decolorization, dietary supplement for shrimp farming, green pesticide, phytoremediation, wastewater treatment

Medicinal Applications: antibacterial, antimicrobial, antioxidant, anti-biofilm, anti-inflammatory, cancer, cardioprotectant, cytotoxic, hepatoprotective, hypotensive, immune-modulating, liver protection, neuroprotective, urease inhibitory

The unique structure of *Salvinia* ferns, which traps an underwater air layer on the fronds, has inspired biomimicry applications. By combining shape memory polymer and hydrophilic silicon dioxide microspheres, researchers have developed a synthetic structure with potential uses in medical, industrial, and biological sectors, particularly for controlled gas containment and release in liquid phases (Tricini et al. 2017; Zhang et al. 2022c). The fern's frond hairs have a peculiar 3D and hierarchical shape that retains oxygen.

Staphylococcus aureus bovine mastitis affects cattle health and dairy production, leading to reduced milk yields and higher mortality rates.

Extracts from the root of eared water moss or butterfly fern (*Salvinia auriculata*) exhibit antimicrobial and anti-biofilm activity. A teat dip formulation shows promising results, equally effective as commercial antimicrobials in reducing bacterial counts (Purgato et al. 2021). The use of antibiotics can restrict milk sales, leading to economic losses. A fern extract herbal soap has been developed to help control bovine mastitis infections. This aquatic fern may also be valuable in post-treatment of dairy industry wastewater (Schwantes et al. 2019).

Salvinia auriculata extracts exhibit liver protection against methotrexate-induced injury in mice. The use of this drug is common in numerous human cancer malignancies. The extracts also exhibit antibacterial activity against *Acinetobacter baumannii* (Attallah et al. 2022). The pathogen is implicated in numerous infections, including pneumonia, sepsis, urinary tract infections, burn and wound infections, necrotizing fasciitis, meningitis, osteomyelitis, and endocarditis. Resistance to carbapenem antibiotics is increasing every year (Ramirez et al. 2020).

Giant or lobed salvinia (*Salvinia biloba*) may help with phytoremediation of carbendazim-contaminated water (Loureiro et al. 2023). Carbendazim is a systemic broad-spectrum fungicide widely used on golf courses and tennis courts. It is also used on various fruit and nut crops, including citrus, bananas, strawberries, and macadamia. High doses of carbendazim can cause infertility and destroy testicles, as shown in laboratory animals (Aire 2005).

Interestingly, carbendazim has completed Phase 1 clinical trials for multidrug-resistant cancer treatment (Goyal et al. 2018). Recent research has also found that vermicomposting with earthworms can help transform this aquatic fern into a benign and safe organic fertilizer (Tabassum et al. 2023).

Asian watermoss (*Salvinia cucullata*) may be useful for phytoremediation of copper-polluted environments (Das and Goswami 2017). This aquatic fern is fast-growing and has a hardy physiology that may be useable in some mine sites and to clean up pulp and paper effluent (Das and Mazumdar 2016).

It may also be a beneficial dietary supplement for white shrimp farming. The enclosed water environments make the shrimp susceptible to the bacteria *Vibrio parahaemolyticus*, and fern extracts as functional feed improves the growth, immune health, and disease resistance of farmed shrimp (Santhosh et al. 2023). The gram-negative bacterium is found in estuary, marine, and coastal environments, and is the leading cause of human acute gastroenteritis following consumption of raw or undercooked seafood. I love shrimp but due to personal ecological and environmental concerns, I restrict my own diet to wild Argentinian shrimp harvested in cold Antarctic waters.

Giant water fern (*Salvinia molesta*) is considered one of the world's worst aquatic weeds. The species name *molesta* gives a hint of its aggressive growth behavior.

This water fern contains glycosides, methyl benzoate, hypogallic acid, caffeic acid, paeoniflorin, pikuroside, saviniol, salviniside I-11, and numerous abietane diterpenes.

Hypogallic acid was shown to decrease blood pressure and induce the dilation of aortic rings in rats. The hypotensive activity is related to the release of nitric oxide from the vascular endothelium, opening of K(ATP) and K(Ca) channels in the vascular smooth muscle cells (Leeya et al. 2010).

Paeoniflorin is found in the root of *Paeonia* species, some of them being extremely important TCM herbs. PubMed lists over 1,400 citations of medicinal benefits of this compound, including cancer, depression, immunity, inflammation, pulmonary fibrosis, neurodegeneration, atherosclerosis, multidrug-resistant microbes, diabetes, colitis, osteoporosis, cholesterol, menopause, and post-operative pain.

Pikuroside is found in the ayurvedic herb *Picrorhiza kurroa*, known as *kurro*, *kutki*, or Indian gentian. Gentian roots have a bitter nature. The plant exhibits hepatoprotective, antioxidant, anti-inflammatory, anticancer, and antimicrobial properties.

Saviniol and several diterpenes show selective cytotoxicity to human cancer cell lines (Li et al. 2013b). A glycopyronase derivative exhibits antioxidant and urease inhibitory activity (Naheed et al. 2021). Urease is involved in numerous pathologies such as urolithiasis, pyelonephritis, urinary catheter encrustation, hepatic encephalopathy, and peptic ulcers.

The fern shows efficacy in the tertiary treatment of domestic wastewater. This suggests investment in the use of green technology to reduce pollution in natural water systems (Mustafa and Hayder 2021).

The fern has been shown to remove 97% of the antibiotic ciprofloxacin from contaminated water, including catfish ponds, which prevents the accumulation of antimicrobials in fish, making them safer for human consumption (Kitamura et al. 2023). Cipro, as it is commonly known, is used in fish and shellfish aquaculture and increases the risk of drug-resistant bacterial infections in humans.

Other potential uses include bio-decolorization of water-containing artificial dyes and the mitigation of glyphosate levels.

Some regions of the world spray this toxic herbicide to kill mosquito larvae, but the compound is also present in various GMO crops including corn, soy, and canola. A study by Gomes et al. (2023) found that the aquatic fern removed up to 49% of glyphosate from water sources. Glyphosate sprayed on wheat, to ripen it faster and dessicate it, removes any dietary benefits from this valuable cereal for millions of people. The turn to gluten-free products, with their own health concerns, may be an intestinal microbiome disruption rather than a true gluten-sensitivity. The thickening agent, carrageenan, found in gluten-free products, can cause intestinal dysbiosis.

Giant water fern or kariba weed (*Salvinia molesta*) and *Salvinia natans* contain methyl benzoate, which has a pleasant odor. In parts of the world, it is used to attract orchid bees for pollination and has shown potential as a green pesticide (Bunch et al. 2020). The compound exhibits mild toxicity to cultured human cell lines.

A 1% spray of methyl benzoate is highly effective as an acaricidal and repellent against spider mites (*Tetranychus urticae*) without affecting bean, cucumber, pepper, or tomato plants in greenhouse settings (Mostafiz et al. 2020).

Blue-green algae (*Microcystis aeruginosa*) blooms are common on ponds and small lakes and are at times associated with agricultural run-off and seasonal warming of water. Work by Zhang et al. (2016) found that an aquaculture of *Salvinia natans* (above) has a powerful inhibitory effect on the blue-green algae by changing the structure of algal cells and enzyme activity.

Floating water moss or water butterfly wings (*Salvinia natans*) hyper-accumulates lithium. With increasing use of lithium batteries, more waste will undoubtably be discharged into ecosystems, making this fern a valuable resource for phytoremediation.

Natansnin, an unusual antioxidant isolated from the fern, has been found to protect rat liver tissue against carbon tetrachloride-induced oxidative stress and cell degeneration (Srilaxmi et al. 2010).

Water splangles or common salvinia (*Salvinia minima*) helps remove metals in coal mine runoff drainage into streams and wetlands (Lindell et al. 2016).

SPHAEROSTEPHANOS

The genus name refers to the yellow glands which fringe the indusium. Various extracts of *Sphaerostephanos unitus* exhibit antibacterial, antioxidant, anti-inflammatory, and antidiabetic properties, depending on the solvent used (Johnson et al. 2020).

STENOCHLAENA

Vine Ferns

The genus *Stenochlaena* includes only a half-dozen species.

The vine fern *Stenochlaena chusanum* syn. *Odontosoria chinensis* is used in TCM, possibly due in part to its high flavonoid content. In temperate climates, flavonoid and phenolic content is highest in February. The fronds are much higher in flavonoid content, but the rhizome extract is slightly higher in phenolics and antioxidant activity. The extracts of both exhibit higher inhibition against tyrosinase than arbutin, the control, and when harvested in February, they exhibit the highest anti-proliferative activity and apoptosis against K562 (human myelogenous leukemia) cell lines (Wu et al. 2017c).

Swamp vine fern (*Stenochlaena palustris*) is a popular vegetable in Malaysia, known as *paku nyai*, and is cooked and eaten like a fiddlehead and flavored with shrimp paste. The Tagalog name for the fern is *dilimán*. The Diliman district in Quezon City, Philippines, is named in honor of this fern. *Palustris* is Latin for "of the marsh."

It is a food enjoyed in India; in parts of Indonesia, it is flavored with garlic. In the southern parts of Indonesia, it is known as *kalakai*. In Vietnam it is known as *dot choai* and served in soups, salads, and stir fry dishes. In Malaysia and India, the fronds are used to treat fever, skin diseases, ulcers, and stomach aches (Benjamin and Manickam 2007). The frond stems are strong and durable, and when soaked in the ocean and then dried, they are used for fish traps, rope, or baskets.

Water fractions of the edible and medicinal *Stenochlaena palustris* possess antioxidant activity and inhibit α-glucosidase, suggestive of benefits in managing blood sugar dysfunction. The water extract contains phenolics and hydroxycinnamic acids (Chai et al. 2015b). Extracts of this fern exhibit antifungal activity against *Aspergillus niger* (Sumathy et al. 2010) and the fronds exhibit activity against gram-positive bacteria.

In Borneo and Sumatra, the fern has been traditionally used to heal infected wounds and is taken internally to treat diabetes.

The fronds extracted with ethyl acetate possess antioxidant, anti-plasmodium, and antibacterial properties. Modest inhibition was noted by Hendra et al. (2022) against *Vibrio parahaemolyticus*, *Listeria monocytogenes*, and *Salmonella typhimurium*.

The young fronds exhibit an anti-butyrylcholinesterase activity, when extracted with hexane, while the mature fronds are more inhibitory when extracted with methanol. This suggests the popular vegetable has potential benefits in the prevention and treatment of Alzheimer's disease (Chear et al. 2016).

TECTARIA

Broad Halberd Fern **Broadleaf Tectaria** **Button Fern**

Geographic Range: Antilles, Caribbean, India, Nepal
Habitat: tropical regions, forests
Practical Uses: breast milk production aid, disinfectant, food, cotton whitefly resistance
Medicinal Applications: antibacterial, antihyperlipidemic, anti-inflammatory, antidiabetic, antioxidant, antiproliferative, antipyretic, antiviral, cytotoxic, dysentery, gums, respiratory issues, rheumatism, wounds

The *Tectaria* genus is quite large with over 200 species, mostly from tropical regions. It is a taxonomically confusing fern genus with movement of species in and out of the genus on a regular basis, due in part to DNA analysis.

Button fern (*Tectaria cicutaria*) is a large fern, reaching over a meter in height. It is native to the Antilles in the Caribbean Sea, as well as India and other tropical regions.

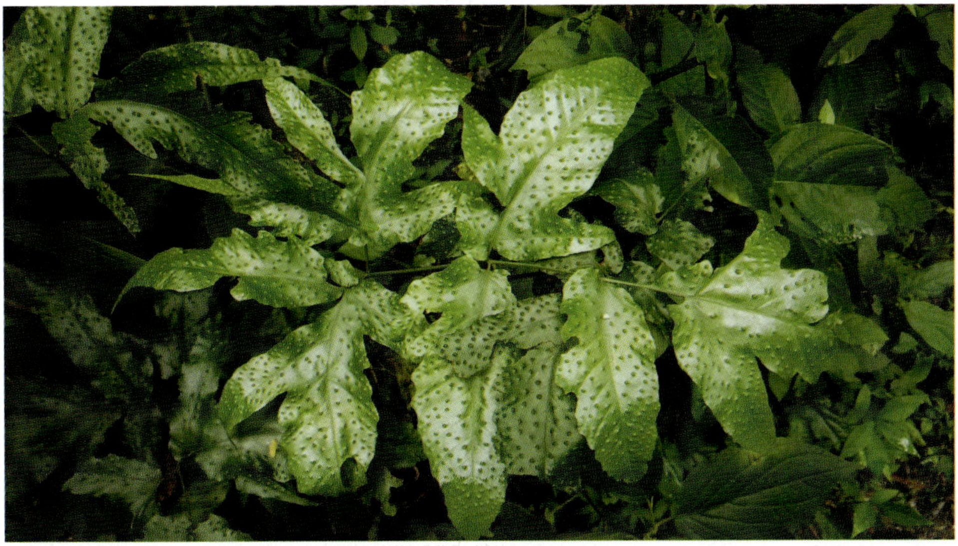

Tectaria heracleifolia (Broad Halberd Fern)
Photo by Alan Rockefeller

In ayurvedic medicine the rhizome has been traditionally used to treat rheumatic pain, chest complaints, breathing issues, burns, sprains, poisonous bites, bee stings, tonsilitis, toothaches, gum infections, cuts, and wounds.

A decoction of the fresh rhizome is used to treat irregular bowel movements, infectious diarrhea, and dysentery. Stomach aches are resolved by ingesting fresh boiled stems.

Water extracts exhibit anti-inflammatory activity both in vitro and in vivo in rodent edema models, with results comparable to diclofenac (Choudhari et al. 2013). Ethanol extracts of the rhizome exhibit antioxidant activity and cytotoxicity against K562 (human leukemia) cell lines by inducing apoptosis (Karade and Jadhav 2017).

The fern *Tectaria coadunata* syn. *T. macrodonta* has been traditionally used in Nepal for medicine, and recent studies by Reddy et al. (2020) suggest numerous medicinal benefits.

The species name *coadunata* means "to unite" or "combine," possibly referring to the contiguous lobes of a leaf united at the base. In parts of India, the fern is known as *kukkutnakhi*. Extracts are used to treat irritable bowel syndrome and inflammatory conditions of the colon. For chest colds, the leaves are combined with honey and foresters use leaf paste to alleviate centipede bites and bee stings.

Extracts show a higher scavenging potential against free radicals than hydrogen peroxide molecules. They exhibit antibacterial activity against *Shigella flexneri*, *Staphylococcus aureus*, and *Salmonella typhi* and show antiproliferative activity against three human leukemia cell lines (KG1, MOLT-3, and K-562) (Reddy et al. 2020).

The ferns contain procyanidin A, eriodictyol-7-O-glucuronide, and luteolin-7-O-glucoronide. Eriodictyol-7-O-glucuronide is a potent inhibitor of dengue virus NS3 protease (Dwivedi et al. 2016). A-type procyanidins may be inhibitors of glycation. Glycation of protein can produce advanced glycation end products (AGEs), and α-dicarbonyl compounds like methylglyoxal. These have potential health risks associated with diabetic complications (Zhao et al. 2022a).

Inhibitory activity against cholinesterase and tyrosinase was observed in a study by Shretha et al. (2019), along with moderate cytotoxicity against OV-2008 (ME-180 derivative) and BxPC3 (pancreas) cancer cell lines.

Rhizome powder exhibits antihyperlipidemic activity in high-fat diet-induced Wistar albino rats. Triglycerides and very low-density lipoproteins were significantly reduced (Mori et al. 2016).

The edible fern *Tectaria macrodontia* syn. *T. coadunata* contains a gene that expresses the protein Tma12, which, when transferred to cotton, makes the plants resistant to whitefly infestation. Tma12 exhibits resistance to whitefly and viral diseases (Yadav et al. 2019). The protein may be a lytic polysaccharide monooxygenase. The species name *macrodontia* means "giant or abnormally large teeth." Filtered water from the rhizome and frond stem is given in India for constipation.

The young fronds of broadleaf tectaria (*Tectaria latifolia*) are lightly boiled and added to the diet of new mothers to ensure adequate production of breast milk (Bourdy and Walter 1992).

Manivannan and Johnson (2020) researched the phenolic, tannin, triterpenoid, flavonoid, and sterol compounds in *Tectaria paradoxa*. Extracts displayed anti-inflammatory, antidiabetic, and cytotoxic properties.

In India, disinfectants are made from the roots of *Tectaria wightii*.

THELYPTERIS

Eastern Marsh Fern
Maiden Ferns
New York Fern
Queen's Veil
Mountain Fern
River Fern

Geographic Range: Caribbean Islands, Central America, Eastern North America, India, Pacific Northwest (U.S.), Southern United States, Washington (U.S.), Aleutian Islands

Habitat: acidic soil, marshes, swamps, stream banks, tropical regions, wastewater ponds

Practical Uses: ground cover, phytoremediation (arsenic, copper, zinc)

Medicinal Applications: abrasions, cancer, Chagas disease, chest conditions, cuts, female reproductive issues, lesions, neutralize poisonwood, parasites, wounds

An endophytic *Nodulisporium* species has been isolated from the broadleaf maiden fern (*Thelypteris angustifolia*) found in a Central American rainforest.

When grown in the lab, the endophyte produces various volatile organic compounds, the most abundant being 1,8-cineole. It also produces the cyclohexane propyl, a common ingredient in diesel fuel.

These volatiles inhibited *Phytophthora cinnamomic* by 100% and caused the death of *Phytophthora palmivora*, *Rhizoctonia solani*, and white mold (*Sclerotinia sclerotiorum*) (Hassan et al., 2013).

Phytophthora cinnamomic is responsible for the sudden death of American chestnut, fraser fir (*Abies fraseri*), grown as Christmas trees, and native oak trees found between South Carolina and Texas. Its pathogenic cousin *Phytophthora palmivora* attacks palm and coconut trees. *Rhizoctonia solani* is destructive to potatoes, and other commercially important crops. White Mold (*Sclerotinia sclerotiorum*) is one of the most damaging and economically problematic pathogens, affecting hundreds of plant species worldwide.

Thelypteris arida syn. *Cyclosorus aridus* leaves and rhizomes are prepared in India into a paste for lesions and abrasions.

The Argentinian, rough hairy maiden fern (*Thelypteris hispidula*) contains polygodial, isopolygodial, drimenin, and isodrimenin.

Polygodial induces changes in mitochondrial membrane permeability in CoN (colon), MCF-7 (breast), and PC-3 (prostate) cancer cell lines (Montenegro et al. 2014).

Isodrimenin exhibits activity against the trypomastigote form of *Trypanosoma cruzi*, the cause of Chagas disease (Muñoz et al. 2013).

Kunth's maiden fern or southern shield fern (*Thelypteris kunthii* syn. *T. macrorhizoma*) is found in swamps and stream banks in the Southern United States and various Caribbean Islands.

The fern was boiled and used to clean and close cuts and wounds, and to counteract poison (Eldridge 1975). The New York fern (*Thelypteris noveboracensis* syn. *Parathelypteris noveboracensis*) is an aggressive ground cover, especially when given lots of water, partial sun, and acidic soil. Its rhizomes emit allelopathic compounds toxic to various trees, especially members of the *Prunus* (cherry) genus. The related river fern (*Thelypteris normalis*) also excretes allelopathic compounds that inhibit the growth of other ferns.

Eastern marsh fern (*Thelypteris palustris*) rhizome was used by the Iroquois of Eastern North America for female reproductive issues (Moerman 1986). *Palustris* means "of the marsh." The Marsh fern moth *Fagitana littera*, feeds exclusively on this fern.

The fern also exhibits potential for phytoremediation of arsenic contamination (Anderson et al. 2011). The fern can be used to remove copper and zinc, up to ten times the legal limit, from wastewater ponds associated with pork production. Copper and zinc are used as feed additives to control enteric bacterial infections (Stroppa et al. 2020).

Queen's veil mountain fern (*Thelypteris quelpaertensis*) is found on the Pacific Northwest from Washington to the Aleutian Islands. The fern has one disjunct population in Gros Morne National Park in Northwestern Newfoundland, thousands of kilometers away. I had the good fortune to travel there in the mid 1970s. The scenery is spectacular, reminiscent of the fjords of Norway.

Protoapigenone, a flavonoid derived from Mariana maiden fern (*Thelypteris torresiana*) inhibits the expression of Epstein-Barr virus lytic proteins by preventing transactivation of Zta (BZLF1, ZEBRA) thereby preventing proliferation (Tung et al. 2011).

The herpes family virus is related to various health conditions. A recent study showed that approximately 20% to 25% of patients with multiple sclerosis (MS) have antibodies in their blood that bind tightly to both a protein from the Epstein-Barr virus (EBV) called EBNA1, and a protein found in the brain and spinal cord called the glial cell adhesion molecule. Infection with EBV increases the risk of developing multiple sclerosis (MS) by 32-fold.

Protoapigenone induces apoptosis in human prostate cancer cells by arresting the S and G2/M phases, both in vitro and in vivo (Chang et al. 2008b). This flavonoid exhibits cytotoxicity against MDAH-2774 and SKOV3 (human ovarian) cancer cell lines, both in vitro and in vivo, with low toxicity in mice (Chang et al. 2008a).

Previous work by Lin et al. (2007) showed that protoapigenone is cytotoxic against five human cancer cell lines: HepG2 (hepatoma), Hep3B (liver), MDA-MB-231 and MCF-7 (breast), and A549 (lung). The fern contains flavotorresin and multiflorin C.

TRICHOMANES

Kidney Fern Killarney Fern Scale Edge Bristle Fern

Scale edge bristle fern (*Trichomanes membranaceum* syn. *Lecanium membranaceum*) is a tiny perennial fern found in the Southern Coastal United States, the Caribbean, and extending from Mexico down to Bolivia.

The Kofan people of Ecuador know the fern as *tusana-si-sehe-pa*. It is boiled and the liquid is used to bathe the head to relieve headaches (Russo 1992).

Fronds from the New Zealand kidney fern (*Trichomanes reniforme*) contain five glycosides, as well mangiferin and 6'-O-acetylmangiferin (Wada et al. 1995).

The latter compound shows anti-inflammatory activity and significantly reduces intracellular lipid accumulation by enhancing lipolysis via AMPK activation, and by upregulating β-oxidation. This suggests potential therapeutic applications for obesity and related conditions (Sim et al. 2019).

The fern also shows in vivo activity against ascitic fibrosarcoma in Swiss mice and in vitro cytotoxicity. Extracts have been found to exhibit in vitro activity against HIV (Guha et al. 1996).

Killarney fern (*Trichomanes speciosum* syn. *Vandenboschia speciosa*) is endemic to Europe but is considered vulnerable and threatened.

VITTARIA

Shoestring Ferns

Narrow stiff shoestring fern (*Vittaria angust-elongata*) contains over thirty compounds.

5,7-dihydroxy-3',4',5'-trimethoxyfavone, found in the fern, exhibits moderate cytotoxicity against the human lung and central nervous system carcinoma cell lines. The closely related eupatilin (5,7-dihydroxy-3,4,6-trimethoxyflavone) attenuates ischemic damage and apoptosis in pancreatic islet cells isolated from Balb/c mice. Islets cultured in eupatilin showed a 1.4-fold increase in glucose-induced insulin secretion compared to those cultured without it. Apoptosis significantly decreased, and GSH levels increased in the eupatilin-pretreated group (Kim et al. 2015).

Vittarilide A and B, as well as ethyl 4-O-caffeoylquinate, exhibit moderate antioxidant activity (Wu et al. 2005b).

Appalachian shoestring fern (*Vittaria appalachiana*) was for a long time mistaken for a liverwort but was correctly identified and named in 1991. It is a very small fern found in dark, moist, non-calcareous rock crevices.

Leaves of stiff shoestring fern (*Vittaria elongata*) are used to treat joint pain in the Andaman and Nicobar Islands (Kumar et al. 2003).

WOODSIA

Cliff Ferns Woodsia Ferns

The genus is named in honor of the English Quaker botanist, author, geologist, and architect Joseph Woods (1776–1864). He was elected a Fellow of both the Linnean Society and the Geological Society for his original research. His early education of home schooling taught him Latin, Greek, Modern Greek, Hebrew, Italian, French, and he initially pursued architecture. By 1818, he turned to his passion for botany and published a book on the genus *Rosa* in 1835. In my province, the wild rose *(Rosa woodsia)* is named in his honor.

This brings up a humorous historical hiccup. In the 1930s, the government of the province of Alberta, where I have resided for over fifty years, asked school children what flower should be named the provincial emblem. The response was overwhelmingly in favor of the wild rose. A politician of the time walked across the High Level Bridge to the University of Alberta (my alma mater) and asked a professor in the Faculty of Education the binomial name of the rose. He replied, "*Rosa acicularis*," the prickly rose, and thus the wild rose province is really associated with the prickly rose. Oops! Should have asked an expert in botany.

The fronds of oblong woodsia, also known as rusty cliff fern (*Woodsia ilvensis*), have been traditionally used in Mongolia and Tibet for diarrhea, soft-tissue injuries, abdominal pain, and external wounds. The fern is also commonly found in North America and Northern Europe, found on sunny cliffs with thin, dry, and acidic soil. It is endangered in the U.K. due to overharvesting during the Victorian fern-collecting era, known as pteridomania or fern-fever.

The fern contains two maleimide N-glycosides, a stilbenoid glycoside, five undescribed acetylated flavonol bisdesmosides, and nineteen other known compounds.

Work by Otgonsugar et al. (2023) notes that veterinarians use the fronds to treat external and internal injuries in livestock, to induce blood coagulation, and promote healing of open wounds. The fern shows plasmin-inhibitory activity, which prevents excessive fibrin degradation.

Blunt lobed woodsia, or cliff fern (*Woodsia obtusa*), got its name for its rounded frond tips. Native to America, this hardy fern is a popular choice for gardening in acidic soil or among calcareous rocks.

Holly fern woodsia (*Woodsia polystichoides*) is not a holly fern but is named for its holly-like fronds. Native to Asia, this winter-hardy fern is a beautiful addition to fern gardens.

Rocky Mountain woodsia fern (*Woodsia scopulina* syn. *Physematium scopulinum*) exhibits broad-spectrum antifungal activity. The fern contains lipophilic flavonoids.

WOODWARDIA

Chain Ferns

Guan zhong was recorded in the ancient Chinese text *Ben Cao Jing*, one of the earliest pharmacopeias of Traditional Chinese Medicine from the Han Dynasty and is believed today to be Asian chain fern (*Woodwardia japonica*).

This edible and medicinal fern contains various flavonoids that contribute to its antioxidant activity. Environmental factors influencing the content and efficacy of this fern have been investigated (Wang et al. 2023).

The total flavonoid content appears to be related to lower temperatures, and antioxidant activity may be influenced by precipitation levels. Flavonol and isoflavone levels may vary with sunshine duration, and flavones appear to be temperature dependent. This suggests the possibility that the climate may greatly influence the content and medicinal activity of all ferns.

Netted chain fern (*Woodwardia areolata* syn. *Lorinseria areolata*) is common throughout the United States but confined to Nova Scotia in Canada. It is hardy to −40° C/F, the same frigid temperature on both scales. Netted chain fern is found in bogs and swamps. The common name derives from the netted veining pattern in the wide green leaflets, and *chain* refers to how the fertile fronds carry spores in chainlike rows. The fern has both sterile and fertile fronds.

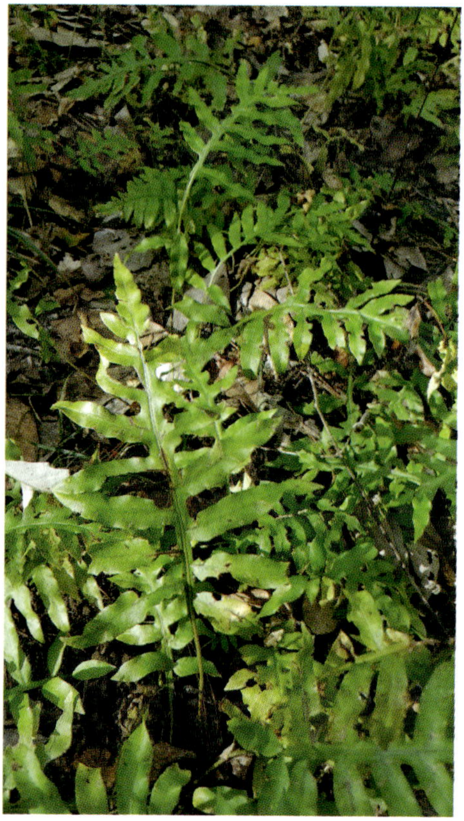

Woodwardia areolata
(Netted Chain Fern)
Photo by Alan Rockefeller

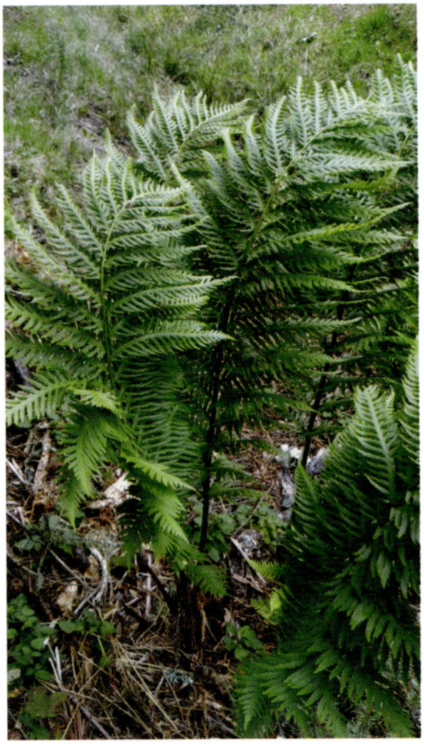

Woodwardia fimbriata
(Giant Chain Fern)
Photo by Alan Rockefeller

The giant chain fern (*Woodwardia fimbriata*) is native to Western North America, from British Columbia down to Baja, California. It is sold in nurseries for natural landscaping and habitat restoration.

Indigenous weavers used the stems, dyed with alder bark, to create red designs. The midrib contains two strands, stripped and used like yarn. The Suiseno used moss to dye fibers a burnt orange (Lloyd 1964).

Woodwardia japonica contains ecdysterone, ponasteroside A, woodwardic acid, and two flavonoids. This fern is both edible and medicinal, exhibiting antioxidant activity (Wang et al. 2023).

Hot water extracts of Oriental chain fern (*Woodwardia orientalis*) reduced the plaque-forming ability of herpes simplex virus type 1 and poliovirus. A new glucoside, woodorien, was isolated from an ethyl acetate extract and exhibited the most potent antiviral activity (Xu et al. 1993).

Chain fern (*Woodwardia radicans*) rhizome decoctions have been used externally for inflammation and internally for intestinal parasites.

The Mexican chain fern (*Woodwardia spinulosa*) stems were used in white basket design by Indigenous weavers.

The Himalayan jeweled chain fern (*Woodwardia unigemmata*) exhibits antioxidant and antibacterial activity against various plant and animal pathogens (Takuli et al. 2020). A full phytochemical analysis was performed, exhibiting a wide range of constituents.

A TCM combination of ferns known as *blechni rhizoma* has been used to treat HIV, hepatitis, measles, swellings, fever, and erysipelas. When combined with other Chinese herbal medicines, a patent (US5837257A) was taken out in 1997 to treat HIV as well as hepatitis virus B and C infections.

Decoctions of the rhizome and fronds were traditionally used for dysentery, the dried rhizome as a purgative tea, and the fronds and rhizome for skin disease and infertility. In India, the rhizome is used to treat abdominal pain and dysentery, and in Nigeria, the leaves are decocted and consumed as tea to treat infertility in women (Nwosu 2002). In China, starch from the rhizomes is used to make noodles, cakes, and liquor.

Virginia chain fern (*Woodwardia virginica*) contains a trinorditerpene glycoside and two cyclohexanone glycosides. The fronds are astringent and were used at one time, in North Carolina, for medicinal purposes (Jacobs and Burlage 1958).

Ferns by Their Common Names

This book is arranged in alphabetical order by genus. The list below is provided for readers who may know a fern by its common name but who do not know its Latin genus and species (binomial). The most current Latin binomial is given. Use the first part of the binomial, the fern's genus, to flip to that section in this book. Older names may be found in the text. Specific varieties are noted with var. An × indicates a cross or hybrid. Occasionally you will see that a common name applies to more than one genus-species.

My hope is that this list will help you find the ferns you wish to explore.

Adder's Fern – *Polypodium vulgare* var. *columbianum*
Adder's-tongue fern – *Ophioglossum peduncolosum*
Akkarghoda lady fern – *Athyrium hohenackerianum*
Alpine lady fern – *Athyrium distentifolium*, *A. yokoscense*
Alpine water fern – *Blechnum penna-marina* ssp. *alpina*
Alpine wood fern – *Dryopteris wallichiana*
Amakusa fern – *Pteris dispar*
American climbing fern – *Lygodium plamatum*
American royal fern – *Osmunda spectabilis*
American walking fern – *Asplenium rhizophyllum*
Angelvein fern – *Polypodium triseriale*
Antilles tongue fern – *Elaphoglossum piloselloides*
Argentinian fern – *Elaphoglossum lindbergii*
Ash leaf fern – *Marattia fraxinea*
Asian beard filmy fern – *Hymenophyllum barbatum*
Asian chain fern – *Woodwardia japonica*
Asian royal fern – *Osmunda japonica*
Asian sword fern – *Nephrolepis multiflora*
Asian walking fern – *Asplenium ruprechtii*
Asian watermoss – *Salvinia cucullata*
Austral bracken – *Pteridium esculentum*
Australian tree fern – *Cyathea cooperi*
Autumn fern – *Dryopteris erythrosora*
Bamboo fern – *Coniogramme japonica*
Bare tongue fern – *Pyrrosia calvata*
Basket fern – *Drynaria rigidula*
Beaded wood fern – *Dryopteris bissetiana*
Bear paw fern – *Aglaomorpha coronans*, *Phlebodium decumanum*
Bear's paw root – *Dryopteris filix-mas*
Big fruit scaly polypody – *Pleopeltis macrocarpa*
Bird foot cliff brake fern – *Pellaea mucronata*
Bird rock brake fern – *Pellaea ornithopus*
Bird's nest fern – *Asplenium australasicum*, *A. nidus*
Bitter fern – *Gleichenia quadripartita*
Black maidenhair – *Asplenium capillus-veneris*, *A. nigrum*, *A. philippense*

Black spleenwort – *Asplenium adiantum-nigrum*
Black tree fern – *Cyathea medullaris*
Blue star fern – *Phlebodium aureum*
Blunt-lobed fern – *Pteris obtusiloba*
Blunt-lobed woodsia – *Woodsia obtusa*
Bog onion – *Osmunda regalis*
Boott's wood fern – *Dryopteris × boottii*
Borrer's scaly male fern – *Dryopteris borreri*
Boston fern – *Nephrolepis exaltata*
Boulder fern – *Dennstaedtia punctilobula*
Bracken fern – *Pteridium aquilinum*
Brake fern – *Pteris vittata*
Branched wood fern – *Dryopteris ramosa*
Braun's holly fern – *Polystichum braunii*
Brazilian blechnum – *Blechnum brasiliense*
Brazilian tree fern – *Cyathea phalerata*
Breadfruit fern – *Microsorum scolopendria*
Brittle maidenhair fern – *Adiantum tenerum*
Broad buckler wood fern – *Dryopteris dilatata*
Broad halberd fern – *Tectaria heracleifolia*
Broadleaf maiden fern – *Thelypteris angustifolia*
Broadleaf maidenhair fern – *Adiantum latifolium*
Broadleaf tectaria – *Tectaria latifolia*
Broad spiny wood fern – *Dryopteris spinulosum* var. *dilatatum*
Broad sword fern – *Nephrolepis falcata*
Brownstem spleenwort – *Asplenium platyneuron*
Buckhorn brake – *Osmunda regalis*
Buckler fern – *Dryopteris aemula*
Bulblet fern – *Cystopteris bulbifera*
Bushman's mattress – *Lygodium articulatum*
Button fern – *Tectaria cicutaria, Pellaea rotundifolia*
Buttonhole – *Asplenium scolopendrium*
California cliff brake fern – *Pellaea mucronata* ssp. *californica*
California fern – *Adiantum shastense*
California maidenhair – *Adiantum jordanii*
California polypody – *Polypodium californicum*
Carrot fern – *Mohria caffrorum, Onychium japonicum*
Caterpillar fern – *Polypodium formosanum*
Centipede fern – *Blechnum orientale*
Chain fern – *Cibotium barometz, Woodwardia radicans*
Champion's wood fern – *Dryopteris championii*
Chick Fern – *Asplenium bulbiferum*
Chinese peng fern – *Abacopteris penangiana, Pronephrium penangianum*
Christmas fern – *Polystichum acrostichoides*
Cinnamon fern – *Osmunda cinnamomea*
Cliff brake fern – *Pellaea andromedifolia*
Cliff fern – *Woodsia obtusa*
Climbing bird's nest fern – *Microsorum punctatum*
Climbing fern – *Lygodium salicifolium*
Climbing shield fern – *Arachniodes adiantiformis*
Clinton's wood fern – *Dryopteris clintoniana*
Clubmoss snake fern – *Microgramma lycopodioides*
Coastal wood fern – *Dryopteris arguta*
Cochinchina fern – *Angiopteris cochinchinensis*
Coffee fern – *Pellaea andromedifolia*
Comb-forked fern – *Gleichenia pectinata*
Common oak fern – *Gymnocarpium dryopteris*
Common polypody – *Polypodium vulgare* var. *columbianum*
Common maidenhair fern – *Adiantum aethiopicum*
Common salvinia – *Salvinia minima*
Common tree fern – *Cyathea dregei*
Countess Dalhousie's spleenwort – *Asplenium dalhousiae*
Cow's tongue – *Asplenium scolopendrium*
Creeping golden polypody – *Phlebodium decumanum*
Creeping spleenwort – *Asplenium serra*
Crested fern – *Microsorum punctatum*
Crested wood fern – *Dryopteris cristata*
Cretan brake – *Pteris cretica*
Crown wood fern – *Dryopteris crassirhizoma*
Curled brake fern – *Pellaea involuta*
Decaying fern – *Athyrium wallichianum*
Deceptive fern – *Dryopteris decipiens*
Deer fern – *Blechnum spicantum*
Deer's tongue – *Asplenium scolopendrium*

Delicate filmy fern – *Hymenophyllum plicatum*
Delta maidenhair fern – *Adiantum cuneatum*
Dense lace fern – *Aspidotis densa*
Devil's hoof – *Pteridium aquilinum*
Diamond maidenhair fern – *Adiantum trapeziforme*
Diliman fern – *Stenochlaena palustris*
Dotted bead fern – *Hypolepis punctata*
Downy maiden – *Christella dentata*
Downy wood fern – *Christella dentata*
Dragon scale fern – *Drymoglossum piloselloides*
Dragon scales fern – *Angiopteris lygodiifolia*
Dragon's scale fern – *Pyrrosia piloselloides*
Dragon's tail fern – *Asplenium ebenoides*
Drooping spleenwort – *Asplenium flaccidum*
Duss' tongue fern – *Elaphoglossum petiolatum*
Dwarf elkhorn fern – *Microsorum punctatum*
Dwarf male fern – *Dryopteris oreades*
Eagle fern – *Pteridium aquilinum*
Eared lady fern – *Athyrium oblitescens*
East Indian holly fern – *Arachniodes simplicior*
Eastern maidenhair fern – *Polystichum woronowii*
Eastern marsh fern – *Thelypteris palustris*
Ebony spleenwort – *Asplenium platyneuron*
Ecklon's lip fern – *Notholaena eckloniana*
Egyptian spleenwort – *Asplenium aethiopicum*
Elephant fern – *Angiopteris evecta*
Elkhorn fern – *Platycerium bifurcatum*
European lady fern – *Athyrium filix-femina* var. *filix-femina*
Evergreen wood fern – *Dryopteris intermedia*
Falcate spleenwort – *Asplenium falcatum*
False hen and chickens fern – *Asplenium × lucrosum*
False shield fern – *Lastreopsis effusa*
False spleenwort – *Dryoathyrium boryanum*
False staghorn fern – *Dicranopteris linearis*
Fancy wood fern – *Dryopteris intermedia*
Fan-leaved maidenhair fern – *Adiantum flabellulatum*
Felt fern – *Pyrrosia davidii*
Fendler's false cloak fern – *Notholaena fendleri*
Filmy fern – *Hymenophyllum caudiculatum*
Finger fern – *Asplenium ceterach*
Fishbone fern – *Nephrolepis cordifolia*
Fishscale fern – *Microgramma squamulosa*
Fishtail fern – *Microsorum punctatum*
Fishtail fern – *Nephrolepis falcata*
Fishtail strap fern – *Microsorum punctatum*
Five-fingered jack – *Adiantum hispidulum*
Five finger Taiwanese tongue fern – *Pyrrosia polydactylis*
Flatfork fern – *Psilotum complanatum*
Flexible climbing fern – *Lygodium flexuosum*
Floating antler-fern – *Ceratopteris pteridoides*
Floating water moss – *Salvinia natans*
Floral fern – *Arachniodes adiantiformis*
Floury cloak fern – *Cheilanthes farinosa*
Flowering fern – *Helminthostachys zeylanica*
Flying spider-monkey tree fern – *Alsophila spinulosa*
Forest shield fern – *Polystichum pungens*
Forked fern – *Dicranopteris dichotoma, D. pedate*
Fortune's holly fern – *Cyrtomium fortunei*
Fountain spleenwort – *Asplenium fontanum* ssp. *pseudofontanum*
Four leaf maidenhair fern – *Adiantum tetraphyllum*
Fox tongue – *Asplenium scolopendrium*
Fragile bladder fern – *Cystopteris fragilis*
Fragile maidenhair fern – *Adiantum fragile*
Fragrant wood fern – *Dryopteris fragrans*
Fuzzy spleenwort – *Alsophila setosa*
Gaston's cliff brake fern – *Pellaea gastonyi*
Gaston's spleenwort – *Asplenium gastonis*
Giant chain fern – *Woodwardia fimbriata*
Giant brake fern – *Pteris tripartita*
Giant holly fern – *Polystichum munitum*
Giant maidenhair fern – *Adiantum trapeziforme*
Giant tree fern – *Alsophila gigantea, Cyathea gigantea*
Giant salvinia – *Salvinia biloba*

Giant sword fern – *Nephrolepis biserrata*
Giant water fern – *Salvinia molesta*
Glabrous-ternate grape fern – *Botrychium ternatum*
Glandular wood fern – *Dryopteris intermedia*
God's hair – *Asplenium scolopendrium*
Goldenback fern – *Pityrogramma triangularis*
Golden chicken – *Cibotium barometz*
Golden leather fern – *Acrostichum aureum*
Golden maidenhair fern – *Polypodium vulgare* var. *columbianum*
Golden polypody – *Polypodium leucotomos*
Golden-scale fern – *Dryopteris affinis*
Golden serpentine fern – *Aspidotis densa*
Gold foot fern – *Phlebodium aureum*
Goldie's fern – *Dryopteris goldiana*
Graceful tongue fern – *Elaphoglossum petiolatum*
Grape fern – *Botrychium* sp.
Grassland fern – *Dryopteris athamantica*
Green cliff brake fern – *Pellaea viridis*
Green marsh fern – *Macrothelypteris viridifrons*
Green mountain maidenhair – *Adiantum viridi-montanum*
Green spleenwort – *Asplenium viride*
Gu sui bu – *Drynaria* spp.
Half-pinnate brake fern – *Pteris semipinnata*
Hairy bracken fern – *Pteridium aquilinum* var. *pubescens*, *P. revolutum*
Hairy lip fern – *Myriopteris lanosa*
Hairy tree fern – *Cyathea crinita*
Hammock fern – *Blechnum occidentale*
Hard fern – *Blechnum spicantum*, *Pellaea calomelanos*
Hard shield fern – *Polystichum aculeatum*
Hardy ribbon fern – *Pteris cretica* var. *nervosa*, *P. laeta*
Hare's foot fern – *Davallia canariensis*, *D. solida*, *Polypodium leucotomos*
Hartford fern – *Lygodium plamatum*
Hart's tongue fern – *Asplenium scolopendrium*
Hay-scented fern – *Dennstaedtia punctilobula*, *Dryopteris aemula*, *Microlepia strigosa*
Hawaii potato fern – *Marattia douglasii*
Heart fern – *Hemionitis arifolia*
Hen and chick(en) fern – *Asplenium bulbiferum*
Hen fern – *Asplenium bulbiferum*
Himalayan jeweled chain fern – *Woodwardia unigemmata*
Himalayan maidenhair fern – *Adiantum venustum*
Hind's tongue – *Asplenium scolopendrium*
Holly fern woodsia – *Woodsia polystichoides*
Horseshoe fern – *Marattia salicina*
Horse tongue – *Asplenium scolopendrium*
Hottentot fern – *Cyclosorus interruptus*
House holly fern – *Cyrtomium falcatum*
Huguenot fern – *Pteris multifida*
Indian male fern – *Dryopteris cochleata*
Indian's dream fern – *Aspidotis densa*
Indian water fern – *Ceratopteris thalictroides*
Interrupted fern – *Osmunda claytoniana*
Irish black spleenwort – *Asplenium onopteris*
Iron fern – *Arachniodes adiantiformis*
Japanese beech fern – *Phegopteris decursive-pinnata*
Japanese bird's nest fern – *Asplenium antiquum*
Japanese claw fern – *Onychium japonicum*
Japanese climbing fern – *Lygodium japonicum*
Japanese holly fern – *Cyrtomium falcatum*
Japanese painted fern – *Athyrium niponicum*
Japanese royal fern – *Osmunda japonica*
Java fern – *Microsorum pteropus*
Jeweled maiden fern – *Cyclosorus extensus*
Kariba weed – *Salvinia molesta*
Kidney fern – *Trichomanes reniforme*
Kidney filmy fern – *Hymenophyllum nephrophyllum*
Killarney fern – *Trichomanes speciosum*
Kimberly queen fern – *Nephrolepis obliterata*
King Charles in the oak – *Pteridium aquilinum*
King fern – *Angiopteris evecta*, *Marattia salicina*

Kiokio – *Blechnum novae-zelandiae*
Korean maiden fern – *Parathelypteris beddomei*
Korean rock fern – *Polystichum tsus-simense*
Kunth's hacksaw fern – *Doodia kunthiana*
Kunth's maiden fern – *Thelypteris kunthii*
Lacy hare's foot fern – *Davallia formosana*
Ladder brake fern – *Pteris vittata*
Ladder fern – *Nephrolepis cordifolia*
Ladder-shape gland fern – *Parathelypteris glanduligera*
Lady fern – *Athyrium filix-femina, A. hohenackerianum*
Lady in red – *Athyrium filix-femina* var. *angustum*
Lance leaf polypody – *Polypodium lanceolatum*
Large-leafed holly fern – *Cyrtomium macrophyllum*
Large marsh fern – *Macrothelypteris oligophlebia*
Large mosquito fern – *Azolla filiculoides*
Leather fern – *Arachniodes adiantiformis*
Leather grape fern – *Botrychium multifidum*
Leatherleaf fern – *Arachniodes adiantiformis (known by* syn. *Rumohra adiantiformis)*
Leathery polypody – *Polypodium scouleri*
Leathery shield fern – *Arachniodes adiantiformis*
Leathery wood fern – *Dryopteris lacera*
Lemon-scented mountain fern – *Oreopteris limbosperma*
Licorice fern – *Polypodium glycyrrhiza*
Limpleaf fern – *Microlepia speluncae*
Lip fern – *Cheilanthes* sp.
Little hard fern – *Blechnum penna-marina*
Lobed basket fern – *Drynaria sparsisora*
Lobed salvinia – *Salvinia biloba*
Long beech fern – *Phegopteris connectilis*
Longstem adder's tongue fern – *Ophioglossum petiolatum*
Long-tail spleenwort – *Asplenium incisum*
Lumbago brake - *Osmunda* sp.
Macho fern – *Nephrolepis biserrata*
Mahogany fern – *Didymochlaena truncatula*
Maidenhair creeper fern – *Lygodium flexuosum*
Maidenhair spleenwort – *Asplenium trichomanes*
Maile-scented fern – *Microsorum scolopendria*
Makino's holly fern – *Polystichum makinoi*
Male fern – *Dryopteris filix-mas*
Manchurian weeping fern – *Lepisorus ussuriensis*
Man fern – *Cibotium* sp., *Dicksonia antarctica*
Mangemange – *Lygodium articulatum*
Mangrove fern – *Acrostichum aureum*
Maquique fern – *Alsophila firma*
Many-leaved fern – *Pteris polyphylla*
Mare's tail fern – *Asplenium polyodon*
Marginal wood fern – *Dryopteris marginalis*
Marginated tongue fern – *Elaphoglossum marginatum*
Mariana maiden fern – *Thelypteris torresiana*
Marsh fern – *Macrothelypteris torresiana*
Mexican chain fern – *Woodwardia spinulosa*
Mexican mosquito fern – *Azolla microphylla*
Mexican stag's tongue fern – *Elaphoglossum paleaceum*
Mole ladder fern – *Asplenium sibiricum*
Molokai twinsorus fern – *Diplazium molokaiense*
Monarch fern – *Microsorum scolopendria*
Mono-sorus maidenhair fern – *Adiantum monochlamys*
Moonwort – *Botrychium lunaria*
Mosquito fern – *Azolla* sp.
Mother fern – *Asplenium bulbiferum*
Mother spleenwort – *Asplenium bulbiferum*
Mountain bladder fern – *Cryopteris bulbifera*
Mountain fern – *Dryopteris oreades*
Mountain hard fern – *Blechnum vulcanicum*
Mountain wood fern – *Dryopteris campyloptera*
Much-divided filmy fern – *Hymenophyllum multifidum*
Mule's foot fern – *Angiopteris evecta*
Multi-toothed lady fern – *Athyrium multidentatum*
Musk fern – *Microsorum grossum, M. scolopendria*
Naked whisk fern – *Psilotum nudum*
Narrow beech fern – *Phegopteris connectilis*

Narrow buckler fern – *Dryopteris carthusiana*
Narrow-leaved felt fern – *Pyrrosia tonkinensis*
Narrow-leaved fern – *Angiopteris angustifolia*
Narrow scaly male fern – *Dryopteris cambrensis*
Narrow spinulose shield fern – *Dryopteris carthusiana*
Narrow spiny wood fern – *Dryopteris carthusiana*
Narrow stiff shoestring fern – *Vittaria angust-elongata*
Narrow wood fern – *Dryopteris carthusiana*
Netted adder's-tongue fern – *Ophioglossum reticulatum*
Netted chain fern – *Woodwardia areolata*
New York fern – *Thelypteris noveboracensis*
Norfolk Island spleenwort – *Asplenium dimorphum*
North American gray royal fern – *Osmunda regalis* var. *spectabilis*
Northeastern maidenhair – *Adiantum pedatum*
Northern buckler fern – *Dryopteris expansa*
Northern holly fern – *Polystichum lonchitis*
Northern lady fern – *Athyrium filix-femina* var. *angustum*
Northern maidenhair fern – *Adiantum pedatum*
Northern oak fern – *Gymnocarpium dryopteris*
Oak fern – *Polypodium vulgare*
Oakleaf basket fern – *Drynaria quercifolia*
Oak leaf fern – *Dryopteris quercifolia*, *D. rigidula*, *D. sparsisora*
Oblong woodsia – *Woodsia ilvensis*
Octopus flower – *Lygodium articulatum*
Old World forked fern – *Dicranopteris linearis*
Oriental chain fern – *Woodwardia orientalis*
Oriental ostrich fern – *Matteuccia orientalis*
Ostrich fern – *Matteuccia struthiopteris*
Palm leaf fern – *Blechnum novae-zelandiae*
Parasitic maiden fern – *Cyclosorus parasiticus*
Parasitic tri-vein fern – *Cyclosorus parasiticus*
Parry's lip fern – *Notholaena parryi*
Parsley fern – *Cryptogramma* sp., *C. crispa*, *Mohria caffrorum*
Peacock's tail fern – *Actiniopteris radiata*
Penny fern – *Drymoglossum piloselloides*
Penther's wood fern – *Dryopteris pentheri*
Pepperwort – *Marsilea quadrifolia*
Piripiri – *Hymenophyllum sanguinolentum*
Plumed maidenhair fern – *Adiantum formosum*
Poison rock fern – *Cheilanthes sieberi*
Prickly shield fern – *Polystichum vestitum*
Prince of Wales feathers fern – *Leptopteris superba*
Protruding filmy fern – *Hymenophyllum exsertum*
Purple cliff brake fern – *Pellaea atropurpurea*
Queen's veil mountain fern – *Thelypteris quelpaertensis*
Rabbit's foot fern – *Davallia sp.*
Rabbit's foot fern – *Davallia griffithiana*
Rasp fern – *Doodia media*, *Sadleria cyatheoides*
Rattlesnake fern – *Botrychium virginianum*
Raw bracken fern – *Pteridium aquilinum*
Ray-fern – *Actiniopteris* radiata
Red-bearded Christmas fern – *Polystichum squarrosum*
Red finger fern – *Lygodium circinnatum*
Red pig fern – *Sadleria pallida*
Redscale scaly polypody – *Pleopeltis polylepis*
Resurrection fern – *Pellaea andromedifolia*, *Polypodium polypodioides*
Ribbon fern – *Ophioglossum pendulum*, *Pteris cretica*
Rigid lace fern – *Microlepia strigosa*
River fern – *Abacopteris* sp., *Thelypteris normalis*
Riverine scrambler fern – *Ampelopteris prolifera*
Rock cap fern – *Polypodium virginianum*
Rock fern – *Cheilanthes tenuifolia*
Rock polypody – *Polypodium vulgare* var. *columbianum*
Rock spleenwort – *Asplenium delavayi*, *A. foreziense*
Rocky Mountain woodsia fern – *Woodsia scopulina*

Rosy maidenhair fern – *Adiantum hispidulum*
Rough hairy maiden fern – *Thelypteris hispidula*
Rough lip fern – *Myriopteris scabra*
Rough maidenhair fern – *Adiantum hispidulum*
Royal fern – *Osmunda* sp., *Osmunda regalis*
Rusty cliff fern – *Woodsia ilvensis*
Rustyback fern – *Asplenium ceterach*
Saw-leaved bracken – *Pteris multifida*
Scale edge bristle fern – *Trichomanes membranaceum*
Scaly fern – *Asplenium ceterach*
Scaly male fern – *Dryopteris affinis*
Scaly sword fern – *Nephrolepis hirsutula*
Scaly tree ferns – *Cyathea* spp.
Scented fern – *Mohria caffrorum*
Scented oak leaf fern – *Polypodium polynesicum*
Schimper's wood fern – *Dryopteris schimperiana*
Scott's spleenwort – *Asplenium ebenoides*
Scrambling fern – *Ampelopteris* sp.
Scurfy sword fern – *Nephrolepis hirsutula*
Sensitive fern – *Onoclea sensibilis*
Serpentine fern – *Aspidotis densa*
Setosa fern – *Alsophila setosa*
Seven weeks fern – *Arachniodes adiantiformis*
Shaggy shield fern – *Dryopteris atrata*
Shaggy wood fern – *Dryopteris cycanida*
Shaking brake fern – *Pteris tremula*
Shearer's felt fern – *Pyrrosia sheareri*
Shiny tree fern – *Alsophila mannianna*
Shield fern – *Dryopteris crassirhizoma*, *Lastreopsis amplissima*
Sickle fern – *Pellaea falcata*
Sickle spleenwort – *Asplenium polyodon*
Silk tree fern – *Metaxya rostrata*
Silverback fern – *Aleuritopteris argentea*
Silver cloak fern – *Aleuritopteris anceps*
Silver fern – *Cheilanthes* sp., *Cyathea dealbata*, *Pityrogramma calomelanos*
Silver cloak fern – *Aleuritopteris anceps*
Silver lace fern – *Pteris ensiformis*
Silver lip fern – *Cheilanthes bicolor*
Silver tree fern – *Cyathea dealbata*
Silvery spleenwort fern – *Deparia acrostichoides*
Single-sorus spleenwort – *Asplenium monanthes*
Slender adder's tongue fern – *Ophioglossum capense*
Slender brake – *Pteris ensiformis*
Slender cliff brake – *Cryptogramma stelleri*
Small kiokio – *Blechnum procerum*
Small-leaf climbing fern – *Lygodium microphyllum*
Smooth cliff brake fern – *Pellaea glabella*
Smooth rock spleenwort – *Asplenium fontanum* ssp. *pseudofontanum*
Snake fern – *Lygodium microphyllum*
Soft shield fern – *Polystichum setiferum*
Soft tree fern – *Dicksonia antarctica*
Southern adder's-tongue – *Ophioglossum vulgatum*
Southern lady fern – *Athyrium asplenioides*
Southern maidenhair fern – *Adiantum capillus-veneris*
Southern shield fern – *Thelypteris kunthii*
Spider bracken fern – *Pteridium arachnoideum*
Spider brake fern – *Pteris multifida*
Spider fern – *Pteris multifida*
Spiny tree fern – *Cyathea manniana*
Spleenwort – *Asplenium appendiculatum*
Split fern – *Gleichenia japonica*
Spreading wood fern – *Dryopteris expansa*
Squirrel's foot fern – *Davallia bullata*
Squirrel's foot fern – *Davallia mariesii*
Scythian lamb – *Cibotium barometz*
Spiny cliff brake – *Pellaea truncata*
Spiny wood fern – *Dryopteris* sp.
Staghorn fern – *Platycerium bifurcatum*
Star cloak fern – *Notholaena standleyi*
Star fern – *Blechnum fluviatile*
Stewart's wood fern – *Dryopteris stewartii*
Stiff shoestring fern – *Vittaria elongata*

Striated maiden fern – *Cyclosorus interruptus* var. *striatus*

Striped brake fern – *Pteris plumula*, *P. quadriaurita*

Subarctic lady fern – *Asplenium cyclosorum*

Swamp fern – *Acrostichum* sp.

Swamp fern – *Blechnum serrulatum*

Swamp shield fern – *Cyclosorus interruptus*

Swamp vine fern – *Stenochlaena palustris*

Sweet fern – *Polypodium vulgare* var. *columbianum*

Sweet root fern – *Polypodium glycyrrhiza*

Sword brake fern – *Pteris ensiformis*

Table fern – *Pteris cretica*

Tailed maidenhair fern – *Adiantum incisum*

Tall marsh fern – *Parathelypteris nipponica*

Tasmanian tree fern – *Dicksonia antarctica*

Tassel fern – *Polystichum polyblepharum*

Terrestrial fern – *Microsorum punctatum*

Thermal adder's tongue fern – *Ophioglossum thermale*

Thick foot tongue fern – *Elaphoglossum crassipes*

Thickleaf brake fern – *Pteris deflexa*

Thick-stemmed wood fern – *Dryopteris crassirhizoma*

Thin-stemmed forest fern – *Dryopteris inaequalis*

Three-finger tongue fern – *Pyrrosia hastata*

Tongue fern – *Pyrrosia lingua*

Toothed midsorus fern – *Blechnum serrulatum*

Trailing maidenhair fern – *Adiantum caudatum*

Tree fern – *Cyathea* spp.

Triangle-lobed moonwort – *Botrychium ascendens*

Triangle staghorn – *Platycerium stemaria*

Tuber sword fern – *Nephrolepis cordifolia*

Turnip fern – *Angiopteris evecta*

Umbrella fern – *Gleichenia cunninghamii*

Uniform wood fern – *Dryopteris uniformis*

Upswept moonwort – *Botrychium ascendens*

Ussuri weeping fern – *Lepisorus ussuriensis*

Vegetable fern – *Diplazium esculentum* syn. *Athyrium esculentum*

Venus maidenhair fern – *Adiantum capillus-veneris*

Verdon spleenwort – *Asplenium jahandiezii*

Vessel fern – *Angiopteris lygodiifolia*

Virginia chain fern – *Woodwardia virginica*

Vogelii maidenhair fern – *Adiantum vogelii*

Walking fern – *Asplenium rhizophyllum*

Walking maidenhair fern – *Adiantum caudatum*, *A. philippense*

Wallich's giant table fern – *Pteris wallichiana*

Wall rue fern – *Asplenium ruta-muraria*

Wart fern – *Microsorum scolopendria*

Water butterfly wings – *Salvinia natans*

Water clover fern – *Marsilea minuta*, *M. quadrifolia*

Water fern – *Azolla* spp., *Ceratopteris*

Water splangles – *Salvinia minima*

Water sprite – *Ceratopteris thalictroides*

Wedge water fern – *Blechnum vulcanicum*

Wedgeleaf spleenwort *Asplenium cuneatum*

Weeping fern – *Pleopeltis thunbergiana*

Western black spleenwort – *Asplenium onopteris*

Western bracken fern – *Pteridium aquilinum* var. *latiusculum*

Western lady fern – *Athyrium filix-femina* var. *cyclosorum*

Western maidenhair fern – *Adiantum aleuticum* var. *aleuticum*

Western oak fern – *Gymnocarpium dryopteris*

Western polypody – *Polypodium vulgare* var. *columbianum*

Western sword fern – *Polystichum munitum*

Whisk Fern – *Psilotum* sp.

White-margined lip fern – *Cheilanthes albomarginata*

White paw fern – *Davallia tyermanii*
White rabbit's foot – *Davallia tyermanii*
Willow-leaved climbing fern – *Lygodium salicifolium*
World-climbing fern – *Lygodium microphyllum*
Wood Fern – *Dryopteris* sp.
Wooton's lace fern – *Cheilanthes wootoni*
Woolly fern – *Cibotium barometz*
Woolly grape fern – *Botrychium lanuginosum*
Woolly tree fern – *Culcita macrocarpa*
Wright's cliff brake fern – *Pellaea wrightiana*

Resources

FERN ESSENCE COMPANIES

Bailey Essences: a product line by Yorkshire Flower Essences. These essences have been around for more than 50 years, and I used them in my clinical practice.

Delta Gardens Flower Essences. New England based company.

Prairie Deva Essences: a product line by Self Heal Distributing. My wife Laurie and I developed this line more than 30 years ago.

The South African Flower and Gem Essences. Reliable and well researched.

First Light Flower Essences of New Zealand. Some of the greatest ferns of the world are found in this country. Very intuitive.

PUBLICATIONS

American Fern Journal is a peer-reviewed journal by the American Fern Society. One of the best!

Fiddlehead Form Newsletter. Informative and timely information.

"Mosses & Ferns" in *Spectrum of Homeopathy* 2021: Vol. 2, Narayana Verlag. A recent account of new insights into homeopathic fern remedies.

ORGANIZATIONS

Each of these fern societies focus on regional ferns:

American Fern Society
British Pteridological Society
The Dutch Fern Association
The Fern Society of Southern Africa

The San Francisco Fern Society
The Ferns of Macronesia
German Fern Group
The Hardy Fern Foundation

BOOKS OF INTEREST

The Complete Book of Ferns: Indoors Outdoors Growing Crafting History & Lore by Mobee Weinstein, Cool Springs Press, 2022. Useful for beginner growers.

Ferns & Allies of the North Woods: A Handy Field Reference to All 86 of Our Ferns and Allies by Joe Walewsk, Kollath-Stensaas Publishing, 2016. Great idea in a handy-to-carry booklet.

Ferns for American Gardens by John T. Mickel, Timber Press, 2003. A timeless classic.

Fern Grower's Manual (revised and expanded edition) by Barbara Joe Hoshizaki and Robbin C. Moran, Timber Press, 2001. Revised edition is excellent.

Ferns: Lessons in Survival from Earth's Most Adaptable Plants by Fay-Wei and J.S. Suissa, Hardie Grant Books, 2025. Newest addition to the subject.

Ferns, Spikemosses, Clubmosses and Quillworts of Eastern North America by Emily B. Sessa, Princeton Field Guides, 2024. Must have for nature lovers.

Identifying Ferns the Easy Way: A Pocket Guide to Common Ferns of the Northeast by Lynn Levine, Cliff Adler, and illustrated by Briony Morrow-Cribbs, Bondcliffe Books, 2019. Great resource for hikers.

Native Ferns, Moss, & Grasses by William Cullina, Houghton Mifflin Harcourt, 2008. One of my favorite books on subject.

A Natural History of Ferns by Robbin C. Moran, Timber Press, 2009. A good compendium on ferns through the ages.

The Plant Lovers' Guide to Ferns by Richie Steffen and Sue Olse, Timber Press, 2015. Beautifully written and illustrated.

The Victorian Fern Craze by Sarah Whittingham, Shire Library, Bloomsbury Publishing, London, 2009. A delightful journey into the fern craze of 18th and 19th centuries.

References

Abdelatty, A. M., M. I. Mandouh, S. A. Mohamed, S. Busato, O. A. M. Badr, M. Bionaz, A. A. Elolimy, M. M. A. Moustafa, O. A. A. Farid, and A. K. Al-Mokaddem. 2021. "Azolla Leaf Meal at 5% of the Diet Improves Growth Performance, Intestinal Morphology and p70S6K1 Activation, and Affects Cecal Microbiota in Broiler Chicken." *Animal* 15 (10): 100362.

Abdel-Azeem, A. M., S. M. Zaki, W. F. Khalil, N. A. Makhlouf, and L. M. Farghaly. 2016. "Anti-Rheumatoid Activity of Secondary Metabolites Produced by Endophytic *Chaetomium globosum.*" *Frontiers in Microbiology* 7: 1477.

Aboul-Soud, M. A. M., R. Siddique, F. Fozia, A. Ullah, Y. Rashid, I. Ahmad, N. S. S. Zaghloul, S.A. Al-Rejaie, and M. Mohany. 2023. "Antiplatelet, Cytotoxic Activities and Characterization of Green-Synthesized Zinc Oxide Nanoparticles Using Aqueous Extract of *Nephrolepis exaltata*." *Environmental Science and Pollution Research International* 30 (29): 73870–80.

Aditama, A. P. R., B. Ma'arif, H. Laswati, and M. Agil. 2021. "In Vitro and In Silico Analysis of Phytochemical Compounds of 96% Ethanol Extract of Semanggi (*Marsilea crenata* Presl.) Leaves as a Bone Formation Agent." *Journal of Basic and Clinical Physiology and Pharmacology* 32 (4): 881–87.

Adnan, M., M. Patel, S. Deshpande, M. Alreshidi, A. J. Siddiqui, M. N. Reddy, N. Emira, and V. De Feo. 2020. "Effect of *Adiantum philippense* Extract on Biofilm Formation, Adhesion with Its Antibacterial Activities against Foodborne Pathogens, and Characterization of Bioactive Metabolites: An In Vitro–In Silico Approach." *Frontiers in Microbiology* 11: 823.

Ahmad, M., N. Jahan, Mahayrookh, Mehjabeen, A. B. Rehman, M. Ahmad, O. Ullah, and N. Mohammad. 2011. "Differential Inhibitory Potencies of Alcoholic Extract of Different Parts of *Dryopteris chrysocoma* on Inflammation in Mice and Rats." *Pakistan Journal of Pharmaceutical Sciences* 24 (4): 559–63.

Ahmed, A., A. Wadud, N. Jahan, A. Bilal, and S. Hajera. 2013. "Efficacy of *Adiantum capillus veneris* Linn in Chemically Induced Urolithiasis in Rats." *Journal of Ethnopharmacology* 146 (1): 411–16.

Ahmed, D., M. M. Khan, and R. Saeed. 2015. "Comparative Analysis of Phenolics, Flavonoids, and Antioxidant and Antibacterial Potential of Methanolic, Hexanic and Aqueous Extracts from *Adiantum caudatum* Leaves." *Antioxidants* 4 (2): 394–409.

Ahmed, S., M. K. Parvez, M. S. Al-Dosari, M. A. S. Abdelwahid, T. A. Alhowiriny, A. J. Al-Rehaily. 2023. "Novel Anti-Hepatitis B Virus Flavonoids Sakuranetin and Velutin from *Rhus retinorrhea." Molecular Medicine Reports* 28 (3): 176.

Aini, N., A. Shukor, and J. Stanslas. 2008. "Cytotoxic Potential on Breast Cancer Cells Using Selected Forest Species Found in Malaysia." *International Journal of Cancer Research* 4: 103–9.

Aire, T. A. 2005. "Short-Term Effects of Carbendazim on the Gross and Microscopic Features of the Testes of Japanese Quails (*Corturnix Coturnix Japonica*)." *Anatomy and Embryology* 210: 43–49.

Ajikumaran Nair, S., B. S. Shylesh, B. Gopakumar, and A. Subramoniam. 2006. "Anti-Diabetes and Hypoglycaemic Properties of *Hemionitis arifolia* (Burm.) Moore in Rats." *Journal of Ethnopharmacology* 106 (2): 192–97.

Ajirioghene, A. E., S. I. Ghasi, L. O. Ewhre, O. G. Adebayo, and J. N. Asiwe. 2021. "Anti-Diabetogenic and *In Vivo* Antioxidant Activity of Ethanol Extract of *Dryopteris dilatata* in Alloxan-Induced Male Wistar Rats." *Biomarkers* 26 (8): 718–25.

Akande, R. T., G. Fouche, I. M. Famuyide, F. N. Makhubu, S. M. Nkadimeng, A. O. Aro, P. N. Kayoka-Kabongo, L. J. McGaw. 2022. "Anthelmintic and Antimycobacterial Activity of Fractions and Compounds Isolated from *Cissampelos mucronate*." *Journal of Ethnopharmacology* 292: 115130.

Akihisa, T., K. Kawashima, M. Orido, H. Akazawa, M. Matsumoto, A. Yamamoto, E. Ogihara, M. Fukatsu, H. Toduka, J. Fuji. 2013. "Antioxidative and Melanogenesis-Inhibitory Activities of Caffeoylquinic Acids and Other Compounds from Moxa." *Chemistry and Biodiversity* 10 (3): 313–27.

Alam, F., S. H. A. Khan, and M. H. H. B. Asad. 2021a. "Phytochemical, Antimicrobial, Antioxidant and Enzyme Inhibitory Potential of the Medicinal Plant *Dryopteris ramosa* (Hope) C. Chr." *BMC Complementary Medicine and Therapies* 21 (1): 197.

Alam, M., N. U. Emon, S. Alam, S. Rudra, N. Akhter, M. M. R. Mamun, A. Ganguly. 2021b. "Assessment of Pharmacological Activities of *Lygodium Microphyllum* Cav. Leaves in the Management of Pain, Inflammation, Pyrexia, Diarrhea and Helminths: In Vivo, in Vitro and in Silico Approaches." *Biomedicine and Pharmacotherapy* 139: 111644.

Al-Assar, N. B., M. N. K. Khattak, Z. U. R. Mashwani, S. Kanan, I. Ullah, U. Ali, and A. A. Khan. 2021. "Phytochemical Prolife and Antiproliferative Activities of Acetone Extracts of *Asplenium polypodioides* Blume. and *A. dalhousiae* Hook. in MDA-MB-231 Breast Cancer Cells." *Saudi Journal of Biological Sciences* 28 (11): 6324–31.

Al-Aubaidy, H. A., A. Dayan, M. A. Deseo, C. Itsiopoulos, D. Jamil, N. R. Hadi, and C. J. Thomas. 2021. "Twelve-Week Mediterranean Diet Intervention Increases Citrus Bioflavonoid Levels and Reduces Inflammation in People with Type 2 Diabetes Mellitus." *Nutrients* 13 (4): 1133.

Alhadrami, H. A., G. Burgio, B. Thissera, R. Orfali, S. E. Jiffri, M. Yaseen, A. M. Sayed, M. E. Rateb. 2022. "Neoechinulin A as a Promising SARS-CoV-2 M^{pro} Inhibitor: In Vitro and In Silico Study Showing the Ability of Simulations in Discerning Active from Inactive Enzyme Inhibitors." *Marine Drugs* 20 (3): 163.

Ali, H. A., A. K. A. Chowdhury, A. K. M. Rahman, T. Borkowski, L. Nahar, S. D. Sarker. 2008. "Pachypodol, a Flavonol from the Leaves of *Calycopteris floribunda*, Inhibits the Growth of CaCo2 Colon Cancer Cell Line in Vitro." *Phytotherapy Research* 22 (12): 1684–87.

Ali, M., A. Rauf, T. B. Hadda, S. Bawazeer et al. 2017. "Mechanisms Underlying Anti-Hyperalgesic Properties of Kaempferol-3,7-di-O-*a*-L-rhamnopyranoside isolated from *Dryopteris cycadina.*" *Current Topics in Medicinal Chemistry* 17 (4): 383–90.

Allen, D. E., and G. Hatfield. 2004. *Medicinal Plants in Folk Tradition. An Ethnobotany of Britain and Ireland.* Portland, OR: Timber Press.

Alqudah, A., R. Y. Athamneh, E. Qnais, O. Gammoh, M. Oqal, R. AbuDalo, H. A. Alshaikh, N. Al-Hashimi, and M. Alqudah. 2023. "The Emerging Importance of Cirsimaritin in Type 2 Diabetes Treatment." *International Journal of Molecular Science* 24 (6): 5749.

Al-Shwilly, H. A. J. 2022. "*Azolla* as a New Dietary Source in Broiler Feed: A Physiological and Production Study." *Archives of Razzi Institute* 77 (6): 2175–80.

Alviz, A. A., R. D. Salas, and L. A. Franco. 2013. "Acute Diuretic Effect of Ethanolic and Aqueous Extracts of *Ceratopteris pteridoides* (Hook) in Normal Rats." *Biomedica* 33 (1): 115–21.

Amagata, T., M. Tanaka, T. Yamada, M. Doi, K. Minoura, H. Ohishi, T. Yamori, and A. Numata. 2007. "Variation in Cytostatic Constituents of a Sponge-Derived *Gymnascella dankaliensis* by Manipulating the Carbon Source." *Journal of Natural Products* 70 (11): 1731–40.

Amin, S., B. Ullah, M. Ali, H. Khan, A. Rauf, S. A. Khan, and E. Sobarzo-Sánchez. 2020. "In Vitro *a*-glucosidase Inhibition and Computational Studies of Kaempferol Derivatives from *Dryopteris cycanida.*" *Current Topics in Medicinal Chemistry* 20 (9): 731–37.

Anacleto-Santos, J., P. López-Camacho, R. Mondragón-Flores, E. Vega-Ávila, G. B. Islas, M. Mondragón-Castelán, E. Carrasco-Ramírez, and N. Rivera-Fernández. 2020. "Anti-Toxoplasma, Antioxidant and Cytotoxic Activities of *Pleopeltis crassinervata* (Fée) T. Moore Hexane Fraction." *Saudi Journal of Biological Sciences* 27 (3): 812–19.

Anacleto-Santos, J., F. Calzada, P. Y. López-Camacho, T. D. J. López-Pérez, E. Carrasco-Ramírez, B. Casarrubias-Tabarez, T. I. Fortoul, M. Rojas-Lemus, N. López-Valdés, and N. Rivera-Fernández. 2023. "Evaluation of the Anti-*Toxoplasma gondii* Efficacy, Cytotoxicity, and GC/MS Profile of *Pleopeltis crassinervata* Active Subfractions." *Antibiotics* 12 (5): 889.

Anderson, L. L., M. Walsh, A. Roy, C. M. Blanchetti, and G. Merchan. 2011. "The Potential of *Thelypteris palustris* and *Asparagus sprengeri* in Phytoremediation of Arsenic Contamination." *International Journal of Phytoremediation* 13 (2): 177–184.

Anderson, S. C. 2017. *Psychobiotic Revolution: The Mood Food of the New Science of the Gut-Brain Connection.* Washington, DC: National Geographic.

Andrade, J. M., C. D. S. Passos, R. R. Dresch, M. A. Kieling-Rubio, P. R. H. Moreno, and A. T. Henriques. 2014. "Chemical Analysis, Antioxidant, Antichemotactic and Monoamine Oxidase Inhibition Effects of Some Pteridophytes from Brazil." *Pharmacognosy Magazine* 10 (Suppl 1): S100–9.

Andrade-Cetto, A., F. Espinoza-Hernández, G. Mata-Torres, and S. Escandón-Rivera. 2021. "Hypoglycemic Effect of Two Mexican Medicinal Plants." *Plants* 10 (10): 2060.

Anggia, V., A. Bakhtiar, and D. Arbain. 2015. "Chemical Constituents and Antibacterial Activities of Leaves of Sumatran King Fern (*Angiopteris evecta* G. Forst Hoffm.)" *Jurnal Farmasi Indonesia* 7 (4): 195.

Angier, B. 1971. *Feasting Free on Wild Edibles*. Harrisburg, PA: Stackpole Books.

Antonysamy, J. M. A., G. Janarthanan, S. Arumugam, J. Narayanan, and N. Mani. 2014. "Antioxidant, Larvicidal, and Cytotoxic Studies on *Asplenium aethiopicum* (Burm. f.) Becherer." *International Scholarly Research Notices* (2014): 876170.

Anuja, G. I., V. J. Shine, P. G. Latha, and S. R. Suja. 2018. "Protective Effect of Ethyl Acetate Fraction of *Drynaria quercifolia* against CCl_4 Induced Rat Liver Fibrosis Via Nrf2/ARE and NFkB Signalling Pathway." *Journal of Ethnopharmacology* 216: 79–88.

Ardila, C. M., J. A. Bedoya-Garcia, and D. González-Arroyave. 2023. "Antimicrobial Resistance in Patients with Endodontic Infections: A Systematic Scoping Review of Observational Studies." *Australian Endodontic Journal* 49 (2): 386–95.

Arif, Y., P. Singh, A. Bajguz, and S. Hayat. 2022. "Phytoecdysteroids: Distribution, Structural Diversity, Biosynthesis, Activity and Crosstalk with Phytohormones." *International Journal of Molecular Science* 23 (15): 8664.

Arokiyaraj, S., R. Bharanidharan, P. Agastian, and H. D. Shin. 2018. "Chemical Composition, Antioxidant Activity and Antibacterial Mechanism of Action from *Marsilea minuta* Leaf Hexane: Methanol Extract." *Chemistry Central Journal* 12 (1): 105.

Arvizu-Espinosa, M. G., G. L. von Poser, A. T. Henriques, A. Mendoza-Ruiz, A. Cardador-Martínez, R. Geesto-Borroto, P. N. Núñez-Aragón, M. L. Villarrel-Ortega, A. Sharma, and A. Cardoso-Taketa. 2019. "Bioactive Dimeric Acylphloroglucinols from the Mexican Fern *Elaphoglossum paleaceum*." *Journal of Natural Products* 82 (4): 785–91.

Assiniwi, B. 1988. *La Médicine des Indiens d'Amérique*. Montreal, QC: Guerin.

Attallah, N. G. M., F. A. Mokhtar, E. Elekhnawy, S. Z. Heneidy, E. Ahmed, S. Magdeldin, W. A. Negm, and A. H. El-Kadem. 2022. "Mechanistic Insights on the In Vitro Antibacterial Activity and In Vivo Hepatoprotective Effects of *Salvinia auriculata* Aubl against Methotrexate-Induced Liver Injury." *Pharmaceuticals* 15 (5): 549.

Awad, R., F. Ahmed, N. Bourbonnais-Spear, M. Mullaly et al. 2009. "Ethnopharmacology of Q'eqchi' Maya Antiepileptic and Anxiolytic Plants: Effects on the GABAergic System." *Journal of Ethnopharmacology* 125 (2): 257–64.

Bahadori, M. B., F. M. Kordi, A. A. Ahmadi, S. Bahadori, and H. Valizadeh. 2015. "Antibacterial Evaluation and Preliminary Phytochemical Screening of Selected Ferns from Iran." *Research Journal of Pharmacognosy* 2 (2): 53–59.

Baharuddin, A. A., R. A. J. Roosli, Z. A. Zakaria, and S. F. M. Tohid. 2018. "*Dicranopteris linearis* Extract Inhibits the Proliferation of Human Breast Cancer Line (MDA-MB-231) via Induction of S-Phase Arrest and Apoptosis." *Pharmaceutical Biology* 56 (1): 422–32.

Baker, J. G. 1868. *Catalogue of the Ferns and Their Allies Cultivated in the Royal Gardens of Kew*. London: Royal Botanic Gardens, Kew.

Balada, C., V. Diaz, M. Castro, M. Echeverria-Bugueno, M. J. Marchant, and L. Guzmán. 2022. "Chemistry and Bioactivity of *Microsorum scolopendria* (Polypodiaceae): Antioxidant Effects on an Epithelial Damage Model." *Molecules* 27 (17): 5467.

Bandyopadhyay, A., and A. Dey. 2022. "Medicinal Pteridophytes: Ethnopharmacological, Phytochemical, and Clinical Attributes." *Beni-Suef University Journal of Basic and Applied Sciences* 11 (113).

Barton, B. H. 1877. *Medicinal Plants of Great Britain*. Thomas Castle, London.

Baskaran, X., A. G. Vigila, and S. Zhang. 2018. "A Review of the Use of Pteridophytes for Treating Human Ailments." *Journal of Zhejiang University Science B* 19: 85–119.

Basnet, P., S. Kadota, M. Shimizu, H. X. Xu, and T. Namba. 1993. "2'-Hydroxymatteucinol, a New C-Methyl Flavanone Derivative from *Matteuccia* [sic] *orientalis*: Potent Hypoglycemic Activity in Streptozotocin (STZ)-Induced Diabetic Rat." *Chemical and Pharmaceutical Bulletin* (Tokyo) 41 (10): 1790–95.

Basnet, P., S. Kadota, K. Hase, and T. Namba. 1995. "Five New C-Methyl Flavonoids, the Potent aldose Reductase Inhibitors from *Matteuccia orientalis* Trev." *Chemical and Pharmaceutical Bulletin* (Tokyo) 43 (9): 1558–64.

Bassey, M. E., E. U. Etuk, M. M. Ibe, and B. A. Ndon. 2001. "*Diplazium sammatii*: Athyraceae ('Nyama idim'): Age-Related Nutritional and Antinutritional Analysis." *Plant Foods for Human Nutrition* 56 (1): 7–12.

Batubara, I., R. I. Astuti, M. E. Prastya, A. Ilmiawati, M. Maeda, M. Suzuki, A. Hamamoto, and H. Takemori. 2020. "The Antiaging Effect of Active Fractions and *Ent*-11α Hydroxy-15-Oxo-Kaur-16-En-19-Oic Acid Isolated from *Adenostemma lavenia* (L.) O. Kuntze at the Cellular Level." *Antioxidants* 9 (8): 719.

Batur, S., S. Ayla, A. A. Sakul, M. E. Okur, A. E. Karadag, B. Daylan, E. M. Ozdemir, N. Kepil, and M. Y. Gunal. 2020. "An Alternative Approach to Wound Healing Field with *Polypodium vulgare*." *Medeniyet Medical Journal* 35 (4): 315–23.

Beerling, D. 2019. *Making Eden*. Oxford University Press.

Benedict, R. C. 1915. "Fern Hats and Fern Cigar Cases." *American Fern Journal* 5: 7–9.

Benjamin, A., and V. S. Manickam. 2007. "Medicinal Pteridophytes from the Western Ghats." *Indian Journal of Traditional Knowledge* 6: 611–18.

Bhadra, S., P. K. Mukherjee, and A. Bandyopadhyay. 2012. "Cholinesterase Inhibition Activity of *Marsilea quadrifolia* Linn. An Edible Leafy Vegetable from West Bengal, India." *Natural Product Research* 26 (16): 1519–22.

Bhattacharya, K., J. Sikdar, I. Hussain, D. Barman, A. K. Shrivastava, B. J. Sahariah, A. Bhattacharjee, N. R. Chanu, and P. Khanal. 2023. "Targeting Melanoma with a Phytochemical Pool: Tailing Makisterone C." *Computers in Biology and Medicine* 166: 107499.

Bhattamisra, S. K., V. K. Khanna, A. K. Agrawal, P. N. Singh, and S. K. Singh. 2008. "Antidepressant Activity of Standardized Extract of *Marsilea minuta* Linn." *Journal of Ethnopharmacology* 117 (1): 51–57.

Bhattamisra, S. K., P. N. Singh, and S. K. Singh. 2012. "Effect of Standardized Extract of *Marsilea minuta* on Learning and Memory Performance in Rat Amnesic Models." *Pharmaceutical Biology* 50 (6): 766–72.

Bhowmick, S., M. Beckmann, J. Y. Shen, and L. A. Mur. 2023. "Identification and Metabolomic Characterization of Potent Anti-MRSA Phloroglucinol Derivatives from *Dryopteris crassirhizoma* Nakai (Polypodiaceae)." *Frontiers in Pharmacology* 14: 1235626.

Bianchi, Nicomede. 1874. *Carlo Matteucci e l'Italia del suo tempo*. Turin: Fratelli Bocca.

Bilal, H. M., A. Sharif, M. N. H. Malik, and H. M. Zubair. 2022. "Aqueous Ethanolic Extract of *Adiantum incisum* Forssk. Protects against Type 2 Diabetes Mellitus via Attenuation of *a*-Amylase and Oxidative Stress." *ACS Omega* 7 (42): 37724–35.

Bilman, F. B., and M. Yetik. 2017. "*Geotrichum candidum*: A Rare Infection Agent in Urinary System: Case Report and Review of the Literature." *Journal of Clinical and Experimental Investigations* 8 (4): 127–29.

Bisht, A., K. K. T. Goh, and L. Matia-Merino. 2023. "The Fate of Mamaku Gum in the Gut: Effect on in Vitro Gastrointestinal Function and Colon Fermentation by Human Faecal Microbiota." *Food and Function* 14 (15): 7024–39.

Bisso, B. N., R. N. E. Nkwelle, R. T. Tchuenteu, and J. P. Dzoyem. 2022. "Phytochemical Screening, Antioxidant, and Antimicrobial Activities of Seven Underinvestigated Medicinal Plants against Microbial Pathogens." *Advances in Pharmacological and Pharmaceutical Sciences* 2022: 1998808.

Blackwood, B. 1935. *Both Sides of the Buka Passage*. Clarendon Press, Oxford.

Boas, F. 2002. *Indian Myths and Legends from the North Pacific Coast of America: A Translation of Franz Boas's 1895 Edition of Indianische Sagen von der Nord Pacifischen Küste Amerikas*. Translated by Gietrich Bertz edited by Randy Bouchard and Dorothy Kennedy. Vancouver, BC: Talonbooks.

Bobach, C., J. Schurwanz, K. Franke, A. Denkert, T. V. Sung, R. Kuster, P. C. Mutiso, B. Seliger, and L. A. Wessjohann. 2014. "Multiple Readout Assay for Hormonal (Androgenic and Antiandrogenic) and Cytotoxic Activity of Plant and Fungal Extracts Based on Differential Prostate Cancer Cell Line Behavior." *Journal of Ethnopharmacology* 155 (1): 721–30.

Boericke, W. 1927. *Pocket Manual of Homeopathic Materia Medica and Repertory* (9th ed.) Delhi, India: B. Jain Publishers (reprint 2008).

Bogale, M., J. M. Sasikumar, and M. C. Egigu. 2023. "An Ethnomedicinal Study in *Tulo* District, West Hararghe Zone, *Oromia* Region, Ethiopia." *Heliyon* 9 (4): e15361.

Bolson, M., S. M. Hefler, E. I. D. O. Chaves, A. Gasparotto Jr., and E. L. Cardozo Jr. 2015. "Ethno-Medicinal Study of Plants Used for Treatment of Human Ailments, with Residents of the Surrounding Region of Forest Fragments of Paraná, Brazil." *Journal of Ethnopharmacology* 161: 1–10.

Boslett, J., C. Hemann, Y. J. Zhao, H. C. Lee, and J. L. Zweier. 2017. "Luteolinidin Protects the Postischemic Heart through CD38 Inhibition with Preservation of NADPH." *Journal of Pharmacology and Experimental Therapeutics* 361 (1): 99–108.

Bouquet, A. 1974. *Plantes Médicinales de la Côte d'Ivoire*. Paris: ORSTOM.

Bourbonnais-Spear, N., R. Awad, Z. Merali, P. Maquin, V. Cal, and J. T. Arnason. 2007. "Ethnopharmacological Investigation of Plants Used to Treat Susto, a Folk Illness." *Journal of Ethnopharmacology* 109 (3): 380–87.

Bourdy, G., and A. Walter. 1992. "Maternity and Medicinal Plants in Vanuatu. I. The Cycle of Reproduction." *Journal of Ethnopharmacology* 37 (3): 179–196.

Boven, A., E. Vlieghe, L. Engstrand, S. Callens, J. Simin, and N. Brusselaers. 2023. "*Clostridioides difficile* Infection-Associated Cause-Specific and All-Cause Mortality: a Population-Based Cohort Study." *Clinical Microbiology and Infection* 29 (11): 1424–30.

Bowen, L., C. Li, L. Bin, T. Ying, L. Shijun, and D. Junxing. 2020. "Chemical Constituents, Cytotoxic and Antioxidant Activities of Extract from the Rhizomes of *Osmunda japonica* Thunb." *Natural Product Research* 34 (6): 847–50.

Braithwaite, M., S. F. Van Vuuren, and A. M. Viljoen. 2008. "Validation of Smoke Inhalation Therapy to Treat Microbial Infections." *Journal of Ethnopharmacology* 119 (3): 501–6.

Breithaupt, A. D., and S. E. Jacob. 2012. "Subacute Cutaneous Lupus Erythematosus: A Case Report of *Polypodium leucotomas* as an Adjuvant Therapy." *Cutis* 89 (4): 183–84.

Bresciani, L. F. V., J. P. Priebe, R. A. Yunes, J. D. Magro, F. D. Monache, F. de Campos, M. M. de Souza, and V. Cechinel-Filho. 2003. "Pharmacological and Phytochemical Evaluation of *Adiantum ceneatum* Growing in Brazil." *Zeitschrift für Naturforschung C* 58 (3–4): 191–94.

Brown, A. R., K. A. Ettefagh, D. A. Todd, P. S. Cole, J. M. Egan, D. H. Foil, E. P Lacey, and N. B. Cech. 2021. "Bacterial Efflux Inhibitors are Widely Distributed in Land Plants." *Journal of Ethnopharmacology* 267: 113533.

Brown, W. H. 1951. "Useful Plants of the Philippines." *Technical Bulletin 10.* Manila, Commonwealth of the Philippines Department of Agriculture and Natural Resources Bureau of Printing.

Brunschwig, H. 1971. *Book of Distillation.* Originally titled *Liber de arte distillandide simplicibus*, in 1500. Johnson Reprint Co. no. 79.

Bunch, H., J. Park, H. Choe, M. M. Mostafiz, J. Kim, and K. Lee. 2020. "Evaluating Cytotoxicity of Methyl Benzoate in Vitro." *Heliyon* 6 (2): e03351.

Buommino, E., A. Vollaro, F. P. Nocera, F. Lembo, M. DellaGreca, L. De Martino, and M. R. Catania. 2021. "Synergistic Effect of Abietic Acid with Oxacillin against Methicillin-Resistant *Staphylococcus pseudintermedius*." *Antibiotics* 10 (1): 80.

Burkill, I. H. 1966. *A Dictionary of the Economic Products of the Malay Peninsula.* Kuala Lumpar Government of Malaysia and Singapore.

Bynigeri, R. R., A. Jakkampudi, R. Jangala, C. Subramanyam, M. Sasikala, G. V. Rao, D. N. Reddy, and R. Talukdar. 2017. "Pancreatic Stellate Cell: Pandora's Box for Pancreatic Disease Biology." *World Journal of Gastroenterology* 23 (3): 382–405.

Cai, Z., Z. Mo, S. Zheng, S. Lan, S. Xie, J. Lu, C. Tang, and Z. Shen. 2022. "Flavaspidic Acid BB Combined with Mupirocin Improves its Anti-Bacterial and Anti-Biofilm Activities against *Staphylococcus epidermidis*." *BMC Microbiology* 22 (1): 179.

Calzada, F., L. Yépez-Mulia, and A. Tapia-Contreras. 2007. "Effect of Mexican Medicinal Plant Used to Treat Trichomoniasis on *Trichomonas vaginalis* Trophozoites." *Journal of Ethnopharmacology* 113 (2): 248–51.

Calzada, F., R. Arista, and H. Pérez. 2010. "Effect of Plants Used in Mexico to Treat Gastrointestinal Disorders on Charcoal-Gum-Acacia-Induced Hyperperistalsis in Rats." *Journal of Ethnopharmacology* 128 (1): 49–51.

Cambie, R. C., and J. Ash. 1994. *Fijian Medicinal Plants.* Melbourne: CSIRO.

Cao, J., X. Xia, X. Dai, J. Xiao, Q. Wang, K. Andrae-Marobela, and H. Okatch. 2013a. "Flavonoids Profiles, Antioxidant, Acetylcholinesterase Inhibition Activities of Extract from *Dryoathyrium boryanum* (Willd.) Ching." *Food and Chemical Toxicology* 55: 121–28.

Cao, J. G., X. Xia, X. F. Chen, J. B. Xiao, and Q. X. Wang. 2013b. "Characterization of Flavonoids from *Dryopteris erythrosora* and Evaluation of Their Antioxidant, Anticancer and Acetylcholinesterase Inhibition Activities." *Food and Chemical Toxicology* 51: 242–50.

Cao, J. G., X. Xia, X. L. Dai, Q. X. Wang, and J. B. Xiao. 2014. "Chemical Composition and Bioactivities of Flavonoids-Rich Extract from *Davallia cylindrica* Ching." *Environmental Toxicology and Pharmacology* 37 (2): 571–79.

Cao, L., R. T. Li, X. Q. Chen, Y. Xue, and D. Liu. 2016. "Neougonin A Inhibits Lipopolysaccharide-Induced Inflammatory Responses via Downregulation of the NF-kB Signaling Pathway in RAW 265.7 Macrophages." *Inflammation* 39 (6): 1939–48.

Cao, S. G., M. M. Radwan, A. Norris, J. S. Miller, F. Ratovoson et al. 2006. "Cytotoxic and Other Compounds from *Didymochlaena truncatula* from the Madagascar Rain Forest." *Journal of Natural Products* 69 (2): 284–86.

Cao, Y., Q. Zhao, F. Liu, L. Zheng, X. Lin, M. Pan, X. Tan, G. Sun, and K. Zhao. 2022. "Drug Value of Drynariae Rhizoma Root-Derived Extracellular Vesicles for Neurodegenerative Diseases Based on Proteomics and Bioinformatics." *Plant Signaling and Behavior* 17 (1): 2129290.

Cárdenas, A., V. Contreras, L. R. Hernández, Z. N. Juárez, E. Sánchez-Arreola, and H. Bach. 2016. "Antimicrobial, Cytotoxic and Anti-inflammatory Activities of *Pleopeltis polylepis.*" *Journal of Ethnopharmacology* 194: 981–86.

Carlson, A. B., C. A. Mathesius, S. Ballou, M. N. Fallers et al. 2022. "Safety Assessment of the Insecticidal Protein IPD079Ea from the Fern, *Ophioglossum pendulum.*" *Food and Chemical Toxicology* 166: 113187.

Castillo, E., M. E. González-Rosende, and I. Martinez-Solis. 2023. "The Use of Herbal Medicine in the Treatment of Vitiligo: An Updated Review." *Planta Medica* 89 (5): 468–83.

Cen, Y. J., X. F. Pang, Q. Zhou, Y. F. Peng, and C. B. Xu. 2004. "Bioassay on Oviposition Repellency on Non-Preferable Plants Extracts against Citrus Red Mite *Panonychus citri.*" *Ying Yong Sheng Tai Xue Bao* 15 (9): 1687–90.

Cha, J. D., E. K. Jung, S. M. Choi, K. Y. Lee, and S. W. Kang. 2017. "Antimicrobial Activity of the Chloroform Fraction of *Drynaria fortunei* against Oral Pathogens." *Journal of Oral Science* 59 (1): 31–38.

Chai, T., L. Yeoh, N. Ismaliza, M. Ismail, F. A. Manan, and F. Wong. 2015a. "Evaluation of Glucosidase Inhibitory and Cytotoxic Potential of Five Selected Edible and Medicinal Ferns." *Tropical Journal of Pharmaceutical Research* 14: 449–54.

Chai, T. T., M. T. Kwek, H. C. Ong, and F. C. Wong. 2015b. "Water Fraction of Edible Medicinal Fern *Stenochlaena palustris* is a Potent *a*-glucosidase Inhibitor with Concurrent Antioxidant Activity." *Food Chemistry* 186: 26–31.

Chai, T. T., S. Elamparuthi, M. L. Yong, and Y. X. Quah. 2013. "Antibacterial, Anti-glucosidase, and Antioxidant Activities of Selected Highland Ferns of Malaysia." *Botanical Studies* 54 (1): 55.

Chai, T. T., L. Y. Yeoh, N. I. Mohd Ismail, H. C. Ong, F. C. Wong. 2015. "Cytotoxicity and Antiglucosidase Potential of Six Selected Edible and Medicinal Fern." *Acta Poloniae Pharmaceutica - Drug Research* 72 (2): 397–401.

Chaity, F. R., M. Khatun, and M. S. Rahman. 2016. "In Vitro Membrane Stabilizing, Thrombolytic and Antioxidant Potentials of *Drynaria quercifolia* L., a Remedial Plant of the Garo Tribal People of Bangladesh." *BMC Complementary and Alternative Medicine* 16: 184.

Chaiwong, S., S. Sretrirutchai, J. K. Sung, and S. Kaewsuwan. 2023. "Antioxidative and Anti-Photooxidative Potential of Interruptins from the Edible Fern *Cyclosorus terminans* in Human Skin Cells." *Current Pharmaceutical Biotechnology* 25 (4): 468–76.

Chakraborty, R., B. De, N. Devanna, and S. Sen. 2013. "Antitussive, Expectorant Activity of *Marsilea minuta* L., an Indian vegetable." *Journal of Advanced Pharmaceutical Technology and Research* 4 (1): 61–64.

Chan, S. M., K. S. Khoo, S. D. Sekaran, and N. W. Sit. 2021. "Mode-Dependent Antiviral Activity of Medicinal Plant Extracts against the Mosquito-Borne Chikungunya Virus." *Plants* 10 (8): 1658.

Chan, Y. S., Y. H. Cheah, P. Z. Chong, H. L. Khor, W. S. Teh, K. S. Khoo, H. C. Ong, and N. W. Sit. 2019. "Antifungal and Cytotoxic Activities of Selected Medicinal Plants from Malaysia." *Pakistan Journal of Pharmaceutical Sciences* 31 (1): 119–27.

Chand Basha, S., M. Sreenivasulu, and N. Pramod. 2013. "Anti-Diabetic Activity of *Actiniopteris radiata* (Linn.)." *Asian Journal of Research in Chemistry and Pharmaceutical Sciences* 1 (1): 1–6.

Chandra, P., E. Yadav, M. Mani, A. K. Ghosh, and M. Sachan. 2015. "Protective Effect of *Lygodium flexuosum* (Family: Lygodiaceae) against Excision, Incision and Dead Space Wound Models in Experimental Rats." *Toxicology and Industrial Health* 31 (3): 274–80.

Chang, H. C., J. C. Chen, J. L. Yang, H. S. Tsay, C. Y. Hsiang, and T. Y. Ho. 2014. "The Suppressive Activities of Six Sources of Medicinal Ferns known as Gusuibu on Heat-Labile Enterotoxin-Induced Diarrhea." *Molecules* 19 (2): 2114–20.

Chang, H. L., J. H. Su, Y. T. Yeh, Y. C. Lee, H. M. Chen, Y. C. Wu, and S. S. F. Yuan. 2008a. "Protoapigenone, a Novel Flavonoid, Inhibits Ovarian Cancer Growth in Vitro and in Vivo." *Cancer Letters* 267 (1): 85–95.

Chang, H. L., Y. C. Wu, J. H. Su, Y. T. Yeh, and S. S. F. Yuan. 2008b. "Protoapigenone, a Novel Flavonoid, Induces Apoptosis in Human Prostate Cancer Cells through Activation of p38 Mitogen-Activated Protein Kinase and c-Jun NH2-terminal Kinase 1/2." *The Journal of Pharmacology and Experimental Therapeutics* 325 (3): 841–49.

Chang, S. H., J. H. Bae, D. P. Hong, K. D. Choi, S. C. Kim, E. Her, S. H. Kim, and C. D. Kang. 2010. "*Dryopteris crassirhizoma* has Anti-Cancer Effects through Both Extrinsic and Intrinsic Apoptotic Pathways and G0/G1 Phase Arrest in Human Prostate Cancer Cells." *Journal of Ethnopharmacology* 130 (2): 248–54.

Chang, T. C., H. Chiang, Y. H. Lai, Y. L. Huang, H. C. Huang, Y. C. Liang, H. K. Liu, and C. Huang. 2019."*Helminthostachys zeylanica* Alleviates Hepatic Steatosis and Insulin Resistance in Diet-Induced Obese Mice." *BMC Complementary and Alternative Medicine* 19 (1): 368.

Chatterjee, A., C. P. Dutta, B. Choudhury, P. K. Dey, C. Chaterjee, S. R. Mukherjee. 1963. "The Chemistry and Pharmacology of Marsiline: A Sedative and Anticonvulsant Principle Isolated from *Marsilea minuata* Linn and *Marsilea rajasthanensis* Gupta." *Journal of Experimental Medical Sciences* 7: 53–67.

Chatterjee, S., S. Bhattacharya, P. R. Choudhury, A. Rahaman, A. Sarkar, A. D. Talukdar, D. P. Mandal, and S. Bhattacharjee. 2022. "*Drynaria quercifolia* Suppresses Paracetamol-Induced Hepatotoxicity in Mice by Inducing Nrf-2." *Bradisklavske Lesarske Listy* 123(2): 110–19.

Chear, N. J. Y., K. Y. Khaw, V. Murugaiyah, and C. S. Lai. 2016. "Cholinesterase Inhibitory Activity and Chemical Constituents of *Stenochlaena palustris* Fronds at Two Different Stages of Maturity." *Journal of Food and Drug Analysis* 24 (2): 358–66.

Chen, C. R., Y. W. Liao, H. T. Wu, W. L. Shih, C. Y. Tzeng, S. Z. Yang, C. E. Hernandez, and C. I. Chang. 2010. "Triterpenoids from *Angiopteris palmiformis*." *Chemical and Pharmaceutical Bulletin* 58 (3): 408–11.

Chen, C. Y., C. C. Huang, K. C. Tsai, W. J. Huang, W. C. Huang, Y. C. Hsu, and F. L. Hsu. 2014a. "Evaluation of the Antihyperuricemic Activity of Phytochemicals from *Davallia formosana* by Enzyme Assay and Hyperuricemic Mice Model." *Evidence Based Complementary and Alternative Medicine* 2014: 873607.

Chen, C. Y., C. H. Yang, Y. F. Tsai, C. C. Liaw, W. Y. Chang, and T. L. Hwang. 2017a. "Ugonin U stimulates NLRP3 Inflammasome Activation and Enhances Inflammasome-Mediated Pathogen Clearance." *Redox Biology* 22: 263–74.

Chen, C. Y., F. Y. Chiu, Y. S. Lin, W. J. Huang, P. S. Hsieh, and F. L. Hsu. 2015. "Chemical Constituents Analysis and Antidiabetic Activity Validation of Four Fern Species from Taiwan." *International Journal of Molecular Sciences* 16 (2): 2497–516.

Chen, G. G., N.-C. Liang, J. F. Y. Lee, U. P. F. Chan, S. H. Wang, B. C. S. Leung, and K. L. Leung. 2004. "Over-Expression of Bcl-2 against *Pteris semipinnata* L-Induced Apoptosis of Human Colon Cancer Cells via a NF-kappa B-Related Pathway." *Apoptosis* 9 (5): 619–27.

Chen, G. Y., J. Luo, Y. Liu, X. B. Yu, X. Y. Liu, and Q. W. Tao. 2022a. "Network Pharmacology Analysis and Experimental Validation to Investigate the Mechanism of Total Flavonoids of Rhizoma *Drynariae* in Treating Rheumatoid Arthritis." *Drug Design Development and Therapy* 16: 1743–66

Chen, G. Y., Y. F. Wang, X. B. Yu, X. Y. Liu, J. Q. Chen, J. Luo, and Q. W. Tao. 2022b. "Network Pharmacology-Based Strategy to Investigate the Mechanisms of *Cibotium barometz* in Treating Osteoarthritis." *Evidence Based Complementary and Alternative Medicine* 2022: 1826299.

Chen, J. F., Y. X. Chen, P. Li, M. Fu, Y. N. Lv, and L. Li. 2011a. "Effect of *Ent*-11-α-hydroxy-15-oxo-kaur-16-en-19-oic-acid on Human Gastric Cancer Cells and its Mechanism." *Nan Fang Yi Ke Da Xue Xue Bao (Journal of Southern Medical University)* 31 (8): 1345–48.

Chen, J. J., T. C. Wang, C. K. Yang, H. R. Liao, P. J. Sung, I. S. Chen, M. J. Cheng, C. F. Peng, and J. F. Chen. 2013. "New Pterosin Sesquiterpenes and Antitubercular Constituents from *Pteris ensiformis*." *Chemistry and Biodiversity* 10 (10): 1903–8.

Chen, J. L., H. P. Song, J. L. Ruan, and Y. F. Lei. 2014b. "Prostatic Protective Nature of the Flavonoid-Rich Fraction from *Cyclosorus acuminatus* on Carrageenan-Induced Non-Bacterial Prostatitis in Rat." *Pharmaceutical Biology* 52 (4): 491–97.

Chen, J. L., X. L. Chen, Y. F. Lei, H. Wei, C. M. Xiong, Y. J. Liu, W. Fu, and J. L. Ruan. 2011b. "Vascular Protective Potential of the Total Flavanol Glycosides from *Abacopteris penangiana* via Modulating Nuclear Transcription Factor-kB Signaling Pathway and Oxidative Stress." *Journal of Ethnopharmacology* 136 (1): 217–23.

Chen, J. L., Y. F. Lei, G. H. Wu, Y. H. Zhang, W. Fu, C. M. Xiong, and J. L. Ruan. 2012a. "Renoprotective Potential of *Macrothelypteris torresiana* via Ameliorating Oxidative Stress and Proinflammatory Cytokines." *Journal of Ethnopharmacology* 139 (1): 207–13.

Chen, J. P., Y. C. Li, J. G. Cao, J. W. Huang, C. Jiang, X. L. Dai, and G. H. Huang. 2022c. "Adiantic Acid, a New Unsaturated Fatty Acid with a Cyclopropane Moiety from *Adiantum flabellulatum* L." *Natural Product Research* 36 (9): 2386–92.

Chen, K., G. W. Plumb, R. N. Bennett, and Y. Bao. 2005. "Antioxidant Activities of Extracts from Five Anti-Viral Medicinal Plants." *Journal of Ethnopharmacology* 96 (1–2): 201–5.

Chen, L., Y. Q. Xiong, J. Xu, J. P. Wang, Z. L. Meng, and Y. Q. Hong. 2017b. "Juglanin Inhibits Lung Cancer by Regulation of Apoptosis, ROS and Autophagy Induction." *Oncotarget* 8 (55): 93878–98.

Chen, L., Z. S. Tao, H. Chen, K. L. Zhou, and D. S. Zhou. 2018. "Combined Treatment with Alendronate and *Drynaria* Rhizome Extracts: Effect on Fracture Healing in Osteoporotic Rats." *Zeitschrift für Gerontologie und Geriatrie* 51 (8): 875–81.

Chen, L. L., D. R. Zhang, J. Li, H. M. Wang, C. H. Song, X. Tang, Y. Guan, Y. Chang, and W. F. Wang. 2021a. "Albicanol Alleviates D-Galactose-Induced Aging and Improves Behavioral Ability Via by Alleviating Oxidative Stress-Induced Damage." *Neurochemical Research* 46 (5): 1058–67.

Chen, N. H., Y. B. Zhang, X. J. Huang, L. Jiang, S. Q. Jiang, G. Q. Li, Y. L. Li, and G. C. Wang. 2016. "Drychampones A-C: Three Meroterpenoids from *Dryopteris championii*." *Journal of Organic Chemistry* 81 (19): 9443–48.

Chen, N. H., Y. R. Qian, W. Li, Y. B. Zhang, Y. D. Zhou, G. Q. Li, Y. L. Li, and G. C. Wang. 2017c. "Six New Acylphloroglucinols from *Dryopteris championii*." *Chemistry and Biodiversity* 14 (7): e1700001.

Chen, Q. X., L. Zhou, T. Long, D. L. Qin, Y. L. Wang, Y. Ye, X. G. Zhou, J. M. Wu, and A. G. Wu. 2022d. "Galangin Exhibits Neuroprotective Effects in 6-OHDA-Induced Models of Parkinson's Disease via the Nrf2/Keap1 Pathway." *Pharmaceuticals* 15 (8): 1014.

Chen, S. Q., W. Liang, X. M. Zhang, X. Li, Z. L. Zhan, L. P. Guo, L. Q. Huang, X. M. Zhang, and W. Y. Gao. 2021b. "Research Progress of Chemical Compositions and Pharmacological Action of *Drynariae* Rhizoma." *Zhongguo Zhong Yao Za Zhi* 46 (11): 2737–45.

Chen, X., Y. Zhang, J. Pei, X. Zeng, Y. Yang, Y. Zhang, F. Li, and Y. Deng. 2022e. "Phellopterin Alleviates Atopic Dermatitis-Like Inflammation and Suppresses IL-4-Induced STAT3 Activation in Keratinocytes." *International Immunopharmacology* 112: 109270.

Chen, Y. F., K. J. Wu, L. R. Siao, and H. Y. Tsai. 2022f. "Trilinolein, a Natural Triacylglycerol, Protects Cerebral Ischemia through Inhibition of Neuronal Apoptosis and Ameliorates Intimal Hyperplasia via Attenuation of Migration and Modulation of Matrix Metalloproteinase-2 and RAS/MEK/ERK Signaling Pathways in VSMCs." *International Journal of Molecular Sciences* 23 (21): 12820.

Chen, Y. F., S. J. Liu, and F. Wang. 2012b. "Sesquiterpenoids of *Coniogramme maxima*." *Zhongguo Zhong Yao Za Zhi* 37 (7): 946–50.

Cheng, A., Y. Zhang, J. Sun, D. Huang et al. 2023. "Pterosin Sesquiterpenoids from *Pteris laeta* Wall. ex Ettingsh. Protects Cells from Glutamate Excitotoxicity by Modulating Mitochondrial Signals." *Journal of Ethnopharmacology* 308: 116308.

Cheng, A. S., W. C. Chang, Y. H. Cheng, K. Y. Chen, K. H. Chen, and T. L. Chang. 2012. "The Effects of Davallic Acid from *Davallia divaricata* Blume on Apoptosis Induction in A549 Lung Cancer Cells." *Molecules* 17 (11): 12938–49.

Cheng, D. D., Y. Y. Zhang, D. M. Gao, and H. M. Zhang. 2014. "Antibacterial and Anti-Inflammatory Activities of Extract and Fractions from *Pyrrosia petiolosa* (Christ et Bar.) Ching." *Journal of Ethnopharmacology* 155 (2): 1300–5.

Cheng, J., M. Cao, S. Yi, Y. Tao et al. 2021. "Anti-Inflammatory and Antibacterial Activities of *Pyrrosia petiolosa* Ethyl Acetate (PPEAE) against *Staphylococcus aureus* in Mice." *Pakistan Journal of Pharmaceutical Sciences* 34 (2): 493–98.

Cheng, J. F., J. X. Guo, Y. N. Bian, Z. L. Chen, C. L. Li, X. D. Li, and Y. H. Li. 2019. "*Sphingobacterium athyrii* sp. nov., a Cellulose- and Xylan-Degrading Bacterium Isolated from a Decaying Fern (*Athyrium wallichianum* Ching)." *International Journal of Systematic and Evolutionary Microbiology* 69 (3): 752–60.

Chi, C., S. S. Giri, J. W. Jun, H. J. Kim, S. Yun, S. G. Kim, and S. C. Park. 2016. "Immunomodulatory Effects of a Bioactive Compound Isolated from *Dryopteris crassirhizoma* on the Grass Carp Ctenopharyngodon Idella." *Journal of Immunology Research* 2016: 3068913.

Chiang, H. C., Y. J. Lo, and F. J. Lu. 1994. "Xanthine Oxidase Inhibitor from the Leaves of *Alsophila spinulosa* (Hook) Tryon." *Journal of Enzyme Inhibition* 8 (1): 61–71.

Chick, C. N., T. Misawa-Suzuki, Y. Suzuki, and T. Usuki. 2020. "Preparation and Antioxidant Study of Silver Nanoparticles of *Microsorum pteropus* Methanol Extract." *Bioorganic and Medicinal Chemistry Letters* 30 (22): 127526.

Chiu, C. C., H. W. Chang, D. W. Chuang, F. R. Chang et al. 2009. "Fern Plant-Derived Protoapigenone Leads to DNA Damage, Apoptosis, and G_2/M Arrest in Lung Cancer Cell Line H1299." *DNA and Cell Biology* 28 (10): 501–6.

Cho, H. J., W. J. Bae, S. J. Kim, S. H. Hong, J. Y. Lee, T. K. Hwang, Y. J. Choi, S. Y. Hwang, and S. W. Kim. 2014. "The Inhibitory Effect of an Ethanol Extract of the Spores of *Lygodium japonicum* on Ethylene Glycol-Induced Kidney Calculi in Rats." *Urolithiasis* 42 (4): 309–15.

Cho, Y. C., B. R. Kim, H. T. T. Le, and S. Cho. 2017. "Anti-Inflammatory Effects on Murine Macrophages of Ethanol Extracts of *Lygodium japonicum* Spores via Inhibition of NF-kB and p38." *Molecular Medicine Reports* 16 (4): 4362–70.

Choi, S. Y. 2013. "Inhibitory Effect of *Cyrtomium fortunei* J. Smith Root Extract on Melanogenesis." *Pharmacognosy Magazine* 9 (35): 227–30.

Chopra, R. N., S. L. Nayar, and I. C. Chopra. 1956. *Glossary of Indian Medicinal Plants.* New Delhi Council of Scientific and Industrial Research.

Chou, P. Y., G. J. Huang, C. H. Pan, Y. C. Chien, Y. Y. Chen, C. H. Wu, M. J. Sheu, and H. C. Cheng. 2011. "Trilinolein Inhibits Proliferation of Human Non-Small Cell Lung Carcinoma A549 through the Modulation of PI3K/Akt Pathway." *American Journal of Chinese Medicine* 39 (4): 803–15.

Choudhari, A. S., P. Raina, M. M. Deshpande, A. G. Wali, A. Zanwar, S. L. Bodhankar, and R. Kaul-Ghanekar. 2013. "Evaluating the Anti-Inflammatory Potential of *Tectaria cicutaria* L. Rhizome Extract in Vitro as Well as in Vivo." *Journal of Ethnopharmacology* 150 (1): 215–22.

Chu, Q., K. Hashimoto, K. Satoh, Q. T. Wang, and H. Sakagami. 2009a. "Effect of Three Herbal Extracts on NO and PGE2 Production by Activated Mouse Macrophage-Like Cells." *In Vivo* 23 (4): 537–44.

Chu, Q., K. Satoh, T. Kanamoto, S. Terakubo, H. Nakashima, Q. Wang, and H. Sakagami. 2009b. "Antitumor Potential of Three Herbal Extracts against Human Oral Squamous Cell Lines." *Anticancer Research* 29 (8): 3211–19.

Chuang, Y. C., M. C. Hsieh, C. C. Lin, Y. S. Lo, H. Y. Ho, M. J. Hsieh, and J. T. Lin. 2021. "Pinosylvin Inhibits Migration and Invasion of Nasopharyngeal Carcinoma Cancer Cells via Regulation of Epithelial-Mesenchymal Transition and Inhibition of MMP-2." *Oncology Reports* 46 (1): 143.

Chumsuwan, N., P. Khongkow, S. Kaewsuwan, and K. Kanokwiroon. 2022. "Interruptin C, a Radioprotective Agent, Derived from *Cyclosorus terminans* Protect Normal Breast MCF-10A and Human Keratinocyte HaCaT Cells against Radiation-Induced Damage." *Molecules* 27 (10): 3298.

Cioffi, G., P. Montoro, O. L. De Ugaz, A. Vassallo, L. Severino, C. Pizza, and N. De Tommasi. 2011. "Antioxidant Bibenzyl Derivatives from *Notholaena nivea* Desv." *Molecules* 16 (3): 2527–41.

Clericuzio, M., B. Burlando, G. Gandini, S. Tinello, E. Ranzato, S. Martinotti, and L. Cornara. 2014. "Keratinocyte Wound Healing Activity of Galactoglycerolipids from the Fern *Ophioglossum vulgatum* L." *Journal of Natural Medicines* 68 (1): 31–37.

Coles, W. 1657. *Adam in Eden: or Natures Paradise.* London: Streater.

Cooke, S. V. G. 2010. "Stone Age Humans Liked Their Burgers in a Bun." *New Scientist,* 18.

Copeland, E. B. 1942. "Edible Ferns." *American Fern Journal* 32: 121–26.

Core, E. L. 1967. "Ethnobotany of S. Appalachian Aborigines." *Economic Botany* 21: 203.

Corzo, M. C. V., M. J. A. Cordero, C. D. T. Galvàn, and D. S. Millán. 2014. "Benefits of Decumanum Phlebodium Intake on the Muscle Damage in the Response to Intense Physical Exercise in Sedentary Subjects." *Nutrición Hospitalaria* 29 (6): 1408–18.

Costa, H. R., I. Simão, H. Silva, P. Silveira, A. M. S. Silva, and D. C. G. A. Pinto. 2021. "*Aglaomorpha quericfolia* (L.) Hovenkamp & S. Linds a Wild Fern Used in Timorese Cuisine." *Foods* 10 (1): 87.

Creasey, W. A. 1969. "Antitumoral Activity of the Fern *Cibotium schiedei*." *Nature* 222 (5200): 1281–82.

Cullina, W. 2008. *Native Ferns Moss & Grasses*. New York: Houghton Mifflin Co.

Culpeper, N. 1652. *The English Physician*. Later appeared in 1653 as *Complete Herbal*. London, England: Peter Cole, Cornhil.

Cuong, N. X., C. V. Minh, P. V. Kiem, H. T. Huong et al. 2009. "Inhibitors of Osteoclast Formation from Rhizomes of *Cibotium barometz*." *Journal of Natural Products* 72 (9): 1673–77.

Dai, G. C., B. Hu, W. F. Zhang, F. Peng, R. Wang, Z. Y. Liu, B. X. Xue, J. Y. Liu, and Y. X. Shan. 2017. "Chemical Characterization, Anti-Benign Prostatic Hyperplasia Effect and Subchronic Toxicity Study of Total Flavonoid Extract of *Pteris multifida*." *Food and Chemical Toxicology* 108 (Pt B): 524–31.

Dall'Acqua, S., F. Tome, S. Vitalini, E. Agradi, and G. Innocenti. 2009. "In Vitro Estrogenic Activity of *Asplenium trichomanes* L. Extracts and Isolated Compounds." *Journal of Ethnopharmacology* 122 (3): 424–29.

Daniyal, M., Y. Jian, F. Xiao, W. Sheng, J. Fan, C. Xiao, Z. Wang, B. Liu, C. Peng, Q. Yuhui, and W. Wang. 2020. "Development of a Nanodrug-Delivery System Camouflaged by Erythrocyte Membranes for the Chemo/Phototherapy of Cancer." *Nanomedicine* (London) 15 (7): 691–709.

da Rocha, M. N., A. M. da Fonseca, A. N. M. Dantas, H. S. Dos Santos, E. S. Marinho, and G. S. Marino. 2023. "In Silico Study in MPO and Molecular Docking of the Synthetic Drynaran Analogues against the Chronic Tinnitus: Modulation of the M1 Muscarinic Acetylcholine Receptor." *Molecular Biotechnology* 66 (2): 254–69.

Darwin, Erasmus. 1791. *The Botanic Garden: A Poem in Two Parts*. London: J. Johnson, St. Paul's Churchyard.

Das, A. J., P. Khawas, D. Seth, T. Miyaji, and S. C. Deka. 2016a. "Optimization of the Extraction of Phenolic Compounds from *Cyclosorus extensa* with Solvents of Varying Polarities." *Preparative Biochemistry and Biotechnology* 46 (8): 755–63.

Das, A. J., T. Miyaji, and S. C. Deka. 2019a. "Bioflavonoids from *Artocarpus heterophyllus* Iam. and *Cyclosorus extensus* (Blume) H. Ito as Preservatives for Increased Storage Stability of Rice Beer." *Natural Product Research* 33 (21): 3161–66.

Das, B., A. Dey, A. D. Talukdar, K. Nongalleima, M. D. Choudhury, and L. Deb. 2014. "Antifertility Efficacy of *Drynaria quercifolia* (L.) J. Smith on Female Wister Albino Rats." *Journal of Ethnopharmacology* 153 (2): 424–29.

Das, G., S. J. Park, and K. H. Baek. 2017. "Diversity of Endophytic Bacteria in a Fern Species *Dryopteris uniformis* (Makino) Makino and Evaluation of Their Antibacterial Potential against

Five Foodborne Pathogenic Bacteria." *Foodborne Pathogens and Disease* 14 (5): 260–68.

Das, K., S. Deb, and T. Karanth. 2019b. "Phytochemical Screening and Metallic Ion Content and Its Impact on the Antipsoriasis Activity of Aqueous Leaf Extracts of *Calendula officinalis* and *Phlebodium decumanum* in an Animal Experiment Model." *Turkish Journal of Pharmaceutical Sciences* 16 (3): 292–302.

Das, S., and K. Mazumdar. 2016. "Phytoremediation Potential of a Novel Fern, *Salvinia cucullata*, Roxb. Ex Bory, to Pulp and Paper Mill Effluent: Physiological and Anatomical Response." *Chemosphere* 163: 62–72.

Das, S., and S. Goswami. 2017. "Copper Phytoextraction by *Salvinia cucullata*: Biochemical and Morphological Study." *Environmental Science and Pollution Research International* 24 (2): 1363–71.

Dascalu, A. E., A. Ghinet, E. Lipka, C. Furman, B. Rigo, A. Fayeulle, and M. Billamboz. 2020. "Design, Synthesis and Antifungal Activity of Pterolactam-Inspired Amide Mannich Bases." *Fitoterapia* 143: 104581.

da Silva, G. C., A. M. de Oliveira, J. C. B. Machado, M. R. A. Ferreira, P. L. de Medeiros, L. A. L. Soares, I. A. de Souza, P. M. G. Paiva, and T. H. Napoleão. 2020. "Toxicity Assessment of Saline Extract and Lectin-Rich Fraction from *Microgramma vacciniifolia* Rhizome." *Toxicon* 187: 65–74.

da Silva, G. C., A. M. de Oliveira, W. K. Costa, A. F. da Silva Filho, M. G. da Rocha Pitta, M. J. B. de Melo Rêgo, I. A. de Souza, P. M. G. Paiva, and T. H. Napoleão. 2022. "Antibacterial and Antitumor Activities of a Lectin-Rich Preparation from *Microgramma vacciniifolia* Rhizome." *Current Research in Pharmacology and Drug Discovery* 3: 100093.

David, M., Q. U. Ain, M. Ahmed, W. Zaman, and S. Jahan. 2019. "A Biochemical and Histological Approach to Study Antifertility Effects of Methanol Leaf Extract of *Asplenium dalhousiae* Hook. in Adult Male Rats." *Andrologia* 51 (6): e13262.

de Albuquerque, L. P., E. V. Pontual, G. M. de Sà Santana, L. R. S. Silva et al. 2014. "Toxic Effects of *Microgramma vacciniifolia* Rhizome Lectin on *Artemia salina*, Human Cells, and the Schistosomiasis Vector *Biomphalaria glabrata*." *Acta Tropica* 138: 23–27.

de Baïracli Levy, J. 1973. *Herbal Handbook for Farm and Stable*. London: Faber & Faber.

de Bellis, R., M. P. Piacentini, M. A. Meli, M. Mattioli, M. Menotta, M. Mari, L. Valentini, L. Palomba, D. Desideri, and L. Chiarantini. 2019. "In Vitro Effects on Calcium Oxalate Crystallization Kinetics and Crystal Morphology of an Aqueous Extract from *Ceterach officinarum*: Analysis of a Potential Antilithiatic Mechanism." *PLoS One* 14 (6): e0218734.

de Boer, H. J., A. Kool, A. Broberg, W. R. Mziray, I. Hedberg, and J. J. Levenfors. 2005. "Anti-Fungal and Anti-Bacterial Activity of Some Herbal Remedies from Tanzania." *Journal of Ethnopharmacology* 96 (3): 461–69.

de Boussac, H., S. Maqdasy, A. Trousson, N. Zelcer, D. H. Volle, J. M. A. Lobaccaro, and S. Baron. 2015. "Enolase is Regulated by Liver X Receptors." *Steroids* 99 (Pt B): 266–271.

Deepa, J., T. R. Parashurama, M. Krishnappa, and S. Nataraja. 2013. "Antimicrobial Efficacy of *Blechnum orientale* L." *International Journal of Pharma and Bio Sciences* 4 (2): (P) 475–79.

DeFilipps, R. A., S. L. Maina, and J. Crepin. 2004. *Medicinal Plants of the Guianas (Guyana, Surinam, French Guiana)*. Washington, DC: Smithsonian.

Deharo, E., M. Sauvain, C. Moretti, B. Richard, E. Ruiz, and G. Massiot. 1992. "Antimalarial Effect of n-Hentriacontanol Isolated from *Cuatresia* sp (Solanaceae)." *Annals de parasitologie humaine et comparée* 67 (4): 126–27.

Dehdari, S., and H. Hajimehdipoor. 2018. "Medicinal Properties of *Adiantum capillus-veneris* Linn. in Traditional Medicine and Modern Phytotherapy: A Review Article." *Iranian Journal of Public Health* 47 (2): 188–97.

de Mello Andrade, J. M., N. Maurmann, P. Pranke, I. C. C. Turatti, N. P. Lopes, and A. T. Henriques. 2017. "Identification of Compounds from Non-Polar Fractions of *Blechnum* spp and a Multitarget Approach involving Enzymatic Modulation and Oxidative Stress." *The Journal of Pharmacy and Pharmacology* 69 (1): 89–98.

Deng, Z., S. Hassan, M. Rafiq, H. Li, Y. He, Y. Cai, X. Kang, Z. Liu, and T. Yan. 2020. "Pharmacological Activity of Eriodictyol: The Major Natural Polyphenolic Flavanone." *Evidence Based Complementary and Alternative Medicine* 2020: 6681352.

Densmore, F. 1928. *Uses of Plant by the Chippewa Indians*. Washington, DC: 44th Annual Report of the Bureau of American Ethnology to the Secretary of the Smithsonian Institution, 1926–1927.

Densmore, F. 1939. *Nootka and Quilete Music*. Bulletin, Bureau of American Ethnology 124.

de Siqueira Patriota, L. L., T. F. Procópio, J. de Santana Brito, V. Sebag et al. 2017. "*Microgramma vacciniifolia* (Polypodiaceae) Fronds Contain a Multifunctional Lectin with Immunomodulatory Properties on Human Cells." *International Journal of Biological Macromolecules* 103: 36–46.

de Siqueira Patriota, L. L. , D. de B. M. Ramos, M. G. e Silva, A. C. L. A. dos Santos et al. 2022. "Inhibition of Carrageenan-Induced Acute Inflammation in Mice by the *Microgramma vacciniifolia* Frond Lectin (MvFL)." *Polymers* 14 (8): 1609.

de Souza, M. M., M. A. Pereira, J. V. Ardenghi, T. C. Mora, L. F. Bresciani, R. A. Yunes, F. D. Monache, and V. Cechinel-Filho. 2009. "Filicene Obtained from *Adiantum cuneatum* Interacts with the Cholinergic, Dopaminergic, Glutamatergic, GABAergic, and Tachykinergic Systems to Exert Antinociceptive Effect in Mice." *Pharmacology Biochemistry and Behavior* 93 (1): 40–46.

Devi, R. K., S. Vasantha, A. Panneerselvam, N. V. Rajesh, and N. Jeyathilakan. 2016. "Phytochemical Constituents and in Vitro Trematocidal Activity of *Blechnum orientale* Linn. against *Gastrothylax crumenifer*." *Annals of Phytomedicine* 5: 127–34.

Dhiman, A. K. 1998. "Ethnomedicinal Uses of Some Pteridophytic Species in India." *Indian Fern Journal* 15 (1–2): 61–64.

Díaz-Castro, J., R. Guisado, N. Kajarabille, C. García, I. M. Guisado, C. De Teresa, and J. J. Ochoa. 2012. "*Phlebodium decumanum* is a Natural Supplement that Ameliorates the Oxidative Stress and Inflammatory Signalling Induced by Strenuous Exercise in Adult Humans." *European Journal of Applied Physiology* 112 (8): 3119–28.

Ding, Z. T., Y. S. Fang, Z. G. Tai, M. H. Yang, Y. Q. Xu, F. Li, and Q. E. Cao. 2008. "Phenolic Content and Radical Scavenging Capacity of 31 Species of Ferns." *Fitoterapia* 79 (7–8): 581–83.

Dion, C., C. Haug, H. Guan, C. Ripoll et al. 2015. "Evaluation of the Anti-Inflammatory and Antioxidative Potential of Four Fern Species from China Intended for Use as Food Supplements." *Natural Product Communications* 10 (4): 597–603.

Dioscorides, P. 50. *De Materia Medica* III.121.

Dissanayake, A. A., K. Georges, and M. G. Nair. 2022. "Cyclooxygenase Enzyme and Lipid Peroxidation Inhibitory Terpenoids and Steroidal Compounds as Major Constituents in *Cleome viscosa* Leaves." *Planta Medica* 88 (14): 1287–92.

Dixit, R. D. 1989. "Ecology and Taxonomy of Pteridophytes of Madhya Pradesh." *Indian Fern Journal* 6: 140–49.

Do, H. J., T. W. Oh, J. H. Yang, K. Park II, and J. Y. Ma. 2017. "*Davallia mariesii* Moore Improves Fc & RI-Mediated Allergic Responses in the Rat Basophilic Leukemia Mast Cell Line RBL-2H3 and Passive Cutaneous Anaphylaxis in Mice." *Mediators of Inflammation* 2017: 8701650.

Dobat, K., and W. Dressendorfer. 2001. *Leonhart Fuchs: The New Herbal of 1543*. Los Angeles: Taschen.

Dodoens, R. 1583. *Stirpium historiae pemptades sex*. Antuerpiae: Ex officina Christophori Plantini.

Dong, G. C., T. Y. Ma, C. H. Li, C. Y. Chi, C. M. Su, C. L. Huang, Y. H. Wang, and T. M. Lee. 2020. "A Study of *Drynaria fortunei* in Modulation of BMP-2 Signalling by Bone Tissue Engineering." *Turkish Journal of Medical Sciences* 50 (5): 1444–53.

Dong, J. W., L. Cai, X. J. Li, L. Peng, Y. Xing, R. F. Mei, J. P. Wang, and Z. T. Ding. 2016. "Two New Peroxy Fatty Acids with Antibacterial Activity from *Ophioglossum thermale* Kom." *Fitoterapia* 109: 212–16.

Dong, Z. Y., Q. H. Zeng, L. Wei, X. Guo, Y. Sun, F. C. Meng, G. W. Wang, X. Z. Lan, Z. H. Liao, and M. Chen. 2022. "Berberisides A-D: Three Novel Prenylated Benzoic Acid Derivatives and a Clerodane Glycoside from *Berberis tsarica* Ahrendt." *Natural Product Research* 36 (8): 1996–2001.

Dotan, I., S. Fishman, Y. Dgani, M. Schwartz et al. 2006. "Antibodies against Laminaribioside and Chitobioside are Novel Serologic Markers in Crohn's Disease." *Gastroenterology* 131 (2): 366–78.

Dowling, A. E. P. 1900. *The Flora of the Sacred Nativity*. London: Kagan Paul, Trench Trubner & Co. Ltd.

Downing, B. P. 1851. *Doctor Downing's Reformed Practice and Family Physician*. New Brunswick, Canada: Roberts and Sherman.

du Bartas, G. de Sulluste. 1587. *La Semaine*. Translated by Henry Lee. 1887. *The Vegetable Lamb of Tartary*. Sampson Low, Marston, Searle and Rivington.

Dutta, A., A. Dahiya, and S. Verma. 2021. "Quercitin-3-rutinoside Protects against Gamma Radiation Inflicted Hematopoietic Dysfunction by Regulating Oxidative, Inflammatory, and Apoptotic Mediators in Mouse Spleen and Bone Marrow." *Free Radical Research* 55 (3): 230–45.

Dwivedi, V. D., I. P. Tripathi, S. Bharadwaj, A. C. Kaushik, and S. K. Mishra. 2016. "Identification of New Potent Inhibitors of Dengue Virus NS3 Protease from Traditional Chinese Medicine Database." *Virusdisease* 27 (3): 220–25.

Eckey, E. W. 1954. *Vegetable Fats and Oils*. New York: Reinhold Publishing Co.

Elasbali, A. M., W. Abu Al-Soud, Z. H. Al-Oanzi, H. Qanash, B. Alharbi, N. K. Binsaleh, M. Alreshidi, M. Patel, and M. Adnan. 2022. "Cytotoxic Activity, Cell Cycle Inhibition, and Apoptosis-Inducing Potential of *Athyrium hohenackerianum* (Lady Fern) with Its Phytochemical Profiling." *Evidence Based Complementary and Alternative Medicine*: 2055773.

Eldridge, J. 1975. "Bush Medicine in the Exumas and Long Island, Bahamas." *Economic Botany* 29: 307–32.

Ellingwood, F. 1919. *American Materia Medica Therapeutics & Pharmacognosy*. Reprinted by Eclectic Medical Publications 1998, Sandy, Oregon.

Elrasoul, A. S. A., A. A. Mousa, S. H. Orabi, M. A. E. Mohamed, S. M. Gad-Allah, R. Almeer, M. M. Abdel-Daim, S. A. M. Khalifa, H. R. El-Seedi, and M. A. A. Eldaim. 2020. "Antioxidant, Anti-inflammatory and Anti-Apoptotic Effects of *Azolla pinnata* Ethanolic Extract against Lead-Induced Hepatotoxicity in Rats." *Antioxidants* 9 (10): 1014.

El-Fadel, M. H. A., H. A. M. Hassanein, H. A. El-Sanafawy. 2020. "Effect of Partial Replacement of Protein Sun Flower Meal by Azolla Meal as Source of Protein on Productive Performance of Growing Lambs." *Journal of Animal and Poultry Production* article 4 11 (4): 149–53.

El-Tantawy, M. E., M. M. Shams, and M. S. Afifi. 2016. "Chemical Composition and Biological Evaluation of the Volatile Constituents from the Aerial Parts of *Nephrolepis exaltata* (L.) and *Nephrolepis cordifolia* (L.) C. Presl Grown in Egypt." *Natural Product Research* 30 (10): 1197–1201.

Erhirhie, E. O., C. N. Emeghebo, E. E. Ilodigwe, D. L. Ajaghaku, B. O. Umeokoli, P. M. Eze, K. G. Ngwoke, and F. B. G. C. Okoye. 2019. "*Dryopteris filix-mas* (L.) Schott Ethanolic Leaf Extract and Fractions Exhibited Profound Anti-Inflammatory Activity." *Avicenna Journal of Phytomedicine* 9 (4): 396–409.

Esteban, S., P. M. Llamas, H. Garcia-Cortés, and M. Catalá. 2016. "The Endocrine Disruptor Nonylphenol Induces Sublethal Toxicity in Vascular Plant Development at Environmental Concentrations: A Risk for Riparian Plants and Irrigated Crops?" *Environmental Pollution* 216: 480–86.

Fan, P. H., L. X. Zhao, K. Hostettmann, and H. X. Lou. 2012. "Chemical Constituents of *Asplenium ruta-muraria* L." *Natural Product Research* 26 (15): 1413–18.

Fan, Y., H. Y. Feng, L. Liu, Y. Y. Zhang, X. W. Xin, and D. M. Gao. 2020a. "Chemical Components and Antibacterial Activity of the Essential Oil of Six *Pyrrosia* Species." *Chemistry and Biodiversity* 17 (10): e2000526.

Fan, Y., X. Xin, L. Liu, H. Feng, P. Wang, Y. Zhang, and D. Gao. 2020b. "Diversity Analysis and Associated Antimicrobial Activity of Essential Oil in *Pyrrosia petiolosa*." *Chemistry and Biodiversity* 17 (12): e2000666.

Fang, J. B., J. C. Chen, and H. Q. Duan. 2010. "Two New Flavan-4-ol Glycosides from *Abacopteris penangiana*." *Journal of Asian Natural Products Research* 12 (5): 355–59.

Fang, W., J. N. Ruan, Z. Wang, Z. X. Zhao, J. Zou, D. Zhou, and Y. L. Cai. 2006. "Acetylated Flavanone Glycosides from the Rhizomes of *Cyclororus acuminatus*." *Journal of Natural Products* 69 (11): 1641–44.

Fang, X., X. Lin, S. Liang, W. D. Zhang, Y. Feng, and K. F. Ruan. 2012. "Two New Compounds from *Hicriopteris glauca* and Their Potential Antitumor Activities." *Journal of Asian Natural Products Research* 14 (12): 1175–79.

Fang, X. H., G. E. Zhou, and N. Lin. 2023. "Total Flavonoids from Rhizoma Drynariae (Gusuibu) Alleviates Diabetic Osteoporosis by Activating BMP2/Smad Signaling Pathway." *Combinatorial Chemistry and High Throughput Screening* 26 (13): 2401–09.

Farnsworth, N. R. (ed.) 1999. "NAPRALERT: Natural Products Alert Database." Program for Collaborative Research in the Pharmaceutical Sciences, Department of Medicinal Chemistry and Pharmacognosy, College of Pharmacy (website), at Chicago: University of Illinois.

Farràs, A., M. Mitjans, F. Maggi, G. Caprioli, M. P. Vinardell, and V. Lopez. 2021. "*Polypodium vulgare* L. (Polypodiaceae) as a Source of Bioactive Compounds: Polyphenolic Prolife, Cytotoxicity and Cytoprotective Properties in Different Cell Lines." *Frontiers in Pharmacology* 12: 727528.

Farràs, A., M. Mitjans, F. Maggi, G. Caprioli, M. P. Vinardell, and V. Lopez. 2022. "Exploring wild *Aspleniaceae* Ferns as Safety Sources of Polyphenols: The Case of *Asplenium trichomanes* L. and *Ceterach officinarum* Willd." *Frontiers in Pharmacology* 9: 994215.

Fasolo, J. M. M. A., A. F. K. Vizuete, E. P. Rico, R. B. S. Rambo, N. S. B. Toson, E. Santos, D. L. de Oliveira, C. A. S. Gonçalves, E. E. S. Schapoval, and A. T. Henriques. 2021. "Anti-Inflammatory Effect of Rosmarinic Acid Isolated from *Blechnum braisiliense* in Adult Zebrafish Brain." *Comparative Biochemistry and Physiology: Toxicology and Pharmacology* 239: 108874.

Femi-Adepoju, A. G., A. O. Dada, K. O. Otun, A. O. Adepoju, and O. P. Fatoba. 2019. "Green Synthesis of Silver Nanoparticles Using Terrestrial Fern (*Gleichenia Pectinata* [Willd.] C. Presl.): Characterization and Antimicrobial Studies." *Heliyon* 5 (4): e01543.

Ferdous, R., M. B. Islam, M. Y. Al-Amin, A. K. Dey, M. O. A. Mondal, M. N. Islam, A. K. Alam, A. A. Rahman, and M. G. Sadik. 2024. "Anticholinesterase and Antioxidant Activity of *Drynaria quercifolia* and Its Ameliorative Effect in Scopolamine-Induced Memory Impairment in Mice." *Journal of Ethnopharmacology* 319 (Pt 1): 117095.

Fernald, M. L., and A. C. Kinsey. 1974. *Edible Plants of Eastern North America*. New York: Harper & Row.

Ferrazzano, G. F., L. Roberto, M. R. Catania, A. Chiaviello, A. De Natale, E. Roscetto, G. Pinto, A. Pollio, A. Ingenito, and G. Palumbo. 2013. "Screening and Scoring of Antimicrobial and Biological Activities of Italian Vulnerary Plants against Major Oral Pathogenic Bacteria." *Evidence Based Complementary and Alternative Medicine* 2013 (1): 316280.

Fiorin, E., L. Sáez, and A. Malgosa. 2018. "Ferns as Healing Plants in Medieval Mallorca, Spain? Evidence from Human Dental Calculus." *International Journal of Osteoarchaeology* 29 (1): 82–90.

Fons, F., D. Froissard, J. M. Bessiere, B. Buatois, S. Rapior. 2010. "Biodiversity of Volatile Organic Compounds from five French Ferns." *Natural Product Communications* 5 (10): 1655–8.

Fosberg, F. R. 1942. "Uses of Hawaiian Ferns." *American Fern Journal* 32: 15–23.

Fu, R. H., Y. C. Wang, S. P. Liu, T. R. Shih et al. 2014. "Dryocrassin Suppresses Immunostimulatory Function on Dendritic Cells and Prolongs Skin Allograft Survival." *Cell Transplantation* 23 (4–5): 641–56.

Fu, W., G. Du, D. Liu, and J. L. Ruan. 2013. "Neuroprotective Effect of a Caffeic Acid Derivative from *Abacopteris penangiana*." *Pharmaceutical Biology* 51 (3): 376–82.

Fu, W., J. Chen, Y. Cai, Y. Lei, L. Chen, L. Pei, D. Zhou, X. Liang, and J. Ruan. 2010a. "Antioxidant, Free Radical Scavenging, Anti-Inflammatory and Hepatoprotective Potential of the Extract from *Parathelypteris nipponica* (Franch et Sav.) Ching." *Journal of Ethnopharmacology* 130 (3): 521–28.

Fu, W., Y. Lei, J. Chen, C. Xiong, D. Zhou, G. Wu, J. Chen, Y. Cai, and J. Ruan. 2010b. "Parathelypteriside Attenuates Cognition Deficits in d-Galactose Treated Mice by Increasing Antioxidant Capacity and Improving Long-Term Potentiation." *Neurobiology of Learning and Memory* 94 (3): 414–21.

Fu, X., P. Wan, P. Li, J. Wang et al. 2021. "Mechanism and Prevention of Ototoxicity Induced by Aminoglycosides." *Frontiers in Cellular Neuroscience* 15 (2021): 692762.

Gan, R. Y., L. Kuang, X. R. Xu, Y. Zhang, E. Q. Xia, F. L. Song, and H. B. Li. 2010. "Screening of Natural Antioxidants from Traditional Chinese Medicinal Plants Associated with Treatment of Rheumatic Disease." *Molecules* 15 (9): 5988–97.

Gao, B. B., Y. F. Ou, Q. F. Zhu, Z. P. Zhou, Z. T. Deng, M. Li, and Q. S. Zhao. 2021. "Clerodane-Type Diterpene Glycosides from *Dicranopteris pedata.*" *Natural Products and Bioprospecting* 11 (5): 557–64.

Gao, C., N. Guo, N. Li, X. Peng, P. Wang, W. Wang, M. Luo, and Y. Fu. 2016. "Investigation of Antibacterial Activity of Aspidin BB against *Propionibacterium acnes*." *Archives of Dermatological Research* 308 (2): 79–86.

Gao, P., X. Huang, T. Liao, G. Li, X. Yu, Y. You, and Y. Huang. 2019. "Daucosterol Induces Autophagic-Dependent Apoptosis in Prostate Cancer via JNK Activation." *Bioscience Trends* 13 (2): 160–67.

Gao, S. Y., P. Wu, J. H. Xue, H. X. Li, and X. Y. Wei. 2022. "Cytochalasans from the Endophytic Fungus *Diaporthe ueckerae* Associated with the Fern *Pteris vittata*." *Phytochemistry* 202: 113295.

Gaur, R. D., and B. P. Bhatt. 1994. "Utilization of Some Pteridophytes of Deoprayag Area in Garhwal Himalaya, India." *Economic Botany* 48: 146–151.

Gee, X., G. Ye, P. Li, W. J. Tang, J. L. Gao, and W. M. Zhao. 2008. "Cytotoxic Diterpenoids and Sesquiterpenoids from *Pteris multifida*." *Journal of Natural Products* 71 (2): 227–31.

Gerard, J. 1597. *The Herball or Generall Historie of Plants*. London: John Norton Pub.

Gleńsk, M., D. Tichaczek-Goska, K. Środa-Pomianek, M. Włodarczyk, C. A. Wesolowski, and D. Wojnicz. 2019. "Differing Antibacterial and Antibiofilm Properties of *Polypodium vulgare* L. Rhizome Aqueous Extract and One of Its Purified Active Ingredients-Osladin." *Journal of Herb Medicine* 17–18: 100261.

Gnanaraj, C., M. D. Shah, T. T. Song, and M. Iqbal. 2017. "Hepatoprotective Mechanism of *Lygodium microphyllum* (Cav.) R. Br. through Ultrastructural Signaling Prevention against Carbon Tetrachloride (CCl_4)-Mediated Oxidative Stress." *Biomedicine and Pharmacotherapy* 92: 1010–22.

Gomes, M. P., M. P. dos Santos, P. L. de Freitas, A. M. Schafaschek, E. N. de Barros, R. S. A. Kitamura, V. Paulete, and M. A. Navarro-Silva. 2023. "The Aquatic Macrophyte *Salvinia molesta* Mitigates Herbicides (Glyphosate and Aminomethylphosphonic Acid) Effects to Aquatic Invertebrates." *Environmental Science and Pollution Research International* 30 (5): 12348–61.

Gonzalez-Jurado, J. A., F. Pradas, E. S. Molina, and C. de Teresa. 2011. "Effect of *Phlebodium decumanum* on the Immune Response Induced by Training in Sedentary University Students." *Journal of Sports Science and Medicine* 10 (2): 315–21.

Gonzalez-Rivera, M. L., J. C. Barragan-Galvez, D. Gasca-Martínez, S. Hidalgo-Figueroa, M. Isiordia-Espinoza, and A. J. Alonso-Castro. 2023. "In Vivo Neuropharmacological Effects of Neophytadiene." *Molecules* 28 (8): 3457.

Goswani, H. K., K. Sen, and R. Mukhopadhyay. 2016. "Pteridophytes: Evolutionary Boon as Medicinal Plants." *Plant Genetic Resources: Characterization and Utilization* 14 (4): 328–55.

Goyal, K., A. Sharma, R. Arya, R. Sharma, G. K. Gupta, and A. K. Sharma. 2018. "Double Edge Sword Behavior of Carbendazim: A Potent Fungicide with Anticancer Therapeutic Properties." *Anticancer Agents in Medicinal Chemistry* 18 (1): 38–45.

Gridling, M., N. Stark, S. Madlener, A. Lackner et al. 2009. "In Vitro Anti-Cancer Activity of Two Ethnopharmacological Healing Plants from Guatemala *Pluchea odorata* and *Phlebodium decumanum*." *International Journal of Oncology* 34 (4): 1117–28.

Grierson, D. S., and A. J. Afolayan. 1999. "Antibacterial Activity of Some Indigenous Plants Used for the Treatment of Wounds in the Eastern Cape, South Africa." *Journal of Ethnopharmacology* 66 (1): 103–6.

Grieve, M. 1971. *A Modern Herbal*. New York: Dover Publications.

Grohmann, G. 1989. *The Plant: A Guide to Understanding Its Nature*. Kimberton, PA: Bio-Dynamic Farming and Gardening Association.

Guan, H. Y., T. Yan, D. Y. Wu, and A. S. Tripathi. 2022. "Epifriedelinol Ameliorates the Neuropathic Pain and Recovers the Function in Spinal Cord Injury by Downregulation of Neuronal Apoptosis and NMDA Receptor." *The Tohoku Journal of Experimental Medicine* 258 (2): 143–48.

Guarrera, P. M., F. Lucchese, and S. Medori. 2008. "Ethnophytotherapeutical Research in the High Molise Region (Central-Southern Italy)." *Journal of Ethnobiology and Ethnomedicine* 4: 7.

Guha, S., S. Ghosal, and U. Chattopadhyay. 1996. "Antitumor, Immunomodulatory and Anti-HIV Effects Mangiferin, a Naturally Occurring Glycosylxanthone." *Chemotherapy* 42 (6): 443–51.

Guil-Guerrero, J. L., and P. Campra. 2009. "Cytotoxicity Screening of Endemic Plants from Guayana Highlands." *Tropical Biomedicine* 26 (2): 149–54.

Gunther, E. 1945. *Ethnobotany of Western Washington: The Knowledge and Use of Indigenous Plants by Native Americans*. University of Washington Press, Seattle.

Guo, G. H., D. G. Zhang, M. Lei, X. M. Wan, J. Yang, H. Wei, and S. Q. Chen. 2023a. "Phytoextraction of As by *Pteris vittate* L. Assisted with Municipal Sewage Sludge Compost and Associated Mechanism." *The Science of the Total Environment* 893: 164705.

Guo, H. W., J. X. Wang, J. Huang, Y. G. Tian, Y. H. Liu, and H. Wei. 2022a. "Two New C21 Steroids from *Lepidogrammitis drymoglossoides* (Bak.) Ching." *Phytochemistry Letters* 49: 56–59.

Guo, J. P., J. Pang, X. W. Wang, Z. Q. Shen, M. Jin, and J. W. Li. 2006. "In Vitro Screening of Traditionally Used Medicinal Plants in China against Enteroviruses." *World Journal of Gastroenterology* 12 (25): 4078–81.

Guo, S., N. Xing, G. Xiang, Y. Zhang, and S. H. Wang. 2023b. "Eriodictyol: A Review of Its Pharmacological Activities and Molecular Mechanisms Related to Ischemic Stroke." *Food and Function* 14 (4): 1851–58.

Guo, W. H., K. Zhang, and L. H. Yang. 2022b. "Potential Mechanisms of *Pyrrosiae folium* in Treating Prostate Cancer Based on Network Pharmacology and Molecular Docking." *Drug Development and Industrial Pharmacy* 48 (5): 189–97.

Gupta, R. S., P. Kumar, A. Sharma, T. N. Bharadwaj, and V. P. Dixit. 2000. "Hypocholesterolemic Activity of *Marsilea minuta* in Gerbils." *Fitoterapia* 71 (2): 112–17.

Gupta, S., H. S. Buttar, G. Kaur, and H. S. Tuli. 2022. "Baicalein: Promising Therapeutic Applications with Special Reference to Published Patents." *Pharmaceutical Patent Analyst* 11 (1): 23–32.

Hai, P., He, Y., Wang, R., Yang, J., Gao, Y., Wu, X., Chen, N., Ye, L., and Li, R. 2023. "Antimicrobial Acylphloroglucinol Meroterpenoids and Acylphoroglucinols from *Dryopteris crassirhizoma*." *Planta Medica* 89 (3): 295–307.

Haider, S., S. Nazreen, M. M. Alam, A. Gupta, H. Hamid, and M. S. Alam. 2011. "Anti-Inflammatory and Anti-Nociceptive Activities of Ethanolic Extract and Its Various Fractions from *Adiantum capillus veneris* Linn." *Journal of Ethnopharmacology* 138 (3): 741–47.

Hamamoto, A., R. Isogai, M. Maeda, M. Hayazaki, E. Horiyama, S. Takashima, M. Koketsu, and H. Takemori. 2020. "The High Content of *Ent*-11α-hydroxy-15-oxo-kaur-16-en-19-oic Acid in *Adenostemma lavenia* (L.) O. Kuntze Leaf Extract: With Preliminary in Vivo Assays." *Foods* 9 (1): 73.

Han, L., F. Zheng, Y. Zhang, E. Liu, W. Li, M. Xia, T. Wang, and X. Gao. 2015. "Triglyceride Accumulation Inhibitory Effects of New Chromone Glycosides from *Drynaria fortunei*." *Natural Products Research* 29 (18): 1703–10.

Han, P., Y. J. Lai, J. Chen, X. N. Zhang, J. L. Chen, and X. Yang. 2016. "Protective Potential of the Methanol Extract of *Macrothelypteris oligophlebia* Rhizomes for Chronic Non-Bacterial Prostatitis in Rats." *Pakistan Journal of Pharmaceutical Sciences* 29 (4): 1217–21.

Han, Q., X. Liu, W. Yao, Z. Cheng, T. Lin, C. Song, and S. Yin. 2012. "Unusual 9,19: 24,32-dicyclotetracyclic Triterpenoids from *Lygodium japonicum*." *Planta Medica* 78 (18): 1971–75.

Han, X. Z., R. Ma, Q. Chen, X. Jin, Y. Z. Jin, R. B. An, X. M. Piao, M. L. Lian, L. H. Quan, and J. Jiang. 2018. "Anti-Inflammatory Action of *Athyrium multidentatum* Extract Suppresses the LPS-Induced TLR4 Signaling Pathway." *Journal of Ethnopharmacology* 217: 220–27.

Hanif, U., C. Raza, I. Liaqat, M. Rani, S. M. Afifi, T. Esatbeyoglu, S. Bahadur, and S. Shahid 2022. "Evaluation of Safety of Stewart's Wood Fern (*Dryopteris stewartii*) and Its Anti-Hyperglycemic Potential in Alloxan-Induced Diabetic Mice." *International Journal of Molecular Sciences* 23 (20): 12432.

Hare, H. A, C. Caspari, and H. Rusby. 1916. *The National Standard Dispensatory*. Philadelphia: Lea & Febiger.

Harinantenaina, L., K. Matsunami, and H. Otsuka. 2008. "Chemical and Biologically Active Constituents of *Pteris multifida*." *Journal of Natural Medicines* 62 (4): 452–55.

Hartley, W. J. 1962. *Handbook of Liberian Ferns*. Kew Bulletin 16: 12. Ganta, Liberia: Ganta Mission.

Hassan, S. R. U., G. Strobel, B. Geary, and J. Sears. 2013. "An Endophytic *Nodulisporium* sp, from Central America Producing Volatile Organic Compounds with Both Biological and Fuel Potential." *Journal of Microbiology and Biotechnology* 23 (1): 29–35.

Hassanein, E. H. M., F. E. M. Ali, M. M. Sayed, A. R. Mahmoud, F. A. Jaber, M. H. Kotob, and T. H. Abd-Elhamid. 2023. "Umbelliferone Potentiates Intestinal Protective Effect of *Lactobacillus acidophilus* against Methotrexate-Induced Intestinal Injury: Biochemical and Histological Study." *Tissue and Cell* 82: 102103.

He, H., Y. Sui, X. Yu, G. Luo, J. Xue, W. Yang, and Y. Long. 2023. "Potential Low Toxic Alternative for Na-Cl Cotransporter Inhibition: A Diuretic Effect and Mechanism Study of *Pyrrosia petiolosa*." *Annales Pharmaceutiques Françaises* S0003–4509(23)00071–8.

He, S., R. Ou, W. Wang, L. Ji et al. 2018. "*Camptosorus sibiricus* rupr Aqueous Extract Prevents Lung Tumorigenesis via Dual Effects against ROS and DNA Damage." *Journal of Ethnopharmacology* 220: 44–56.

He, T. P., Z. H. He, L. Mo, and N. C. Liang. 2005. "Study on the Effect and Its Mechanisms of 5F from *Pteri semipinnata* L. on the Cell Cycle of Highly Metastatic Ovarian Carcinoma HO-8910PM Cells." *Zhong Yao Cai* 28 (8): 672–76.

He, X. M., N. Ji, X. C. Xiang, P. Luo, and J. K. Bao. 2011. "Purification, Characterization, and Molecular Cloning of a Novel Antifungal Lectin from the Roots of *Ophioglossum pedunculosum*." *Applied Biochemistry and Biotechnology* 165 (7–8): 1458–72.

Hellwege, J. N., S. B. Russell, S. M. Williams, T. L. Edwards, D. R. V. Edwards. 2018. "Gene-Based Evaluation of Low-Frequency Variation and Genetically-Predicted Gene Expression Impacting Risk of Keloid Formation." *Annals of Human Genetics* 82 (4): 206–215.

Hendra, R., R. Khodijah, M. Almurdani, Y. Haryani, A. S. Nugraha, N. Frimayanti, H. Y. Teruna, and R. Abdulah. 2022. "Free Radical Scavengin, Anti-infectious, and Toxicity Activities from *Stenochlaena palustris* (Burm.f.) Bedd. Extracts." *Advances in Pharmacological and Pharmaceutical Sciences* 2022: 5729217.

Hernández-López, J., S. Crockett, O. Kunert, E. Hammer, W. Schuehly, R. Bauer, K. Crailsheim, and U. Riessberger-Gallé. 2014. "In Vitro Growth Inhibition by *Hypericum* Extracts and Isolated Pure Compounds of *Paenibacillus larvae*, a Lethal Disease Affecting Honeybees Worldwide." *Chemistry and Biodiversity* 11 (5): 695–708.

Hewagama, S. P., and R. P. Hewawasam. 2022. "Antiurolithiatic Potential of Three Sri Lankan Medicinal Plants by the Inhibition of Nucleation, Growth, and Aggregation of Calcium Oxalate Crystals in Vitro." *The Scientific World Journal* 2022: 8657249.

Hill, J. 1789. *The Useful Family Herbal.* London: Wilson and French.

Hirono, I., H. Mori, K. Kato, Y. Ushimaru, T. Kato, and M. Haga. 1978. "Safety Examination of Some Edible Plants, Part 2." *Journal of Environmental Pathology and Toxicology* 1 (1): 71–74.

Hirose, T., K. Ozaki, Y. Saito, R. Takai-Todaka et al. 2023. "Studies on the Catechin Constituents of Bark of *Cinnamomum sieboldii*." *Chemical and Pharmaceutical Bulletin* 71 (5): 374–79.

Ho, R., T. Teai, A. Meybeck, and P. Raharivelomanana. 2015. "UV-Protective Effects of Phytoecdysteroids from *Microsorum grossum* Extracts on Human Dermal Fibroblasts." *Natural Product Communications* 10 (1): 33–36.

Ho, R., T. Teai, J. P. Bianchini, R. Lafont, P. Raharivelomanana, A. Kumar, and M. A. Revilla (eds). 2010. "Ferns: From Traditional Uses to Pharmaceutical Development, Chemical Identification of Active Principles." In *Working with Ferns: Issues and Applications*, edited by A. Kumar, H. Fernández, and M. A. Revilla. New York: Springer Science. 321–346.

Ho, S. T., M. S. Yang, T. S. Wu, and C. H. Wang. 1985. "Studies on the Taiwan Folk Medicine; III. A Smooth Muscle Relaxant from *Onychium siliculosum*, Onitin." *Planta Medica* (2): 148–150.

Hoa, N. K., D. V. Phan, N. D. Thuan, and C. G. Ostenson. 2009. "Screening of the Hypoglycemic Effect of Eight Vietnamese Herbal Drugs." *Methods and Findings in Experimental and Clinical Pharmacology* 31 (3): 165–69.

Hoang, T. T. T., L. T. C. Tu, P. L. Nga, and Q. P. Dao. 2013. "A Preliminary Study on the Phytoremediation of Antibiotic Contaminated Sediment." *International Journal of Phytoremediation* 15 (1): 65–76.

Holdsworth, D. K. 1980. "Traditional Medicinal Plants of the Central Province of Papua New Guinea." *Science in New Guinea* 7: 132–47.

Holmlund, H. I., S. D. Davis, F. W. Ewers, N. M. Aguirre, G. Sapes, A. Sala, and J. Pittermann. 2020. "Positive Root Pressure is Critical for Whole-Plant Desiccation Recovery in Two Species of Terrestrial Resurrection Ferns." *Journal of Experimental Botany* 71 (3): 1139–50.

Hort, M. A., I. M. C. Brighente, M. G. Pizzolatti, and R. M. Ribeiro-do-Valle. 2019. "Mechanisms Involved in the Endothelium-Dependent Vasodilatory Effect of an Ethyl

Acetate Fraction of *Cyathea phalerata* Mart. in Isolated Rats' Aorta Rings." *Journal of Traditional and Complementary Medicine* 10 (4): 360–65.

Hort, M. A., S. DalBó, I. M. C. Brighente, M. G. Pizzolatti, R. C. Pedrosa, and R. M. Ribeiro-do-Valle. 2008. "Antioxidant and Hepatoprotective Effects of *Cyathea phalerata* Mart. (Cyatheaceae)." *Basic and Clinical Pharmacology and Toxicology* 103 (1): 17–24.

Hoseinifar, S. H., M. A. Jahazi, R. Mohseni, M. Raeisi, M. Bayani, M. Mazandarani, M. Yousefi, H. Van Doan, and M. Torfi Mozanzadeh. 2020. "Effects of Dietary Fern (*Adiantum capillus-veneris*) Leaves Powder on Serum and Mucus Antioxidant Defence, Immunological Responses, Antimicrobial Activity and Growth Performance of Common Carp (*Cyprinus carpio*) Juveniles." *Fish and Shellfish Immunology* 106: 959–66.

Hosseini, E. K., P. Derakhshi, M. Rabbani, and N. Mooraki. 2021. "Pollutant Removal from Dairy Wastewater Using Live *Azolla filiculoides* in Batch and Continuous Bioreactors." *Water Environment Research* 93 (10): 2122–34.

Hou, B., Z. Liu, X. B. Yang, W. F. Zhu, J. Y. Li, L. Yang, F. C. Reng, Y. F. Lv, J. M. Hu, G. Y. Liao, and J. Zhou. 2019. "Total Synthesis of Dryocrassin ABBA and Its Analogues with Potential Inhibitory Activity against Drug-Resistant Neuraminidases." *Bioorganic and Medicinal Chemistry* 27 (17): 3846–52.

Hou, B., Y. M. Zhang, H. Y. Liao, L. F. Fu et al. 2022. "Target-Based Virtual Screening and LC/MS-Guided Isolation Procedure for Identifying Phloroglucinol-Terpenoid Inhibitors of SARS-CoV-2." *Journal of Natural Products* 85 (2): 327–36.

Hou, M., W. Hu, Z. Xiu, Y. Shi, K. Hao, D. Cao, Y. Guan, and H. Yin. 2020. "Efficient Enrichment of Total Flavonoids from *Pteris ensiformis* Burm. Extracts by Microporous Adsorption Resins and in Vitro Evaluation of Antioxidant and Antiproliferative Activities." *Journal of Chromatography. B, Analytical Technologies in the Biomedical and Life Sciences* 1138: 121960.

Hsiao, H. B., J. B. Wu, and W. C. Lin. 2019. "Anti-Arthritic and Anti-Inflammatory Effects of (-)-Epicatechin-3-O-b-d-allopyranoside, a Constituent of *Davallia formosana*." *Phytomedicine* 52: 12–22.

Hsieh, H.-L., S.-H. Yang, T.-H. Lee, J.-Y. Fang, and C.-F. Lin. 2016. "Evaluation of Anti-Inflammatory Effects of *Helminthostachys zeylanica* Extracts via Inhibiting Bradykinin-Induced MMP-9 Expression in Brain Astrocytes." *Molecular Neurobiology* 53 (9): 5995–6005.

Hsieh, P. F., W. P. Jiang, S. Y. Huang, P. Basavaraj, J. B. Wu, H. Y. Ho, G. J. Huang, and W. C. Huang. 2020. "Emerging Therapeutic Activity of *Davalllia formosana* on Prostate Cancer Cells through Coordinated Blockade of Lipogenesis and Androgen Receptor Expression." *Cancers* 12 (4): 914.

Hsu, C. Y. 2008. "Antioxidant Activity of *Pyrrosia petiolosa*." *Fitoterapia* 79 (1): 64–66.

Hsu, F. L., C. F. Huang, Y. W. Chen, Y. P. Yen, C. T. Wu, B. J. Uang, R. S. Yang, and S. H. Liu. 2013. "Antidiabetic Effects of Pterosin A, a Small-Molecular-Weight Natural Product, on Diabetic Mouse Models." *Diabetes* 62 (2): 628–38.

Hu, J., X. D. Shi, and J. G. Chen. 2012. "Four New Antioxidant Phenylpropanoid Glycosides from *Microlepia pilosissima*." *Archives of Pharmacal Research* 35 (12): 2127–33.

Hu, J., Y. Song, H. Li, X. Mao, Y. M. Zhao, and X. D. Shi. 2015. "Antimicrobial and Cytotoxic Isopimarane Diterpenoid Glycosides from *Microlepia pilosissima* Ching." *Fitoterapia* 101: 27–33.

Hu, J. P., S. P. Liu, Y. Long, N. Tao, B. Yang, and L. Y. Zhang. 2022. "Ptercresions A-C: Three New Terpenes with Hepatoprotective Activity from *Pteris cretica* L." *Natural Product Research* 36 (24): 6252–58.

Hu, Q. Y., L. L. Chen, and R. F. Wang. 2010. "Traditional Chinese Medicine *Drynaria fortunei* J. Smith Naringin Promotes Proliferation and Differentiation of Human Periodontal Ligament Cells." *Zhejiang Da Xue Bao Yi Xue Ban* 39 (1): 79–83.

Hua, X., Q. Yang, W. Zhang, Z. Dong, S. Yu, S. Schwarz, and S. Liu. 2018. "Antibacterial Activity and Mechanism of Action of Aspidinol against Multi-Drug-Resistant Methicillin-Resistant *Staphylococcus aureus*." *Frontiers in Pharmacology* 9: 619.

Huang, W. C., N. C. Ting, Y. L. Huang, and L. C. Chen et al. 2020. "*Helminthostachys zeylanica* Water Extract Ameliorates Airway Hyperresponsiveness and Eosinophil Infiltration by Reducing Oxidative Stress and Th2 Cytokine Production in a Mouse Asthma Model." *Mediators of Inflammation* 2020: 1702975.

Huang, X. F., S. J. Yuan, and C. Yang. 2012. "Effects of Total Flavonoids from *Drynaria fortunei* on the Proliferation and Osteogenic Differentiation of Rat Dental Pulp Stem Cells." *Molecular Medicine Reports* 6 (3): 547–552.

Huang, X. H., P. C. Xiong, C. M. Xiong, Y. L. Cai, A. H. Wei, J. P. Wang, X. F. Liang, and J. L. Ruan. 2010a. "In Vitro and in Vivo Antitumor Activity of *Macrothelypteris torresiana* and Its Acute/Subacute Oral Toxicity." *Phytomedicine* 17 (12): 930–34.

Huang, Y. C., T. L. Hwang, Y. L. Yang, S. H. Wu, M. H. Hsu, J. P. Wang, S. C. Chen, L. J. Huang, and C. C. Liaw. 2010b. "Acetogenin and Prenylated Flavonoids from *Helminthostachys zeylanica* with Inhibitory Activity on Superoxide Generation and Elastase Release by Neutrophils." *Planta Medica* 76 (5): 447–53.

Huang, Y. H., W. M. Zeng, G. Y. Li, G. Q. Liu, D. D. Zhao, J. Wang, and Y. L. Zhang. 2014. "Characterization of a New Sesquiterpene and Antifungal Activities of Chemical Constituents from *Dryopteris fragrans* (L.) Schott." *Molecules* 19(1): 507–513.

Huang, Y. L., C. C. Shen, Y. C. Shen, W. F. Chiou, and C. C. Chen. 2017. "Anti-Inflammatory and Antiosteoporosis Flavonoids from the Rhizomes of *Helminthostachys zeylanica*." *Journal of Natural Products* 80 (2): 246–53.

Huang, Y. L., P. Y. Yeh, C. C. Shen, and C. C. Chen. 2003. "Antioxidant Flavonoids from the Rhizomes of *Helminthostachys zeylanica*." *Phytochemistry* 64 (7): 1277–83.

Hwang, J. Y., K. J. Youn, G. Lim, J. Y. Lee, D. H. Kim, and M. Jun. 2021. "Discovery of Natural Inhibitors of Cholinesterases from *Hydrange*a: In Vitro and in Silico Approaches." *Nutrients* 13 (1): 254.

Ibraheim, Z. Z., A. S. Ahmed, and Y. G. Gouda. 2011. "Phytochemical and Biological Studies of *Adiantum capillus-veneris* L." *Saudi Pharmaceutical Journal* 19 (2): 65–74.

Ibrakaw, A. S., S. I. Omoruyi, O. E. Ekpo, and A. A. Hussein. 2020. "Neuroprotective Activities of *Boophone haemanthoides* (Amaryllidaceae) Extract and Its Chemical Constituents." *Molecules* 25 (22): 5376.

Imran, M., M. S. Arshad, M. S. Butt, J. H. Kwon, M. U. Arshad, and M. T. Sultan. 2017. "Mangiferin: A Natural Miracle Bioactive Compound against Lifestyle Related Disorders." *Lipids in Health and Disease* 16 (1): 84.

Ionson, B. 1631. *The Nevv Inne, or The Light Heart, A Comoedy*. London: Thomas Harper.

Iqbal, I., F. Saqib, M. F. Latif, H. Shahzad, L. Dima, B. Sajer, R. Manea, C. Pojala, and R. Necula. 2023. "Pharmacological Basis for Antispasmodic, Bronchodilator and Antidiarrheal Potential of *Dryopteris ramosa* (Hope) C. via in Vitro, in Vivo, and in Silico Studies." *ACS Omega* 8 (3): 26982–27001.

Isenmann, E., G. Ambrosio, J. F. Joseph, M. Mazzarino, X. de la Torre, P. Zimmer, R. Kazlauskas, C. Goebel, F. Botrè, P. Diel, and M. K. Parr. 2019. "Ecdysteroids as Non-Conventional Anabolic Agent: Performance Enhancement by Ecdysterone Supplementation in Humans." *Archives of Toxicology* 93 (7): 1807–16.

Ishaq, M. S., M. M. Hussain, M. S. Afridi, G. Ali, M. Khattak, S. Ahmad, and Shakirullah. 2014. "In Vitro Phytochemical, Antibacterial, and Antifungal Activities of Leaf, Stem and Root Extracts of *Adiantum capillus veneris*." *The Scientific World Journal* 2014: 269793.

Ishaque, M., Y. Bibi, S. Al Ayoubi, S. Masood, S. Nisa, and A. Qayyum. 2022a. "Iriflophenone-3-C-b-d Glucopyranoside from *Dryopteris ramosa* (Hope) C. Chr. with Promising Future as Natural Antibiotic from Gastrointestinal Tract Infections." *Antibiotics* 10 (9): 1128.

Ishaque, M., Y. Bibi, S. Masood, S. Al Ayoubi, A. Qayyum, S. Nisa, and W. Ahmed. 2022b. "Xanthone C-glycosides Isomers Purified from *Dryopteris ramosa* (Hope) C. Chr. with Bacterial and Cytotoxic Prospects." *Saudi Journal of Biological Sciences* 29 (2): 1191–96.

Islam, M. 1983. "Utilization of Certain Ferns and Fern Allies in the North-East Region of India." *Journal of Economic and Taxonomic Botany* 4: 861–67.

Ismail, N. A., N. S. Shamsahal Din, S. S. Mamat, Z. Zabidi, W. N. W. Zainulddin, F. H. Kamisan, F. Yahya, N. Mohtarrudin, M. N. M. Desa, and Z. A. Zakaria. 2014. "Effect of Aqueous Extract against Paracetamol and Carbon Tetrachloride-Induced Toxicity in Rats." *Pakistan Journal of Pharmaceutical Sciences* 27 (4): 831–35.

Ito, H., T. Muranaka, K. Mori, Z. X. Jin, H. Toduka, H. Nishino, and T. Yoshida. 2000. "Ichthyotoxic Phloroglucinol Derivatives from *Dryopteris fragrans* and Their Anti-Tumor Promoting Activity." *Chemical and Pharmaceutical Bulletin* (Tokyo) 48: 1190–95.

Itzhaki, R. F. 2017. "Herpes Simplex Virus Type 1 and Alzheimer's Disease: Possible Mechanisms and Signposts." *FASEB Journal* 31 (8): 3216–26.

Jabet, A., S. Dellière, S. Seang, A. Chermak et al. 2023. "Sexually Transmitted Trichophyton Mentagrophytes Genotype VII Infection among Men Who Have Sex with Men." *Emerging Infectious Diseases Journal* 29 (7): 1411.

Jacobs, M. L., and H. M. Burlage. 1958. *Index of Plants of North Carolina with Reputed Medicinal Uses*. Chapel Hill, NC: Burlage.

Jafari, N., S. J. Zargar, M. R. Deinavazi, and N. Yassa. 2018. "Cell Cycle Arrest and Apoptosis Induction of Phloroacetophenone Glycosides and Caffeolyquinic Acid Derivatives in Gastric Adenocarcinoma (AGS) Cells." *Anti-Cancer Agents in Medicinal Chemistry* 18 (4): 610–16.

Jain, S. K. 1991. *Dictionary of Indian Folk Medicine and Ethnobotany*. New Delhi: Deep Publications.

Janakiraman, N., and M. Johnson. 2016. "Ethanol Extracts of Selected *Cyathea* Species Decreased Cell Viability and Inhibited Growth in MCF 7 Cell Line Cultures." *Journal of Acupuncture and Meridian Studies* 9 (3): 151–55.

Jang, B. K., K. Park, S. Y. Lee, H. Lee, S. H. Yeon, B. Ji, C. H. Lee, and J. S. Cho. 2021. "Screening of Particulate Matter Reduction Ability of 21 Indigenous Korean Evergreen Species for Indoor Use." *International Journal of Environmental Research and Public Health* 18 (18): 9803.

Jang, J., S. M. Kim, S. M. Yee, and E. M. Kim et al. 2019. "Daucosterol Suppresses Dextran Sulfate Sodium (DSS)-Induced Colitis in Mice." *International Immunopharmacology* 72: 124–30.

Jang, S. A., Y. H Hwang, H. Yang, J. A. Ryuk, D. R. Gu, and H. Ha. 2022a. "Ethanolic Extract of *Pyrrosia lingua* (Thunb.) Farw. Ameliorates OVX-Induced Bone Loss and RANKL-Induced Osteoclastogenesis." *Biomedicine and Pharmacotherapy* 147: 112640.

Jang, W. Y., H. P. Lee, S. A. Kim, L. Huang, J. H. Yoon, C. Y. Shin, A. Mitra, H. G. Kim, and J. Y. Cho. 2022b. "*Angiopteris cochinchinensis* de Vriese Ameliorates LPS-Induced Acute Lung Injury via Src Inhibition." *Plants* 11 (10): 1306.

Jansen, P. C. M. 2004. *Plant Resource of Tropical Africa 2. Vegetables*. In Grubben G. J. H. and Denton O. A. (eds.). Netherlands: PROTA Foundation, Backhuys Publishers, CTA Wageningen.

Ji, X., X. Wei, J. Qian, X. Mo, G. Kai, F. An, and Y. Lu. 2019. "2',4'-Dihydroxy-6'-methoxy-3',5'-Dimethylchalcone Induced Apoptosis and G1 Cell Cycle Arrest through PI3K/AKT Pathway in BEL-7402/5-FU Cells." *Food and Chemical Toxicology* 131: 110533.

Jia, S., Y. Zhang, and J. G Yu. 2017. "Antinociceptive Effects of Isosakuranetin in a Rat Model of Peripheral Neuropathy." *Pharmacology* 100 (3–4): 201–7.

Jiang, B., Y. Xing, B. Zhang, R. Cai, D. Zhang, and G. Sun. 2018. "Effective Phytoremediation of Low-Level Heavy Metals by Native Macrophytes in a Vanadium Mining Area, China." *Environmental Science and Pollution Research International* 25 (31): 31272–82.

Jiang, J. S., Z. L. Zhan, Z. M. Feng, Y. N. Yang, and P. C. Zhang. 2012. "Study on the Chemical Constituents from *Cyathea spinulosa*." *Zhong Yao Cai* 35 (4): 568–70.

Jin, Y. H., S. Jeon, J. Lee, S. Kim, M. S. Jang, C. M. Park, J. H. Song, H. R. Kim, and S. Kwon. 2022. "Anticoronaviral Activity of the Natural Phloroglucinols, Dryocrassin ABBA and Filixic Acid ABA from the Rhizome of *Dryopteris crassirhizoma* by Targeting the Main Proteases of SARS-CoV-2." *Pharmaceutics* 14 (2): 376.

Jin, Z., W. F. Wang, J. P. Huang, H. M. Wang, H. X. Ju, and Y. Chang. 2016. "Dryocrassin ABBA Induces Apoptosis in Human Hepatocellular Carcinoma HepG2 Cells through a Caspase-Dependent Mitochondrial Pathway." *Asian Pacific Journal of Cancer Prevention* 17 (4): 1823–28.

Jing, L., J. R. Jiang, D. M. Liu, J. W. Sheng, W. F. Zhang, Z. J. Li, and L. Y. Wei. 2019. "Structural Characterization and Antioxidant Activity of Polysaccharides from *Athyrium multidentatum* (Doll.) Ching in D-Galactose-Induced Aging Mice via PI3K/AKT Pathway." *Molecules* 24: 3364.

Johnson, M. A. A., C. X. Madona, R. S. Almeida, N. Martins, and H. D. M. Coutinho. 2020. "In Vitro Toxicity, Antioxidant, Anti-Inflammatory, and Antidiabetic Potential of *Sphaerostephanos unitus* (L.) Holttum." *Antibiotics* 9 (6): 333.

Johnson M. (alias Antonysame), V. George, S. J. Iruthayamani, S. Balasundaram. 2023. "Bioactive Compounds and Biological Activities of *Cyathea* Species," edited by H. N. Murty, *Bioactive Compounds in Bryophytes and Pteridophytes. Reference Series in Phytochemistry.* New York: Springer.

Johnson, T. (ed.) 1975. Revised edition of John Gerard's 1633 *The Herbal or General History of Plants*. New York: Dover.

Joshi, B., S. K. Panda, R. S. Jouneghani, M. Liu, N. Parajuli, P. Leyssen, J. Neyts, and W. Luyten. 2020. "Antibacterial, Antifungal, Antiviral and Anthelmintic Activities of Medicinal Plants of Nepal Selected Based on Ethnobotanical Evidence." *Evidence Based Complementary and Alternative Medicine* 2020: 1043471.

Jun, H. J., J. S. Kim, J. Y. Bang, H. Y. Kim, L. R. Beuchat, and J. H. Ryu. 2013. "Combined Effects of Plant Extracts in Inhibiting the Growth of *Bacillus cereus* in Reconstituted Infant Rice Cereal." *International Journal of Food Microbiology* 160 (3): 260–66.

Junejo, J., G. Gogoi, J. Islam, M. Rudrapal, P. Mondal, H. Hazarika, and K. Zaman. 2018. "Exploration of Antioxidant, Antidiabetic and Hepatoprotective Activity of *Diplazium esculentum*—A Wild Edible Plant from North Eastern India." *Future Journal of Pharmaceutical Sciences* 4 (1): 93–101.

Kadakol, A., N. Sharma, Y. A. Kulkarni, and A. B. Gaikwad. 2016. "Esculetin: A Phytochemical Endeavor Fortifying Effect against Non-Communicable Diseases." *Biomedicine and Pharmacotherapy* 84: 1442–48.

Kaewsuwan, S., A. Plubrukarn, M. Utsintong, S.-H. Kim, J.-H. Jeong, J. G. Cho, S. G. Park, and J.-H. Sung. 2016. "Interruptin B Induces Brown Adipocyte Differentiation and Glucose Consumption in Adipose-Derived Stem Cells." *Molecular Medicine Reports* 13 (3): 2078–86.

Kainz, K. P., L. Krenn, Z. Erdem, H. Kaehlig, M. Zehl, W. Bursch, W. Berger, and B. Marian. 2013. "2-Deprenyl-rheediaxanthone B Isolated from *Metaxya rostrata* Induces Active Cell Death in Colorectal Tumor Cells." *PLoS One* 8 (6): e65745.

Kakadia, N. P., M. A. Amin, and S. S. Deshpande. 2020. "Hepatoprotective and Antioxidant Effect of *Adiantum lunulatum* Burm. F. Leaf in Alcohol-Induced Rat Model." *Journal of Complementary and Integrative Medicine* 17 (3).

Kalpana, D. R., N. V. Rajesh, S. Vasantha, and N. Jeyathilakan. 2020. "Screening of in Vitro Antitrematodal Activities of Compounds and Secondary Metabolites Isolated from Selected Pteridophytes." *Veterinaria Italiana* 56 (4): 271–87.

Kamaraj, C., P. Deepak, G. Balasubramani, S. Karthi et al. 2018. "Target and Non-Target Toxicity of Fern Extracts against Mosquito Vectors and Beneficial Aquatic Organisms." *Ecotoxicology and Environmental Safety* 161: 221–30.

Kaneta, Y., M. A. Arai, N. Ishikawa, K. Toume, T. Koyano, T. Kowithayakorn, T. Chiba, A. Iwama, and M. Ishibashi. 2017. "Identification of MMI-1 Promotor Inhibitors from *Beaumontia murtonii* and *Eugenia operculate*." *Journal of Natural Products* 80 (6): 1853–59.

Kang, J. D., C. J. Myers, S. C. Harris, G. Kakiyama, I. K. Lee, B. S. Yun, K. Matsuzaki et al. 2019. "Bile Acid 7α-dehydroxylating Gut Bacteria Secrete Antibiotics that Inhibit *Clostridium difficile*: Role of Secondary Bile Acids." *Cell Chemical Biology* 26 (1): 27–34.e4.

Kang, P. Y., and S. Li. 2022. "Makisterone A Attenuates Experimental Cholestasis by Activating the Farnesoid X Receptor." *Biochemical and Biophysical Research Communications* 623: 162–69.

Kang, S. W., J. L. Kim, G. T. Kwon, Y. J. Lee, J. H. Yoon Park, S. S. Lim, and Y. H. Kang. 2011. "Sensitive Fern (*Onoclea sensibilis*) Extract Suppresses Proliferation and Migration of Vascular Smooth Muscle Cells Inflamed by Neighboring Macrophages." *Biological and Pharmaceutical Bulletin* 34 (11): 1717–23.

Kantari, S. A. K., R. P. Biswal, P. Kumar, M. Dharanikota, and A. Agraharam. 2023. "Antioxidant and Antidiabetic Activities, and UHPLC-ESI-QTOF-MS-Based Metabolite Profiling of an Endophytic Fungus *Nigrospora sphaerica* BRN 01 Isolated from *Bauthinia purpurrea* L." *Applied Biochemistry and Biotechnology* 195 (12): 7465–82.

Kantemir, I., G. Akder, and O. Tulunay. 1976. "Preliminary Report on an Unexpected Effect of an Extract from *Dryopteris filix mas*." *Arzneimittelforschung* 26 (2): 261–62.

Kanwal, Q., A. Qadir, Amina, Asmatullah, H. H. Iqbal, and B. Munir. 2018. "Healing Potential of *Adiantum capillus-veneris L.* Plant Extract on Bisphenol A-Induced Hepatic Toxicity in Male Albino Rats." *Environmental Science and Pollution Research International* 25 (12): 11884–92.

Kao, S. F., H. L. Kuo, Y. C. Lee, H. C. Chiang, and Y. S. Lin. 1994. "Immunostimulation by *Alsophila spinulosa* Extract Fraction VII of Both Humoral and Cellular Immune Responses." *Anticancer Research* 14 (6B): 2439–43.

Kapadia, G. J., H. Tokuda, T. Konoshima, M. Takasaki, J. Takayasu, and H. Nishino. 1996. "Anti-Tumor Promoting Activity of *Dryopteris* Phlorophenone Derivatives." *Cancer Letters* 105 (2): 161–65.

Karade, P. G., and N. R. Jadhav. 2017. "In Vitro Studies of the Anticancer Action of *Tectaria cicutaria* in Human Cancer Cell Lines: G_o/G_1p53-Associated Cell Cycle Arrest-Part I." *Journal of Traditional and Complementary Medicine* 8 (4): 459–64.

Karmakar, J., and S. K. Mukhopadhyay. 2011. "Study of Antimicrobial Activity and Root Symbionts of *Hemionitis arifolia*." *Physiology and Molecular Biology of Plants* 17 (2): 199–202.

Karthik, V., K. Raju, M. Ayyanar, K. Gowrishankar, and T. Sekar. 2011. "Ethnomedicinal Uses of Pteridophytes in Kolli Hills, Eastern Ghats of Tamil Nadu, India." *Journal of Natural Product Plant Resources* 1 (2): 50–55.

Kasabri, V., E. K. Al-Hallaq, Y. K. Bustanji, K. K. Abdul-Razzak, I. F. Abaza, and F. U. Afifi. 2017. "Antiobesity and Antihyperglycaemic Effects of *Adiantum capillus-veneris* Extracts: in Vitro and in Vivo Evaluations." *Pharmaceutical Biology* 55 (1): 164–72.

Kashiwada, Y., G. Nonaka, I. Nishioka, J. J. Chang, and K. H. Lee. 1992. "Antitumor Agents, 129. Tannins and Related Compounds as Selective Cytotoxic Agents." *Journal of Natural Products* 55 (8): 1033–43.

Kashkooe, A., F. A. Sardari, and M. M. Mehrabadi. 2021. "A Review of Pharmacological Properties and Toxicological Effects of *Adiantum capillus-veneris L.*" *Current Drug Discovery Technologies* 18 (2): 186–93.

Kaur, P., M. Kumar, A. P. Singh, and S. Kaur. 2017. "Ethyl Acetate Fraction of *Pteris vittate* L. Alleviates 2-Acetylaminofluorene Induced Hepatic Alterations in Male Wistar Rats." *Biomedicine and Pharmacotherapy* 88: 1080–89.

Kaur, P., M. Kumar, S. Kaur, A. Kumar, and S. Kaur. 2023. "In Vitro Modulation of Genotoxicity and Oxidative Stress by Polyphenol-Rich Fraction of Chinese Ladder Brake (*Pteris vittata* L.)." *Applied Biochemistry and Biotechnology* 196 (2): 774–89.

Kaur, P., V. Kaur, M. Kumar, and S. Kaur. 2014. "Suppression of SOS Response in *E. coli* PQ37, Antioxidant Potential and Antiproliferative Action of Methanolic Extract of *Pteris vittata* L. on Human MCF-7 Breast Cancer Cells." *Food and Chemical Toxicology* 74: 326–33.

Kazmi, Z., N. Safdar, and A. Yasmin. 2019. "Biological Screening of Three Selected Folklore Medicinal Plants from Pakistan." *Pakistan Journal of Pharmaceutical Sciences* 32 (4): 1477–84.

K'Eogh, J. 1735. *An Irish Herbal: The Botanalogia Universalis Hibernica*. Reprint Aquarian Press 1987.

Kernou, O. N., Z. Azzouz, K. Madani, and P. Rijo. 2023. "Application of Rosmarinic Acid with Its Derivatives in the Treatment of Microbial Pathogens." *Molecules* 28 (10): 4243.

Kervran, L. C. 1972. *Biological Transmutations*. Translated by M. Abehsera. Brooklyn, New York: Swan House Publishing.

Khajuria, V., S. Gupta, N. Sharma, A. Kumar, N. A. Lone, M. Khullar, P. Dutt, P. R. Sharma, A. Bhagat, and Z. Ahmed. 2017. "Anti-Inflammatory Potential of Hentriacontane in LPS Stimulated RAW 264.7 Cells and Mice Model." *Biomedicine and Pharmacotherapy* 92: 175–86.

Khamis, T., A. A. Abas Diab, M. H. Zahra, S. E. El-Dahmy et al. 2023. "The Antiproliferative Activity of *Adiantum pedatum* Extract and/or Piceatannol in Phenylhydrazine-Induced Colon Cancer in Male Albino Rats: The miR-145 Expression of the PI-3K/ Akt/ p53 and Oct4/ Sox2/ Nanog Pathways." *Molecules* 28 (14): 5543.

Khan, M. A., D. Singh, M. Jameel, S. K. Maurya, S. Singh, K. Akhtar, H. R. Siddique. 2023. "Lupeol, an Androgen Receptor Inhibitor, Enhances the Chemosensitivity of Prostate Cancer Stem Cells to Antiandrogen Enzalutamie-Based Therapy." *Toxicology and Applied Pharmacology* 478: 116699.

Khan, M. F., H. Tang, J. T. Lyles, R. Pineau, Z.-ur-R. Mashwani, and C. L. Quave. 2018. "Antibacterial Properties of Medicinal Plants from Pakistan against Multidrug-Resistant ESKAPE Pathogens." *Frontiers in Pharmacology* 9: 815.

Khan, M. R., and A. D. Omoloso. 2008. "Antibacterial and Antifungal Activities of *Angiopteris evecta*." *Fitoterapia* 79 (5): 366–69.

Khoja, A. A., S. M. Haq, M. Maheed, M. Hassan et al. 2022. "Diversity, Ecological and Traditional Knowledge of Pteridophytes in the Western Himalayas." *Diversity* 14: 628.

Khoramian, L., S. E. Sajjadi, and M. Minaiyan. 2020. "Anti-Inflammatory Effect of *Adiantum capillus-veneris* Hydroalcoholic and Aqueous Extracts on Acetic Acid-Induced Colitis in Rats." *Avicenna Journal of Phytomedicine* 10 (5): 492–503.

Kim, H. M., Y. M. Lee, E. H. Kim, and S. W. Eun. 2022a. "Anti-Wrinkle Efficacy of Edible Bird's Nest Extract: A Randomized, Double-Blind, Placebo-Controlled, Comparative Study." *Frontiers in Pharmacology* 13: 843469.

Kim, J., S. R. Kim, Y. H. Choi, J. Y. Shin, C. D. Kim, N. G. Kang, B. C. Park, and S. Lee. 2020. "Quercetrin Stimulates Hair Growth with Enhanced Expression of Growth Factors via Activation of MAPK/CREB Signaling Pathway." *Molecules* 25 (17): 4004.

Kim, J. W., H. P. Kim, and S. H. Sung 2017. "Cytotoxic Pterosins from *Pteris multifida* Roots against HCT116 Human Colon Cancer Cells." *Bioorganic and Medicinal Chemistry Letters* 27 (14): 3144–47.

Kim, J. W., J. Y. Seo, W. K. Oh, and S. H. Sung. 2016. "Anti-Neuroinflammatory *ent*-Kaurane Diterpenoids from *Pteris multifida* roots." *Molecules* 22 (1): 27.

Kim, J. Y., S. S. Kim, H. J. Jang, M. Y. Oh et al. 2015. "5,7-dihydroxy-3,4,6-Trimethoxyflavone Attenuates Ischemic Damage and Apoptosis in Mouse Islets." *Transplantation Proceedings* 47 (4): 1073–78.

Kim, M. K., J. S. Kang, A. Kundu, H. S. Kim, and B. M. Lee. 2023a. "Risk Assessment and Risk Reduction of Ptaquiloside in Bracken Fern." *Toxics* 11 (2): 115.

Kim, N. Y., J. Y. Lee, and C. Y. Kim. 2023b. "Protecctive Role of Ethanol Extract of *Cibotium barometz* (Cibotium Rhizome) against Dexamethasone-Induced Muscle Atrophy in C2C12 Myotubes." *International Journal of Molecular Sciences* 24 (19): 14798.

Kim, S. J., Y. G. Kim, D. S. Kim, Y. D. Jeon et al. 2011. "*Oldenlandia diffusa* Ameliorates Dextran Sulphate Sodium-Induced Colitis through Inhibition of NF-kappaB Activation." *American Journal of Chinese Medicine* 39 (5): 957–69.

Kim, S. S., J. Y. Kim, N. H. Lee, and C. G. Hyun. 2008. "Antibacterial and Anti-Inflammatory Effects of Jeju Medicinal Plants against Acne-Inducing Bacteria." *The Journal of General and Applied Microbiology* 54 (2): 101–6.

Kim, Y. S., D. J. Lim, J. S. Song, J. A. Kim, B. H. Lee, and Y. K. Son. 2022b. "Identification and Comparison of Bioactive Components of Two *Dryopteris* sp. Extract Using LC-QTOF-MS." *Plants* 11 (23): 3233.

Felter, H. W., and J. U. Lloyd. 1898. *King's American Dispensatory*. Cincinnatti: Ohio Valley Co.

Kingsley, C. 1890. *Glaucus, The Wonders of the Shore*. London, New York: Macmillan & Co.

Kiran, P. M., A. V. Raju, and B. G. Rao. 2012. "Investigation of Hepatoprotective Activity of *Cyathea gigantea* (Wall. ex. Hook.) Leaves against Paracetamol-Induced Hepatoxicity in Rats." *Asian Pacific Journal of Tropical Biomedicine* 2 (5): 352–56.

Kitamura, R. S. A., M. Vicentini, V. Bitencourt, T. Vicari, W. Motta, J. C. M. Brito, M. M. Cestari, M. M. Prodocimo, H. C. Silva de Assis, and M. P. Gomes. 2023. "*Salvinia molesta*

Phytoremediation Capacity as a Nature-Based Solution to Prevent Harmful Effects and Accumulation of Ciprofloxacin in Neotropical Catfish." *Environment Science and Pollution Research International* 30 (14): 41848–63.

Ko, Y. J., J. B. Wu, H. Y. Ho, and W. C. Lin. 2012. "Antiosteoporotic Activity of *Davallia formosana*." *Journal of Ethnopharmacology* 139 (2): 558–65.

Koch, C. D., C. M. Lee, and S. S. Apte. 2020. "Aggrecan in Cardiovascular Development and Disease." *The Journal of Histochemistry and Cytochemistry* 68 (11): 777–95.

Kohli, I., R. Shafi, R. P. Isedeh, J. L. Griffth, M. S. Al-Jamal et al. 2017. "The Impact of Oral *Polypodium leucotomas* Extract on Ultraviolet B Response: A Human Clinical Study." *Journal of the American Academy of Dermatology* 77 (1): 33–41.

Komala, I., S. Sitorus, R. Fitri, Dewi, N. Nurmeilis, and L. A. Hendarmin. 2022. "Cytotoxic Activity of the Indonesian Fern *Angiopteris angustifolia* C. Presl and Liverwort *Mastigophora diclados* (Birs. ex Web) Nees against Breast Cancer Cell Lines (MCF-7)." *Journal Kimia Vanensi* 8: 79–84.

Kong, Y., Z. Feng, A. Chen, Q. Qi et al. 2019. "The Natural Flavonoid Galangin Elicits Apoptosis, Pyroptosis and Autophagy in Glioblastoma." *Frontiers in Oncology* 9: 942.

Konoshima, T., M. Takasaki, H. Tokuda, K. Masuda, Y. Arai, K. Shiojima, and H. Ageta. 1996. "Anti-Tumor-Promoting Activities of Triterpenoids from Ferns." *Biological and Pharmaceutical Bulletin* 19 (7): 962–65.

Koptur, S., V. Rico-Gray, and M. Palacios-Rios. 1998. "Ant Protection of the Nectaried Fern *Polypodium plebeium* in Central Mexico." *American Journal of Botany* 85 (5): 736–39.

Kösesakal, T., and M. Seyhan. 2023. "Phenanthrene Stress Response and Phytoremediation Potential of Free-Floating Fern *Azolla filiculoides* Lam." *International Journal of Phytoremediation* 25 (2): 207–20.

Kösesakal, T., M. Ünal, O. Kulen, A. Memon, and B. Yüksel. 2016. "Phytoremediation of Petroleum Hydrocarbons by Using a Freshwater Fern Species *Azolla filiculoides* Lam." *International Journal of Phytoremediation* 18 (5): 467–76.

Kräuterman, V. 1725. *Der Curieuse und vernünfftige Zauber-Arzt*. Frankfurt and Leipzig: Niedt.

Kumar, D. G., A. M. Syafiq, Y. Ruhaiyem, and M. Shahnaz. 2015. "*Blechnum orientale* Linn. An Important Edible Medicinal Fern." *International Journal of Pharmaceutical and Phytopharmacological Research* 7: 723–26.

Kumar, M., M. Ramesh, and S. Sequiera. 2003. "Medicinal Pteridophytes of Kerala, South India." *Indian Fern Journal* 21: 1–28.

Kumar, R. P., and S. Siddique. 2022. "22-Hydroxyhopane, a Novel Multitargeted Phytocompound against SARS-CoV-2 from *Adiantum latifolium* Lam." *Natural Product Research* 36 (16): 4276–81.

Kumari, S., B. Pal, S. K. Sahu, P. K. Prabhakar, and D. Tewari. 2023. "Adverse Events of Clenbuterol among Athletes: A Systematic Review of Case Reports and Case Series." *International Journal of Legal Medicine* 137 (4): 1023–37.

Kumudhavalli, M. V., and B. Jaykar. 2012. "Pharmacological Screening on Leaves of the Plant *Hemionitis arifolia* (Burm.) T. Moore." *Research Journal of Pharmaceutical, Biological and Chemical Sciences* 3 (2): 79–83.

Kunkeaw, T., U. Suttisansanee, D. Trachootham, J. Karinchai, B. Chantong, S. Potikanond, W. Inthachat, P. Pitchakarn, and P. Temviriyanukul. 2021. "*Diplaziium esculentum* (Retz.) Sw. Reduces BACE-1 Activities and Amyloid Peptides Accumulation in *Drosophila* Models of Alzheimer's Disease." *Scientific Reports* 11 (1): 23796.

Künzle, John. 1975. *Herbs and Weeds: A Useful Booklet on Medicinal Herbs.* Itengen, Switzerland: Kräuterpfarrer Künzle.

Kuroi, A., K. Sugimura, A. Kumagai, A. Kohara, Y. Nagaoka, H. Kawahara, M. Yamahara, N. Kawahara, H. Takemori, and H. Fuchino. 2017. "The Importance of 11*a*-OH,15-oxo, and 16-en Moieties of 11*a*-Hydroxy-15-oxo-kaur-16-en-19-oic Acid in Its Inhibitory Activity of Melanogenesis." *Skin Pharmacology and Physiology* 30 (4): 205–15.

Labrude, P. 2010. "*Le docteur Garrus et son élixir—d'hier à aujourd'hui* [The Elixir of Doctor Garrus. Drug or Liquor? Original Formula or Imitation?]" *Bulletin Cercle Benelux d'Histoire de la Pharmacie* 118 (April): 14–31.

La Croix, D. 1791. *Connubia florum latino carmine demostrata.* Bath, UK: Bathoniae Publisher.

Lai, H. Y., Y. Y. Lim, and K. H. Kim. 2010. "*Blechnum orientale* Linn—A Fern with Potential as Antioxidant, Anticancer and Antibacterial Agent." *BMC Complementary and Alternative Medicine* 10: 15.

Lai, H. Y., Y. Y. Lim, and K. H. Kim. 2017. "Isolation and Characterisation of a Proanthocyanidin with Antioxidative, Antibacterial and Anti-Cancer Properties from Fern *Blechnum orientale.*" *Pharmacognosy Magazine* 13 (49): 31–37.

Lai, J. C. Y., H. Y. Lai, K. R. Nalamolu, and S. F. Ng. 2016. "Treatment for Diabetic Ulcer Wounds Using a Fern Tannin Optimized Hydrogel Formulation with Antibacterial and Antioxidative Properties." *Journal of Ethnopharmacology* 189: 277–89.

Lai, M. C., W. Y. Liu, S. S. Liou, and I. M. Liu. 2022. "Diosmetin Targeted at Peroxisome Proliferator-Activated Receptor Gamma Alleviates Advanced Glycation End Products Induced Neuronal Injury." *Nutrients* 14 (11): 2248.

Lamichhane, R., P. R. Pandeya, K. H. Lee, S. G. Kim, H. P. Devkota, and H. J. Jung. 2020. "Anti-Adipogenic and Anti-Inflammatory Activities of (-)-*epi*-Osmundalactone and Angiopteroside from *Angiopteris helferiana* C. Presl." *Molecules* 25 (6): 1337.

Lamichhane, R., S. G. Kim, A. Poudel, D. Sharma, K. H. Lee, and H. J. Jung. 2014. "Evaluation of in Vitro and in Vivo Biological Activities of *Cheilanthes albomarginata* Clarke." *BMC Complementary and Alternative Medicine* 14: 342.

Lang, T. Q., Y. Zhang, F. Chen, G. Y. Luo, and W. D. Yang. 2021. "Characterization of Chemical Components with Diuretic Potential from *Pyrrosia petiolosa.*" *Journal of Asian Natural Products Research* 23 (8): 764–71.

Lans, C. A. 2006. "Ethnomedicines used in Trinidad and Tobago for Urinary Problems and Diabetes Mellitus." *Journal of Ethnobiology and Ethnomedicine* 2: 45.

Lee, C. H., Y. L. Huang, J. F. Liao, and W. F. Chiou. 2011. "Ugonin K Promotes Osteoblastic Differentiation and Mineralization by Activation of p38 MAPK- and ERK-Mediated Expression of Runx2 and Osterix." *European Journal of Pharmacology* 668 (3): 383–89.

Lee, D., K. H. Kim, J., G. S. Hwang, H. L. Lee, D. H. Hahm, C. K. Huh, S. C. Lee, S. Lee, and K. S. Kang. 2017. "Protective Effect of Cirsimaritin against Streptozotocin-Induced Apoptosis in Pancreatic Beta Cells." *Journal of Pharmacy and Pharmacology* 69 (7): 875–83.

Lee, H., and J. Y. Lin. 1988. "Antimutagenic Activity of Extracts from Anti-Cancer Drugs in Chinese Medicine." *Mutation Research* 204 (2): 229–34.

Lee, H. B., J. C. Kim, and S. M. Lee. 2009a. "Antibacterial Activity of Two Phloroglucinols, Flavaspidic Acids AB and PB, from *Dryopteris crassirhizoma*." *Archives of Pharmacal Research* 32 (5): 655–59.

Lee, J., H. Kwon, E. Cho, J. Jeon, I. K. Lee, W. S. Cho, S. J. Park, S. Lee, D. H. Kim, and J. W. Jung. 2022a. "*Hydrangea macrophylla* and Thunberginol C Attenuate Stress-Induced Anxiety in Mice." *Antioxidants* 11 (2): 234.

Lee, J. K., W. S. Choi, J. Y. Song, O. S. Kwon, Y. J. Lee, J. S. Lee, S. Lee, S. R. Choi, C. H. Lee, and J. Y. Lee. 2022b. "Anti-Inflammatory Effects of *Athyrium yokoscense* Extract via Inhibition of the Erk1/2 and NF-kB Pathways in Bisphenol A-Stimulated A549 Cells." *Toxicological Research* 39 (1): 135–46.

Lee, J. S., H. Miyashiro, N. Nakamura, and M. Hattori. 2008. "Two New Triterpenes from the Rhizome of *Dryopteris crassirhizoma*, and Inhibitory Activities of Its Constituents on Human Immunodeficiency Virus-1 Protease." *Chemical and Pharmaceutical Bulletin* 56 (5): 711–14.

Lee, S. M., M. K. Na, R. B. An, B. S. Min, and H. K. Lee. 2003. "Antioxidant Activity of Two Phloroglucinol Derivatives from *Dryopteris crassirhizoma*." *Biological and Pharmaceutical Bulletin* 26 (9): 1354–56.

Lee, Y. L., M. H. Lee, H. J. Chang, P. Y. Huang, I. J. Huang, K. T. Cheng, and S. J. Leu. 2009b. "Taiwanese Native Plants Inhibit Matrix Metalloproteinase-9 Activity after Ultraviolet B Irradiation." *Molecules* 14 (3): 1062–71.

Leeya, Y., M. J. Mulvany, E. F. Queiroz, A. Marston, K. Hostettmann, and C. Jansakul. 2010. "Hypotensive Activity of an n-Butanol Extract and Their Purified Compounds from Leaves of *Phyllanthus acidus* (L.) Skeels in Rats." *European Journal of Pharmacology* 649 (1–3): 301–13.

Lei, Y. F., J. L. Chen, H. Wei, C. M. Xiong, Y. H. Zhang, and J. L. Ruan. 2011a. "Hypolipidemic and Anti-Inflammatory Properties of Abacopterin A from *Abacopteris penangiana* in High-Fat Diet-Induced Hyperlipidemic Mice." *Food and Chemical Toxicology* 49 (12): 3206–10.

Lei, Y. F., W. Fu, J. L. Chen, C. M. Xiong, G. H. Wu, H. Wei, and J. L. Ruan. 2011b. "Neuroprotective Effects of Abacopterin E from *Abacopteris penangiana* against Oxidative Stress-Induced Neurotoxicity." *Journal of Ethnopharmacology* 134 (2): 275–80.

Leighton, A. L. 1985. "Wild Plant Use by the Woods Cree (Nihithawak) of East-Central Saskatchewan." *Canadian Ethnology Service Paper No. 101*, Ottawa, ON: National Museum of Man, Mercury Series, National Museums of Canada.

Li, B., Y. Jin, H. Xiang, D. Mu et al. 2019a. "An Inhibitory Effect of Dryocrassin ABBA on *Staphylococcus aureus* vWbp That Protects Mice from Pneumonia." *Frontiers in Microbiology* 10: 7.

Li, B., Y. Ni, L. J. Zhu, F. B. Wu, F. Yan, X. Zhang, and X. S. Yao. 2015a. "Flavonoids from *Matteuccia struthiopteris* and Their Anti-Influenza Virus (H1N1) Activity." *Journal of Natural Products* 78 (5): 987–95.

Li, B. F., T. T. Duan, and L. Fan. 2013a. "On the Inhibitory Effect of *Drynaria fortunei* Extract on Human Myeloma SP20 Cells." *African Journal of Traditional and Complementary and Alternative Medicines* 10 (5): 375–79.

Li, F., A. B. Chen, Y. C. Duan, R. Liao, Y. W. Xu, and L. L. Tao. 2020. "Multiple Organ Dysfunction and Rhabdomyolysis Associated with Moonwort Poisoning: Report of Four Cases." *World Journal of Clinical Cases* 8 (2): 479–86.

Li, F. W., J. C. Villarreal, S. Kelly, C. Rothfels et al. 2014. "Horizontal Transfer of an Adaptive Chimeric Photoreceptor from Bryophytes to Ferns." *Proceedings of the National Academy of Sciences* 111 (18): 6672–77.

Li, F. W., K. M. Pryer, and M. D. Windham. 2012. "*Gaga*, a New Fern Genus Segregated from *Cheilanthes* (Pteridaceae)." *Systematic Botany* 37 (4): 845–60.

Li, H. M., D. Z. Jiang, L. Zhang, J. Z. and Wu. 2017a. "Inhibition of Tumor Growth of Human Hepatocellular Carcinoma HepG2 Cells in a Nude Mouse Xenograft Model by the Total Flavonoids from *Arachniodes exilis*." *Evidence Based Complementary and Alternative Medicine* 2017: 5310563.

Li, J., N. Liang, L. Mo, X. Zhang, and C. He. 1998. "Comparison of the Cytotoxicity of Five Constituents from *Pteris semipinnata* L. in Vitro and the Analysis of Their Structure-Activity Relationships." *Acta Pharmaceutica Sinica* 33 (9): 641–44.

Li, J., Z. H. Wang, C. T. Wang, C. X. Cao, Q. F. Dong, and T. Z. Jia. 2008a. "Influence of *Cibotium barometz* and Its Processed Samples on Haemorheology Index in Mice with Adjuvant Arthritis." *Zhongguo Zhong Yao Za Zhi* 22 (17): 2170–73.

Li, L., M. P. Xie, H. Sun, A. Q. Lu, B. Zhang, D. Zhang, and S. J. Wang. 2019b. "Bioactive Phenolic Acid-Substituted Glycoses and Glycosides from Rhizomes of *Cibotium barometz*." *Journal of Asian Natural Products Research* 21 (10): 947–53.

Li, L., W. J. Li, X. R. Zheng, Q. L. Liu, Q. Du, Y. J. Lai, and S. Q. Liu. 2022a. "Eriodictyol Ameliorates Cognitive Dysfunction in APP/PS1 Mice by Inhibiting Ferroptosis via Vitamin D Receptor-Mediated Nrf2 Activation." *Molecular Medicine* 28 (1): 11.

Li, L., Y. Liu, Y. N. Lv, K. F. Wu, G. Chen, and N. C. Liang. 2010. "Apoptosis Effect and Mechanism of 5F from *Pteris semipinnata* on HepG2 Cells." *Acta Pharmaceutica Sinica* 33 (1): 77–80.

Li, L., Z. Zeng, and G. P. Cai. 2011a. "Comparison of Neoeriocitrin and Naringin on Proliferation and Osteogenic Differentiation in MC3T3-E1." *Phytomedicine* 18 (11): 985–89.

Li, M. C., Z. Yao, Y. Takaishi, S. A. Tang, and H. Q. Duan. 2011b. "Isolation of Novel Phenolic Compounds with Multidrug Resistance (MDR) Reversal Properties from *Onychium japonicum*." *Chemistry and Biodiversity* 8 (6): 1112–20.

Li, N., X. Li, B. L. Hou, and D. L. Meng. 2008b. "New Disaccharoside from *Camptosorus sibiricus* Rupr." *Natural Product Research* 22 (15): 1379–83.

Li, R. P., M. L. Guo, G. Zhang, X. F. Xu, and Q. Li. 2006. "Neuroprotection of Nicotiflorin in Permanent Focal Cerebral Ischemia and in Neuronal Cultures." *Biological and Pharmaceutical Bulletin* 29 (9): 1868–72.

Li, S. Y., P. Wang, G. G. Deng, W. Yuan, and Z. S. Su. 2013b. "Cytotoxic Compounds from Invasive Giant Salvinia (*Salvinia molesta*) against Human Tumor Cells." *Bioorganic and Medicinal Chemistry Letters* 23 (24): 6682–87.

Li, X., L. J. Zhu, J. P. Chen, and C. Y., Shi. 2019c. "C-Methylated Flavanones from the Rhizomes of *Matteuccia intermedia* and Their *a*-Glucosidase Inhibitory Activity." *Fitoterapia* 136: 104147.

Li, X. J., X. H. Song, S. Q. Tang, K. X. Wie et al. 2023. "Phytochemical Constituents from Rhizomes of *Dryopteris crassirhizoma* and Their Anti-Inflammatory Activity." *Natural Product Research* 2023: 1–7.

Li, X. L., L. M. Yang, Y. Zhao, R. R. Wang, G. Xu, Y. T. Zheng, L. Tu, L. Y. Peng, X. Cheng, and Q. S. Zhao. 2007. "Tetranorclerodanes and Clerodane-Type Diterpene Glycosides from *Dicranopteris dichotoma*." *Journal of Natural Products* 70 (2): 265–68.

Li, W. F., J. Wang, J. J. Zhang, X. Song, C. F. Ku, J. Zou, J. X. Li, L. J. Rong, L. T. Pan, and H. J. Zhang. 2015b. "Henrin A: A New Anti-HIV *Ent*-Kaurane Diterpene from *Pteris henryi*." *International Journal of Molecular Sciences* 16 (11): 27978–87.

Li, Y., K. Li, J. Y. Duan, C. P. Zhang, and H. K. Yao. 2018. "A Novel Heterodimer of Coumaric Acid Glucosides from the Chinese Fern *Polypodium hastatum*." *Chemistry of Natural Compounds* 54 (6): 1041–43.

Li, Y., W. Li, W. Deng, Y. Gan, K. Wu, and J. Sun. 2017b. "Synergistic Anti-Proliferative and Pro-Apoptotic Activities of 5F and Cisplatin in Human Non-Small Cell Lung Cancer NCI-H23 Cells." *Oncology Letters* 14 (5): 5347–53.

Li, Y., Z. Zhou, Y. Xia, X. Zhang, Z. X. Ye, Y. Zhang, F. Yang, and H. Yao. 2022b. "Polypodiside Attenuates Inflammation Induced by High Glucose in Mesangial Cells via MAPK/NF-*a*B pathway." *Latin American Journal of Pharmacy* 41 (7): 1433–39.

Lihui, X., G. Jinming, G. Yalin, W. Hemeng, W. Hao, and C. Ying. 2022. "Albicanol Inhibits the Toxicity of Profenofos to Grass Carp Hepatocytes Cells through the ROS/PTEN/PI3K/AKT Axis." *Fish and Shellfish Immunology* 120: 325–36.

Lin, A. S., K. Nakagawa-Goto, F. R. Chang, D. Yu, S. L. Morris-Natschke, C. C. Wu, S. L. Chen, Y. C. Wu, and K. H. Lee. 2007. "First Total Synthesis of Protoapigenone and Its Analogues as Potent Cytotoxic Agents." *Journal of Medicinal Chemistry* 50 (16): 3921–27.

Lin, C., Z. Zeng, Y. Lin, P. Wang et al. 2022. "Naringenin Suppresses Epithelial Ovarian Cancer by Inhibiting Proliferation and Modulating Gut Microbiota." *Phytomedicine* 106: 154401.

Lin, C. H., J. B. Wu, J. Y. Jian, and C. C. Shih. 2017. "(-)-Epicatechin-3-O-b-D-allopyranoside from *Davallia formosana* Prevents Diabetes and Dyslipidemia in Streptozotocin-Induced Diabetic Mice." *PLoS One* 12(3): e0173984.

Lin, H., X. Liu, Z. Shen, W. Cheng, Z. Zeng, Y. Chen, C. Tang, and T. Jiang. 2019. "The Effect of Isoflavaspidic Acid PB Extracted from *Dryopteris fragrans* (L.) Schott on Planktonic and Biofilm Growth of Dermatophytes and the Possible Mechanism of Antibiofilm." *Journal of Ethnopharmacology* 241: 111956.

Lin, T. H., R. S. Yang, K. C. Wang, D. H. Lu, H. C. Liou, Y. Ma, S. H. Chang, and W. M. Fu. 2013. "Ethanol Extracts of Fresh *Davallia formosana* (WL1101) Inhibit Osteoclast Differentiation by Suppressing RANKL-Induced Nuclear Factor-kB Activation." *Evidence Based Complementary and Alternative Medicine* 2013: 647189.

Lin, Y. C., Y. C. Huang, S. C. Chen, C. C. Liaw, S. C. Kuo, L. J. Huang, and P. W. Gean. 2009. "Neuroprotective Effects of Ugonin K on Hydrogen Peroxide-Induced Cell Death in Human Neuroblastoma SH-SY5Y Cells." *Neurochemical Research* 34 (5): 923–30.

Lin, Y. L., C. C. Shen, Y. J. Huang, and Y. Y. Chang. 2005. "Homoflavonoids from *Ophioglossum petiolatum*." *Journal of Natural Products* 68 (3): 381–84.

Lin, Y. T., S. W. Peng, Z. Imtiyaz, C. W. Ho, and W. F. Chiou. 2021. "In Vivo and in Vitro Evaluation of the Osteogenic Potential of *Davallia mariesii* T. Moore ex Baker." *Journal of Ethnopharmacology* 264: 113126.

Lindell, A. H., R. C. Tuckfield, and J. V. McArthur. 2016. "Differences in the Effect of Coal Pile Runoff (Low pH, High Metal Concentrations) Versus Natural Carolina Bay Water (Low pH, Low Metal Concentrations) on Plant Condition and Associated Bacterial Epiphytes of *Salvinia minima*." *Bulletin of Environmental Contamination and Toxicology* 96 (5): 602–7.

Liou, C. J., Y. L. Huang, W. C. Huang, K. W. Yeh, T. Y. Huang, and C. F. Lin. 2017. "Water Extract of *Helminthostachys zeylanica* Attenuates LPS-Induced Acute Lung Injury in Mice by Modulating NF-kB and MAPK Pathways." *Journal of Ethnopharmacology* 199: 30–38.

Liu, C. L., T. L. Ho, S. Y. Fang, J. H. Guo, C. Y. Wu, Y. C. Fong, C. C. Liaw, and C. H. Tang. 2023a. "Ugonin L Inhibits Osteoclast Formation and Promotes Osteoclast Apoptosis by Inhibiting the MAPK and NF-kB Pathways." *Biomedicine and Pharmacotherapy* 166: 115392.

Liu, C. T., K. W. Bi, C. C. Huang, H. T. Wu, H. Y. Ho, J. H. S. Pang, and S. T. Huang. 2017a. "*Davallia bilabiate* Exhibits Anti-Angiogenic Effect with Modified MMP-2/TIMP-2 Secretion and Inhibited VEGF Ligand/Receptors Expression in Vascular Endothelial Cells." *Journal of Ethnopharmacology* 196: 213–24.

Liu, D. M., J. W. Sheng, S. H. Wang, W. F. Zhang, W. Zhang, and D. J. Zhang. 2016. "Cytoproliferative and Cytoprotective Effects of Striatisporolide A Isolated from Rhizomes of *Athyrium multidenatatum* (Doell.) Ching on Human Umbilical Vein Endothelial Cells." *Molecules* 21 (10): 1280.

Liu, F., S. Lin, C. Zhang, J. Ma, Z. Han, F. Jia, W. Xie, and X. Li. 2019a. "The Novel Nature Microtubule Inhibitor Ivalin Induces G2/M Arrest and Apoptosis in Human Hepatocellular Carcinoma SMMC-7721 Cells In Vitro." *Medicina* (Kaunas) 55 (8): 470.

Liu, H. B., C. Y. Jiang, C. M. Xiong, and J. L. Ruan. 2012. "DEDC, a New Flavonoid Induces Apoptosis via a ROS-Dependent Mechanism in Human Neuroblastoma SH-SY5Y Cells." *Toxicology in Vitro* 26 (1): 16–23.

Liu, J. J., J. Y. Chen, B. X. Xu, L. Lin, S. Q. Liu, X. Y. Ma, and J. W. Liu. 2022a. "3,4,5-O-Tricaffeoylquinic Acid with Anti-Radiation Activity Suppresses LPS-Induced NLRP3 Inflammasome Activation via Autophagy in THP-1 Macrophages." *Molecular Immunology* 147: 187–98.

Liu, J. Q., J. C. Shu, R. Zhang, and W. Zhang. 2011. "Two New Pterosin Dimers from *Pteris multifida* (sic) Poir." *Fitoterapia* 82 (8): 1181–84.

Liu, M., G. G. Xiao, P. Rong, J. Dong et al. 2013. "Semen Astragali Complanti- and Rhizoma Cibotii-Enhanced Bone Formation in Osteoporosis Rats." *BMC Complementary and Alternative Medicine* 13: 141.

Liu, M., W. Zhang, W. Zhang, X. Zhou, M. Li, and J. Miao. 2017b. "Prenylflavonoid Isoxanthohumol Sensitizes MCF-7/ADR Cells to Doxorubicin Cytotoxicity via Acting as a Substrate of ABCB1." *Toxins* 9 (7): 208.

Liu, R. Y., Y. C. Zhang, S. Li, C. M. Liu, and S. Y. Zhuang. 2022b. "Receptor-Ligand Affinity-Based Screening and Isolation of Water-Soluble 5-Lipoxygenase Inhibitors from *Phellinus igniarius*." *Journal of Chromatography B, Analytical Technologies in the Biomedical and Life Sciences* 1209: 123415.

Liu, X., J. Liu, T. Jiang, L. Zhang, Y. Huang, J. Wan, G. Song, H. Lin, Z. Shen, and C. Tang. 2018a. "Analysis of Chemical Composition and in Vitro Antidermatophyte Activity of Ethanol Extracts of *Dryopteris fragrans* (L.) Schott." *Journal of Ethnopharmacology* 226: 36–43.

Liu, X. L., W. P. Lu, L. L. Wang, and L. Feng. 2018b. "Effects of Flavonoids from *Pyrrosiae folium* on Pathological Changes and Inflammatory Response of Diabetic Nephropathy." *Zhongguo Zhong Yao Za Zhi* 43 (11): 2352–57.

Liu, Y., L. Zhou, J. Tan, W. Q. Xu, G. L. Huang, and J. Ding. 2021a. "*Ent*-11*a*-hydroxy-15-oxo-kaur-16-en-19-oic Acid Loaded Onto Fluorescent Mesoporous Silica Nanoparticles for the Location and Therapy of Nasopharyngeal Carcinoma." *Analyst* 146 (5): 1596–1603.

Liu, Y. J., Y. W. Zhang, S. L. Zheng, X. C. Zheng, H. Y. Ding, W. X. Xin, J. Sun, L. Li, and P. Huang. 2021b. "*Botrychium schaffneri* Underw. Extract Acts via DIABLO to Induce Apoptosis and Inhibit Proliferation of Non-Small Cell Lung Carcinoma in Vitro and in Vivo." *Annals of Translational Medicine* 9 (22): 1676.

Liu, Z., C. L. Xia, N. Wang, J. G. Cao, G. Z. Huang, and L. Ma. 2023b. "Synthesis and Evaluation of Piperazine-Tethered Derivatives of Alepterolic Acid as Anticancer Agents." *Chemistry and Biodiversity* 20(5): e202300208.

Liu, Z. D., D. D. Zhao, S. Jiang, B. Xue, Y. L. Zhang, and X. F. Yan. 2018c. "Anticancer Phenolics from *Dryopteris fragrans* (L.) Schott." *Molecules* 23 (3): 680.

Liu, Z. M., G. G. Chen, A. C. Vlantis, N. C. Liang, Y. F. Deng, and C. A. van Hasselt. 2005. "Cell Death Induced by *ent*-11alpha-hydroxy-15-oxo-kaur-16-en-19-oic-acid in Anaplastic Thyroid Carcinoma Cells Is Via a Mitochondrial-Mediated Pathway." *Apoptosis* 10 (6): 1345–56.

Liu, Z. M., L. Li, X. Y. Zhu, and F. Z. Song. 2009. "Molecular Mechanism of Apoptosis Induced by PsL5F in Human Anaplastic Thyroid Carcinoma FRO Cells." *Sichuan Da Xue Xue Bao Yi Xue Ban* 40 (6): 1015–20.

Liu, Z. W., S. Cao, C. Jin, Y. He, X. S. Zhou, H. Zhang, and Z. M. Liu. 2019b. "The Antagonism between Apigenin and Protoapigenone to the PDK-1 Target in *Macrothelypteris torresiana*." *Fitoterapia* 134: 12–22.

Lloyd, R. M. 1964. "Ethnobotanical Uses of California Pteridophytes by Western Indians." *American Fern Journal* 54: 76–82.

Long, M., D. Qui, F. R. Li, F. Johnson, and B. Luft. 2005. "Flavonoid of *Drynaria fortunei* Protects against Acute Renal Failure." *Phytotherapy Research* 19 (5): 422–27.

Long, M., E. E. Smouha, D. Qui, F. R. Li, F. Johnson, and B. Luft. 2004. "Flavanoid of *Drynaria fortunei* Protects against Gentamicin Ototoxicity." *Phytotherapy Research* 18 (8): 609–14.

Loureiro, D. B., L. D. Lario, M. S. Herrero, L. M. Salvatierra, L. A. B. Novo, and L. M. Pérez. 2023. "Potential of *Salvinia biloba* Raddi for Removing Atrazine and Carbendazim from Aquatic Environments." *Environmental Science and Pollution Research International* 30 (8): 22089–99.

Lu, J., C. Y. Peng, S. Cheng, J. Q. Liu, Q. G. Ma, and J. C. Shu. 2019. "Four New Pterosins from *Pteris cretica* and Their Cytotoxic Activities." *Molecules* 24 (15): 2767.

Lu, L., Z. Wang, H. Q. Zhang, T. G. Liu, and H. Fang. 2022. "*Drynaria fortunei* Improves Lipid Profiles of Elderly Patients with Postmenopausal Osteoporosis via Regulation of Notch1-NLRP3 Inflammasome-Mediated Inflammation." *Gynecological Endocrinology* 38 (2): 176–80.

Luciano-Montalvo, C., I. Boulogne, and J. Gavillávan-Suárez. 2013. "A Screening for Antimicrobial Activities of Caribbean Herbal Remedies." *BMC Complementary and Alternative Medicine* 13: 126.

Luetragoon, T., R. P. Sranujit, C. Noysang, Y. Thongsri, P. Potup, N. Suphrom, N. Nuengchamnong, and K. Usuwanthim. 2020. "Anti-Cancer Effect of 3-Hydroxy-b-Ionone Identified from *Moringa oleifera* Lam. Leaf on Human Squamous Cell Carcinoma 15 Cell Line." *Molecules* 25 (16): 3563.

Luschiim, A. C., and N. J. Turner. 2021. *Luschiim's Plants: Traditional Indigenous Foods, Materials and Medicines*. Madiera Park, B.C., Canada: Harbour Publishing.

Luo, X. K., C. J. Li, P. Luo, X. Lin, H. Ma, N. P. Seeram, C. Song, J. Xu, and Q. Gu. 2016. "Pterosin Sesquiterpenoids from *Pteris cretica* as Hypolipidemic Agents via Activating Liver X Receptors." *Journal of Natural Products* 79 (12): 3014–21.

Ma, J. H., J. Qi, F. Y. Liu, S. Q. Lin, C. Y. Zhang, W. D. Xie, H. Y. Zhang, and X. Li. 2018. "Ivalin Inhibits Proliferation, Migration and Invasion by Suppressing Epithelial Mesenchymal Transition in Breast Cancer Cells." *Nutrition and Cancer* 70 (8): 1330–38.

Ma, J., R. Y. Li, F. Xu, F. Zhu, and X. W. Xu. 2023. "Dehydrovomifoliol Alleviates Nonalcoholic Fatty Liver Disease via the E2F1/AKT/mTOR Axis: Pharmacophore Modeling and

Molecular Docking Study." *Evidence Based Complementary and Alternative Medicine* 2023: 9107598.

Ma, S. N., S. L. Duan, M. N. Jin, and H. Q. Duan. 2013. "A New Flavanol Glycoside from *Phymatopteris hastata* with Effect on Glucose Metabolism." *Zhongguo Zhong Yao Za Zhi* 38 (6): 831–34.

Ma'arif, B., D. M. Mirza, M. Hasanah, H. Laswati, and M. Agil. 2020a. "Antineuroinflammation Activity of n-Butanol Fraction of *Marsilea crenata* Presl. In Microglia HMC3 Cell Line." *Journal of Basic and Clinical Physiology and Pharmacology* 30 (6): 20190255.

Ma'arif, B., M. Agil, and H. Laswati. 2020b. "The Enhancement of Arg1 and Activated ERb Expression in Microglia HMC3 by Induction of 96% Ethanol Extract of *Marsilea crenata* Presl. Leaves." *Journal of Basic and Clinical Physiology and Pharmacology* 30 (6): 20190284.

Madboli, A. E. A., and M. M. Seif. 2021. "*Adiantum capillus-veneris* Linn Protects Female Reproductive System against Carbendazim Toxicity in Rats: Immunohistochemical, Histopathological, and Pathophysiological studies." *Environmental Science and Pollution Research International* 28 (16): 19768–82.

Magalhães, L. G., G. J. Kapadia, L. R. da Silva Tonuci, S. C. Caixeta, N. A. Parreira, V. Rodrigues, and A. A. Da Silva Filho. 2010. "In Vitro Schistosomicidal Effects of Some Phloroglucinol Derivatives from *Dryopteris* Species against *Schistosoma mansoni* Adult Worms." *Parasitology Research* 105 (2): 395–401.

Mak, K. K., S. Zhang, J. S. Low, M. K. Balijepalli, R. Sakirolla, A. T. Dinkova-Kostova, O. Epemolu, Z. Mohd, and M. R. Pichika. 2022. "Anti-Inflammatory Effects of Auranamide and Patriscabratine-Mechanism and in Silico Studies." *Molecules* 27 (15): 4992.

Mala, P., G. A. Khan, R. Gopalan, D. Gedefaw, and K. Soapi. 2022. "Fijian Medicinal Plants and Their Role in the Prevention of Type 2 Diabetes Mellitus." *Bioscience Reports* 42 (11): BSR20220461.

Malomane, M. T., K. Kondiah, and M. H. Serepa-Diamini. 2023. "Genetic Engineering of *Escherichia coli* BL21 (DE3) with a Codon-Optimized Insecticidal Toxin Complex Gene *tccZ*." *Access Microbiology* 5(1): acmi000426.

Manivannan, V., and M. Johnson. 2020. "Total Accepted Phenolic, Tannin, Triterpenoid, Flavonoid and Sterol Contents, Anti-Diabetic, Anti-Inflammatory and Cytotoxic Activities of *Tectaria paradoxa* (Fee.) Sledge." *Toxicology Reports* 7: 1465–68.

Manna, S. K., C. Bueso-Ramos, F. Alvarado, and B. B. Aggarwal. 2003. "Calagualine Inhibits Nuclear Transcription Factors-kappaB Activated by Various Inflammatory and Tumor Promoting Agents." *Cancer Letters* 190 (2): 171–82.

Mannan, A., R. A. Khan, and M. Asif. 1989. "Pharmacodynamic Studies on *Polypodium vulgare* (Linn.)." *Indian Journal of Experimental Biology* 27 (6): 556–60.

Mannan, M. M., M. Maridass, and B. Victor. 2008. "A Review on the Potential Uses of Ferns." *Ethnobotanic Leaflets* 12: 281–85.

Manubolu, M., L. Goodla, B. G. N. Chandar, S. Ravilla, and V. R. Obulum. 2013. "Chemical Composition and Antibacterial Activity of Wax from *Actiniopteris radiata* (Sw.) Link." *Journal of Essential Oil Bearing Plants* 16 (3): 87–392.

Manubolu, M., L. Goodla, S. Ravilla, J. Thanasekaran, P. Dutta, K. Malmlöf, and V. R. Obulum. 2014. "Protective Effect of *Actiniopteris radiata* (Sw.) Link. against CCl_4 Induced Oxidative Stress in Albino Rats." *Journal of Ethnopharmacology* 153 (3): 744–52.

Maran, B. A. V., K. Palaniveloo, T. Mahendran, D. K. Chellappan et al. 2023. "Antimicrobial Potential of Aqueous Extract of Giant Sword Fern and Ultra-High-Performance Liquid Chromatography-High-Resolution Mass Spectrometry Analysis." *Molecules* 28 (16): 6075.

Marisass, M. 2009. "Antibacterial Activity of *Mecodium exsertum* (Wall. ex Hook) Copel—A Rare Fern." *Pharmacology Online* 1: 1–7.

Marimuthu, J., S. Thangaiah, A. Santhanam, and V. George. 2021. "Evaluation of Cytotoxic Effect of Silver Nanoparticles (AgNP) Synthesized from *Phlebodium aureum* (L.) J. Smith Extracts." *Anti-cancer Agents in Medicinal Chemistry* 21 (18): 2603–9.

Marles, R. J., C. Clavelle, L. Monteleone, N. Tays, and D. Burns. 2000. *Aboriginal Plant Use in Canada's Northwest Boreal Forest*. Vancouver: UBC Press.

Maroyi, A. 2014. "Not Just Minor Wild Edible Forest Products: Consumption of Pteridophytes in Sub-Saharan Africa." *Journal of Ethnobiology and Ethnomedicine* 10 (2014): 1–9.

Martin, M. 1703. *A Description of the Western Islands of Scotland*. London: Andrew Bell.

Mas-Capdevila, A., J. Teichenne, C. Domenech-Coca, A. Caimari, J. M. Del Bas, X. Escoté, and A. Crescenti. 2020. "Effect of Hesperidin on Cardiovascular Risk Factors: The Role of Intestinal Microbiota on Hesperidin Bioavailability." *Nutrients* 12 (5): 1488.

Mashamba, T. G., I. J. Adeosun, I. T. Baloyi, E. T. Tshikalange, and S. Cosa. 2022. "Quorum Sensing Modulation and Inhibition in Biofilm Forming Foot Ulcer Pathogens by Selected Medicinal Plants." *Heliyon* 8 (4): e09303.

Masuda, S., Y. Makioka-Itaya, T. Ijichi, and T. Tsukahara. 2022. "Edible Bird's Nest Extract Downregulates Epidermal Apoptosis and Helps Reduce Damage by Ultraviolet Radiation in Skin of Hairless Mice." *Journal of Clinical Biochemistry and Nutrition* 70 (1): 33–36.

Masuda, T., T. Inouchi, A. Fujimoto, Y. Shingai, M. Inai, M. Nakamura, and S. Imai. 2012. "Radical Scavenging Activity of Spring Mountain Herbs in the Shikoku Mountain Area and Identification of Antiradical Constituents by Simple HPLC Detection and LC-MS Methods." *Bioscience Biotechnology and Biochemistry* 76 (4): 705–11.

Matchide, M. G. T., S. Y. Y. Hnin, Y. M. M. Nguekeu, E. G. Matheuda et al. 2023. "Dryoptkirbioside, A New Fructofuranoside Glycerol, and Other Constituents from *Dryopteris kirbi* Hook et Grav Rhizomes." *Chemistry and Biodiversity* 20 (9): e202301127.

Matsuda, H., M. Yamazaki, S. Naruo, Y. Asanuma, and M. Kubo. 2002. "Anti-Androgenic and Hair Growth Promoting Activities of Lygodii spora (spore of *Lygodium japonicum*) I. Active Constituents Inhibiting Testosterone 5-Alpha-reductase." *Biological and Pharmaceutical Bulletin* 25 (5): 622–26.

Mawang, C. I., Y. Y. Lim, K. S. Ong, A. Muhamad, and S. M. Lee. 2017. "Identification of *a*-Tocopherol as a Bioactive Component of *Dicranopteris linearis* with Disrupting Property against Preformed Biofilm of *Staphylococcus aureus*." *Journal of Applied Microbiology* 123 (5): 1148–59.

May, L. W. 1978. "The Economic Uses and Associated Folklore of Ferns and Fern Allies." *The Botanical Review* 44: 491–528.

McCutcheon, A. R., T. E. Roberts, E. Gibbons, S. M. Ellis, L. A. Babiuk, R. E. W. Hancock, and G. H. N. Towers. 1995. "Antiviral Screening of British Columbian Medicinal Plants." *Journal of Ethnopharmacology* 49 (2): 101–10.

Medeiros-Fonseca, B., A. L. Abreu-Silva, R. Medeiros, P. A. Oliveira, and R. M. G. da Costa. 2021. "*Pteridium* spp. and Bovine Papillomavirus: Partners in Cancer." *Frontiers in Veterinary Science* 8: 758720.

Meigs, T. E., S. W. Sherwood, and R. D. Simoni. 1995. "Farnesyl Acetate, a Derivative of an Isoprenoid of the Mevalonate Pathway, Inhibits DNA Replication in Hamster and Human Cells." *Experimental Cell Research* 219 (2): 461–70.

Mello, E. B., M. P. Vilela, G. C. Maugé, and D. M. Malheiro. 1978. "Oral Treatment of Human Taeniasis by Ethereal Extract of Male-Fern (Aspidium) Preceded by the Administration of Hypertonic Solution of Magnesium Sulphate." *Zentralblatt für Bakteriologie, Parasitenkunde, Infektionskrankheiten und Hygiene* 241 (3): 384–87.

Mességué, M. 1972. *Des Hommes et des plantes.* London: Weidenfield and Nicolson Ltd.

Metwaly, A. M., H. A. Kadry, A. A. El-Hela, A. E. I. Mohammad, G. Ma, S. J. Cutler, S. A. Ross et al. 2014. "Nigrosphaerin A - A new Isochromene Derivative from the Endophytic Fungus *Nigrospora sphaerica*." *Phytochemistry Letters* 7: 1–5.

Miao, M. S., and L. L. Xiang. 2020. "Pharmacological Action and Potential Targets of Chlorogenic Acid." *Advances in Pharmacology* 87: 71–88.

Micheloud, J. F., L. A. Colque-Caro, O. G. Martinez, E. J. Gimeno, D. da Silva, F. Ribeiro, and B. S. Blanco. 2017. "Bovine Enzootic Haematuria Form Consumption of *Pteris deflexa* and *Pteris plumula* in Northwestern Argentina." *Toxicon* 134: 25–29.

Mitsuhashi, H. 1976. "Medicinal Plants of the Ainu of Hokkaido." *Economic Botany* 30: 209–17.

Mittermair, E., H. Kählig, A. Tahir, S. Rindler, X. Hudec, H. Schueffl, P. Heffeter, B. Marian, and L. Krenn. 2020. "Methylated Xanthones from the Rootlets of *Metaxya rostrata* Display Cytotoxic Activity in Colorectal Cancer Cells." *Molecules* 25 (19): 4449.

Mittermair, E., L. Krenn, and B. Marian. 2019. "Prenylated Xanthones from *Metaxya rostrata* Suppress FoxM1 and Induce Active Cell Death by Distinct Mechanisms." *Phytomedicine* 50: 152912.

Miyazawa, M., E. Horiuchi, and J. Kawata. 2007. "Components of the Essential Oil from *Matteuccia struthiopteris*." *Journal of Oleo Science* 56 (9): 457–461.

Mizushina, Y., I. Watanabe, K. Ohta, M. Takemura et al. 1998. "Studies on Inhibitors of Mammalian DNA Polymerase a and b: Sulfolipids from a Pteridophyte, *Athyrium niponicum*." *Biochemical Pharmacology* 55 (4): 537–541.

Modak, D., S. Paul, S. Sarkar, S. Thakur, and S. Bhattacharjee. 2021. "Validating Potent Anti-Inflammatory and Anti-Rheumatoid Properties of *Drynaria quercifolia* Rhizome Methanolic Extract through in Vitro, in Vivo, in Silico and GC-MS-Based Profiling." *BMC Complementary Medicine and Therapies* 21 (1): 89.

Moerman, D. E. 1986. *Medicinal Plants of Native America. Volume One. Research Reports in Ethnobotany, Contribution 2*. Ann Arbor: University of Michigan Museum of Anthropology Technical Reports Number 19.

Moerman, D. E. 2004. *Native American Ethnobotany*. Portland, OR: Timber Press.

Moerman, D. E. 2010. *Native American Food Plants: An Ethnobotanical Dictionary*. Portland, OR: Timber Press.

Mohamad, S., N. M. Zin, H. A. Wahab, P. Ibrahim, S. F. Sulaiman, A. S. M. Zahariluddin, and S. S. M. Noor. 2011. "Antituberculosis Potential of Some Ethnobotanically Selected Malaysian Plants." *Journal of Ethnopharmacology* 133 (3): 1021–26.

Mohany, K. M., A. B. Abdel Shakour, S. I. Mohamed, R. S. Hanna, and A. Y. Nassar. 2023. "Cytotoxic n-Hexane Fraction of the Egyptian *Pteris vittate* Functions as Anti-breast Cancer through Coordinated Actions on Apoptotic and Autophagic Pathways." *Applied Biochemistry and Biotechnology* 195 (11): 6927–41.

Molina, M., V. Reyes-García, and M. Pardo-de-Santayana. 2009. "Local Knowledge and Management of the Royal Fern (*Osmunda regalis* L.) in Northern Spain: Implications for Biodiversity Conservation." *American Fern Journal* 99 (1): 45-55.

Mondal, S., D. Ghosh, S. Ganapaty, S. V. G. Chekuboyina, and M. Samal. 2017. "Hepatoprotective Activity of *Macrothelypteris torresiana* (Gaudich.) Aerial Parts against CCl_4-Induced Hepatoxicity in Rodents and Analysis of Polyphenolic Compounds by HPTLC." *Journal of Pharmaceutical Analysis* 7 (3): 181–89.

Montenegro, I., G. Tomasoni, C. Bosio, N. Quiñones, A. Madrid, H. Carrasco, A. Olea, R. Martinez, M. Cuellar, and J. Villena. 2014. "Study on the Cytotoxic Activity of Drimane Sesquiterpenes and Nordrimane Compounds against Cancer Cell Lines." *Molecules* 19 (11): 18993–9006.

Moon, S. H., J. L. Son, S. J. Shin, S. H. Oh, S. H. Kim, and J. M. Bae. 2021. "Inhibitory Effect of *Asplenium incisum* on Bacterial Growth, Inflammation, and Osteoclastogenesis." *Medicina* (Kaunas) 57 (7): 641.

Moore, M. 2003. *Medicinal Plants of the Mountain West*. Santa Fe: Museum of New Mexico Press.

Morais-Braga, M. F. B., T. M. Souza, K. K. A. Santos, and G. M. M. Guedes. 2013. "Phenol Composition, Cytotoxic and Anti-Kinetoplastidae Activities of *Lygodium venustum* SW. (Lygodiaceae)" *Experimental Parasitology* 134 (2): 178–82.

Morais-Braga, M. F. B., T. M. Souza, K. K. A. Santos, G. M. M. Guedes, J. C. Andrade, S. R. Tintino, C. E. Sobral-Souza, J. G. M. Costa, A. A. F. Saraiva, and H. D. M. Coutinho. 2012. "Phenolic Compounds and Interaction between Aminoglycosides and Natural Products of *Lygodium venustum* SW against Multiresistant Bacteria." *Chemotherapy* 58 (5): 337–40.

Morais-Braga, M. F. B., T. M. Souza, K. K. A. Santos, G. M. M. Guedes, J. C. Andrade, S. R. Tintino, C. E. Sobral-Souza, J. G. M. Costa, A. A. F. Saraiva, and H. D. M. Coutinho. 2016. "Additive Effect of *Lygodium venustum* SW. in Association with Gentamicin." *Natural Product Research* 30 (16): 1851–53.

Mori, H., K. Nishteswar, B. R. Patel, and M. Nariya. 2016. "Acute Toxicity and Antihyperlipidemic Activity of Rhizome of *Tectaria coadunata* (Kukkutnakhi): A Folklore Herb." *Ayu* 37 (3–4): 238–43.

Mostafiz, M., J. K. Shim, H. S. Hwang, and H. Y. Bunch. 2020. "Acaricidal Effects of Methyl Benzoate against *Tetranychus urticae* Koch (Acari: Tetranychidae) on Common Crop Plants." *Pest Management Science* 76 (7): 2347–54.

Mottaghipisheh, J., H. Taghrir, A. Boveiri Dehsheikh, K. Zomorodian, C. Irajie, M. Mahmoodi Sourestani, and A. Iraji. 2021. "Linarin, a Glycosylated Flavonoid, with Potential Therapeutic Attributes: A Comprehensive Review." *Pharmaceuticals* 14 (11): 1104.

Müller-Ebeling, C., C. Rätsch, and W. D. Storl. 1998. *Witchcraft Medicine: Healing Arts, Shamanic Practices, and Forbidden Plants*. Rochester VT: Inner Traditions.

Muñoz, O. M., J. D. Maya, J. Ferreira, P. Christen, J. San Martin, R. López-Muñoz, A. Morello, and U. Kemmerling. 2013. "Medicinal Plants of Chile: Evaluation of Their *Trypanosoma cruzi* activity." *Zeitschrift für Naturforschung C* 68 (5–6): 198–202.

Mustafa, H. M., and G. Hayder. 2021. "Performance of *Salvinia molesta* Plants in Tertiary Treatment of Domestic Wastewater." *Heliyon* 7 (1): e06040.

Mustapha, M., and C. N. M. Taib. 2023. "Beneficial Role of Vitexin in Parkinson's Disease." *The Malaysian Journal of Medical Sciences* 30 (2): 8–25.

Na, M. K., J. P. Jang, B. S. Min, S. J. Lee, M. S. Lee, B. Y. Kim, W. K. Oh, and J. S. Ahn. 2006. "Fatty Acid Synthase Inhibitory Activity of Acylphloroglucinols Isolated from *Dryopteris crassirhizoma*." *Bioorganic and Medicinal Chemistry Letters* 16 (18): 4738–42.

Naheed, N., S. Maher, F. Saleem, A. Khan et al. 2021. "New Isolate from *Salvinia molesta* with Antioxidant and Urease Inhibitory Activity." *Drug Development Research* 82 (8): 1169–81.

Naik, J. B., and D. R. Jadge. 2010. "Evaluation of Analgesic Activity of *Actiniopteris radiata*." *Journal of Pharmacy Research* 3 (7): 1556–57.

Namazi, M. R., and A. K. Shotorbani. 2015. "Evaluation of the Efficacy of Topical Ethyl Vanillate in Enhancing the Effect of Narrow Band Ultraviolet B against Vitiligo: A Double Blind Randomized, Placebo-Controlled Clinical Trial." *Iranian Journal of Medical Sciences* 40 (6): 478–84.

Nath, K., A. D. Talukdar, M. K. Bhattacharya, D. Bhowmik, S. Chetri, D. Choudhury, A. Mitra, and N. A. Choudhury. 2019. "*Cyathea gigantea* (Cyatheaceae) as an Antimicrobial Agent against Multidrug Resistant Organisms." *BMC Complementary and Alternative Medicine* 19 (1): 279.

Nazifi, S. M. R., M. H. Asgharshamsi, M. M. Dehkordi, and K. K. Zborowski. 2019. "Antioxidant Properties of *Aloe vera* Components: a DFT Theoretical Evaluation." *Free Radical Research* 53 (8): 922–31.

Nazir, S., H. Khan, S. A. Khan, W. Alam. R. Ghaffar, S. H. A. Khan, and M. Daglia. 2021. "In Vivo Acute Toxicity, Laxative and Antiulcer Effect of the Extract of *Dryopteris ramose* (sic)." *Cellular and Molecular Biology* (Noisy-le-grand) 67 (1): 9–16.

Neef, H., P. Declercq, and G. Lackeman. 1995. "Hypoglycaemic Activity of Selected European Plants." *Phytotherapy Research* 9 (1): 45–48.

Nekrasov, E. V., V. I. Svetashev, O. V. Khrapko, and M. V. Vyssotski. 2019. "Variability of Fatty Acid Profiles in Ferns: Relation to Fern Taxonomy and Seasonal Development." *Phytochemistry* 162: 47–55.

Netto, J. B., E. S. A. Melo, A. G. S. Oliveira, L. R. Sousa et al. 2022. "Matteucinol Combined with Temozolmide Inhibits Glioblastoma Proliferation, Invasion and Progression: An in Vitro, in Silico, and in Vivo Study." *Brazilian Journal of Medical and Biological Research* 55: e12076.

Newcombe, C. F. 1897. *Unpublished Notes on Haida Plants*. C. F. Newcombe Accession 1897–47. New York: Department of Anthropology, American Museum of Natural History.

Newcombe, C. F. 1898–1913. *Unpublished Papers*. Victoria, BC, Canada: Provincial Archives of British Columbia.

Ngobeni, B., S. S. Mashele, N. J. Malebo, E. van der Watt, and I. T. Manduna. 2020. "Disruption of Microbial Cell Morphology by *Buxus macowanii*." *BMC Complementary Medicine and Therapies* 20 (1): 266.

Ngouana, V., E. Z. Menkem, D. Y. Youmbi, L. V. Yimgang, R. M. Kouipou Toghueo, and F. F. Boyom. 2021. "Serial Exhaustive Extraction Revealed Antimicrobial and Antioxidant Properties of *Platycerium stemaria* (Beauv) Desv." *BioMed Research International* 2021: 1584141.

Ni, G., N. J. Fu, D. Zhang, H. Z. Yang, X. G. Chen, and D. Q. Yu. 2015. "An Unusual Dihydrobenzofuroisocoumarin and *ent*-kaurane Diterpenoids from *Pteris multifida*." *Journal of Asian Natural Products Research* 17 (5): 423–29.

Nicole, B., A. Murdock, and E. Harris. 2006. "Medical Ethnobotany, Phytochemistry and Bioactivity of the Ferns of Moorea, French Polynesia." Senior Honors Thesis. Department of Integrative Biology, University of California, Berkeley.

Nilforoushzadeh, M. A., S. H. Javanmard, M. Ghanadian, G. Asghari, F. Jaffary, A. Fallah Yakhdani, N. Dana, and S. A. Fatemi. 2014. "The Effects of *Adiantum capillus-veneris* on Wound Healing: An Experimental In Vitro Evaluation." *International Journal of Preventative Medicine* 5 (10): 1261–68.

Nobel, P. S. 1978. "Microhabitat, Water Relations, and Photosynthesis of a Desert fern, *Notholaena parryi*." *Oecologia* 31 (3): 293–309.

Nonato, F. R., T. A. A. Barros, A. M. Lucchese, C. E. C. Oliveira, R. R. dos Santos, M. B. P. Soares, and C. F. Villarreal. 2009. "Anti-Inflammatory and Antinociceptive Activities of *Blechnum occidentale* L. Extract." *Journal of Ethnopharmacology* 125 (1): 102–7.

Nonato, F. R., T. M. O. Nogueira, T. A. de Almeida Barros, A. M. Lucchese, C. E. Cordeiro Oliveira, R. R. dos Santos, M. B. P. Soares, and C. F. Villarreal. 2011. "Antinociceptive and Anti-Inflammatory Activities of *Adiantum latifolium* Lam.: Evidence for a Role of IL-1b Inhibition." *Journal of Ethnopharmacology* 136 (3): 518–24.

Norhayati, I., K. Getha, J. M. Haffiz, A. M. Ilham, H. L. Sahira, M. M. S. Syarifah, and A. M. Syamil. 2013. "In Vitro Anti-Trypanosomal Activity of Malaysian Plants." *Journal of Tropical Forest Science* 25 (1): 52–59.

Noro, T., A. Ueno, M. Mizutani, T. Hashimoto, T. Miyase, M. Kuroyanagi, and S. Fukushima. 1984. "Inhibitors of Xanthine Oxidase from *Athyrium mesosorum*." *Chemical and Pharmaceutical Bulletin* (Tokyo) 32 (11): 4455–59.

Noubarani, M., H. Rostamkhani, M. Erfan, M. Kamalinejad, M. R. Eskandari, M. Babaeian, and J. Salamzadeh. 2014. "Effect of *Adiantum capillus veneris* Linn on an Animal Model of Testosterone-Induced Hair Loss." *Iranian Journal of Pharmaceutical Research* 13 (suppl): 113–18.

Núñez, V., R. Otero, J. Barona, M. Saldarriaga, R. G. Osorio, R. Fonnegra, S. L. Jiménez, A. Díaz, and J. C. Quintana. 2004. "Neutralization of the Edema-Forming, Defibrinating and Coagulant Effects of *Bothrops asper* Venom by Extracts of Plants Used by Healers in Columbia." *Brazilian Journal of Medical and Biological Research* 37 (7): 969–77.

Nwiloh, B. I., C. C. Monago, and A. A. Uwakwe. 2014. "Chemical Composition of Essential Oil from the Fiddleheads of *Pteridium aquilinum* L. Kuhn Found in Ogoni." *Journal of Medicinal Plants Research* 8 (1): 77–80.

Nwosu, M. O. 2002. "Ethnobotanical Studies of Some Pteridophytes of Southern Nigeria." *Economic Botany* 56: 255–59.

O'Day, D. H. 2023. "Phytochemical Interactions with Calmodulin and Critical Calmodulin Binding Proteins Involved in Amyloidogenesis in Alzheimer's Disease." *Biomolecules* 13 (4): 678.

Ofsoské-Wyber, F. 2009. *The Sacred Plant Medicine of Aotearoa*. Christchurch, NZ: Vanterra House Publishing.

Oh, H. C., D. H. Kim, J. H. Cho, and Y. C. Kim. 2004. "Hepatoprotective and Free Radical Scavenging Activities of Phenolic Petrosins and Flavonoids Isolated from Equisetum Arvense." *Journal of Ethnopharmacology* 95 (2–3): 421–24.

Oh, S. Y., M. J. Jang, Y. H. Choi, H. Hwang, H. Rhim, B. Lee, C. W. Choi, and M. S. Kim. 2021. "Central Administration of Afzelin Extracted from *Ribes fasciculatum* Improves Cognitive and Memory Function in a Mouse Model of Dementia." *Scientific Reports* 11 (1): 9182.

Ojo, O. O., A. O. Ajayi, and I. I. Anibijuwon. 2007. "Antibacterial Potency of Methanol Extracts of Lower Plants." *Journal of Zhejiang University Science*. B 8 (3): 189–91.

Oliveira, C. da C., C. de C. Veloso, R. C. M. Ferreira, G. A. Lage, L. P. S. Pimenta, I. D. G. Duarte, T. R. L. Romero, and A. de C. Perez. 2017. "Peltatoside Isolated from *Annona crassiflora* Induces Peripheral Antinociception by Activation of the Cannabinoid System." *Planta Medica* 83 (3–4): 261–67.

Osman, S. M., N. A. Ayoub, S. A. Hafez, H. A. Ibrahim, M. A. El Raey, S. Z. El-Emam, A. A. Seada, and A. M. Saadeldeen. 2020. "Aldose Reductase Inhibitor Form (sic) *Cassia glauca*: A Comparative Study of Cytotoxic Activity with AG Nanoparticles (NPs) and Molecular Docking Evaluation." *PLoS One* 15 (10): e0240856.

Otgonsugar, P., B. Buyankhishig, T. Undrakhbayar, B. Bilguun, K. Sasaki et al. 2023. "Phytochemical Investigation of Aerial Parts of *Woodsia ilvensis* and its Plasmin-Inhibitory Activity *in Vitro*." *Phytochemistry* 215: 113826.

Ouyang, D. W., X. Ni, H. Y. Xu, J. Chen, P. M. Yang, and D. Y. Kong. 2010. "Pterosins from *Pteris multifida*." *Planta Medica* 76 (16): 1896–1900.

Owumi, S. E., A. I. Kazeem, B. Wu, L. O. Ishokare, U. O. Arunsi, and A. K. Oyelere. 2022. "Apigeninidin-Rich *Sorghum bicolor* (L. Moench) Extracts Suppress A549 Cells Proliferation and Ameliorate Toxicity of Aflatoxin B1-Mediated Liver and Kidney Derangement in Rats." *Scientific Reports* 12 (1): 7438.

Oyen, L. P. A. 2010. "*Cyclosorus interruptus* (Willd.) H. Itô." Prota 16: In *Fibres/Plantes à fibres*," edited by M. Y. Brink and E. G. Achigan-Dako. Netherlands: PROTA Wageningen.

Pacifico, A., G. Damiani, P. Iacovelli, R. R. Z. Conic, Young Dermatologists Italian Network (YDIN), S. Gonzalez, and A. Morrone. 2021. "NB-UVB Plus Oral *Polypodium leucotomos* Extract Display Higher Efficacy than NB-UVB Alone in Patients with Vitiligo." *Dermatological Therapy* 34 (2): e14776.

Pan, P. C., J. Cheng, Y. Si, W. Chen et al. 2021. "A Stop-Flow Comprehensive Two-Dimensional HK-2 and HK-2/CIKI Cell Membrane Chromatography Comparative Analysis System for Screening the Active Ingredients from *Pyrrosia calvata* (Bak.) Ching against Crystal-Induced Kidney Injury." *Journal of Pharmaceutical and Biomedical Analysis* 195: 113825.

Panda, S. K., S. D. Rout, N. Mishra, and T. Panda. 2011. "Phytotherapy and Traditional Knowledge of Tribal Communities of Mayurbhanj District, Orrisa." *Indian Journal of Pharmacognosy and Phytotherapy* 3 (7): 101–13.

Pandey, L. K., and K. R. Sharma. 2022. "Analysis of Phenolic and Flavonoid Content, *a*-Amylase Inhibitory and Free Radical Scavenging Activities of Some Medicinal Plants." *The Scientific World Journal* 2022 (1): 4000707.

Parihar, P., and L. Parihar. 2006. "Some Pteridophytes of Medicinal Importance from Rajasthan." *Natural Product Radiance* 5 (4): 297–302.

Park, M., S. Park, J. Y. Yoo, Y. Kim, K. M. Lee, D. Y. Hwang, and H. J. Son. 2022. "Enzyme-Mediated Biocalcification of a Novel Alkaliphilic *Bacillus psychrodurans* LC40 and Its Eco-Friendly Application as a Biosealant for Crack Healing." *The Science of the Total Environment* 802: 149841.

Parkinson, J. 1629. *Paradisi in sole paradisus terrestris*. London: Methuen & Co. Facsimile reprint 1904.

Parrado, C., M. Mascaraque, Y. Gilaberte, A. Juarranz, and S. Gonzalez. 2016. "Femblock (*Polypodium leucotomas* extract): Molecular Mechanisms and Pleiotropic Effects in Light-Related Skin Conditions, Photoaging, and Skin Cancers, a Review." *International Journal of Molecular Science* 17 (7): 1026.

Patel, D. K. 2022. "Medicinal Importance, Pharmacological Activities and Analytical Aspects of a Flavonoid Glycoside 'Nicotiflorin' in the Medicine." *Drug Metabolism and Bioanalysis Letters* 15 (1): 2–11.

Patel, M., and M. N. Reddy. 2018. "Discovery of the World's Smallest Terrestrial Pteridophyte." *Scientific Reports* 8 (1): 5911.

Pathak, G., S. Singh, P. Kumari, W. Raza, Y. Hussain, and A. Meena. 2021. "Cirsimaritin, a Lung Squamous Carcinoma Cells (NCIH-520) Proliferation Inhibitor." *Journal of Biomolecular Structure and Dynamics* 39 (9): 3312–23.

Paul, R. K., V. Irudayaraj, M. Johnson, and R. D. Patric. 2011. "Phytochemical and Anti-Bacterial Activity of Epidermal Glands Extract of *Christella parasitica* (L.) H. Lev." *Asian Pacific Journal of Tropical Biomedicine* 1 (1): 8–11.

Paul, T., B. Das, K. G. Apte, S. Banerjee, and R. C. Saxena. 2012. "Evaluation of Anti-Hyperglycemic Activity of *Adiantum Philippense* Linn., a Pteridophyte in Alloxan Induced Diabetic Rats." *Journal of Diabetes and Metabolic Disorders* 3 (9): 1–8.

Paul, T., K. G. Apte, P. B. Parab, and B. Das. 2017. "Role of *Adiantum philippense* L. on Glucose Update in Isolated Pancreatic Cells and Inhibition of Adipocyte Differentiation in 3T3-L1 Cell Line." *Pharmacognosy Magazine* 13 (suppl. 2): S334–38.

Pavičić, A., M. Zajíčková, M. Šadibolová, G. Svobodová, P. Matoušková, B. Szotáková, L. Langhansová, P. Maršík, and L. Skálová. 2023. "Anthelmintic Activity of European Fern Extracts against *Haemonchus contortus*." *Veterinary Research* 54 (1): 59.

Pechey, J. 1694. *The London Dispensatory.*

Pei, X., Y. Lou, Q. Ren, Y. Liu, X. Dai, M. Ye, G. Huang, and J. Cao. 2023. "Anti-Inflammatory Activities of Several Diterpenoids Isolated from *Hemionitis albofusca*." *Naunyn-Schmiedeberg's Archive of Pharmacology* 397 (1): 437–47.

Pei, Y. H., N. N. Yan, H. F. Zhang, S. T. Zhang et al. 2022. "Physicochemical Characterization of a Fern Polysaccharide from *Alsophila spinulosa* Leaf and Its Anti-Aging Activity in *Caenorhabditis elegans*." *Chemistry and Biodiversity* 19 (10): e202200156.

Pellacani, G., K. Peris, S. Ciardo, C. Pezzini, S. Tambone, F. Farnetani, C. Longo, C. Chello, and S. González. 2023. "The Combination of Oral and Topical Photoprotection with a Standardized *Polypodium leucotomos* Extract is Beneficial against Actinic Keratosis." *Photodermatology Photoimmunology & Photomedicine* 39 (4): 384–91.

Peng, B., R. F. Bai, P. Li, X. Y. Han, H. Wang, C. C. Zhu, Z. P. Zeng, and X. Y. Chai. 2016. "Two New Glycosides from *Dryopteris fragrans* with Anti-Inflammatory Activities." *Journal of Asian Natural Product Research* 18 (1): 59–64.

Peng, B., X. Y. Han, H. Wang, W. J. Zhang, and Z. P. Zeng. 2022a. "Two New Cadinane-Type Sesquiterpenoid Glycosides from *Dryopteris fragrans* with Anti-Inflammatory Activities." *Journal of Asian Natural Product Research* 24 (11): 1064–70.

Peng, C. H., W. Y. Lin, C. Y. Li, K. K. Dharini, C. Y. Chang, J. T. Hong, and M. D. Lin. 2022b. "Gui Sui Bu (*Drynaria fortunei* J. Sm.) Antagonizes Glucocorticoid-Induced Mineralization Reduction in Zebrafish Larvae by Modulating the Activity of Osteoblasts and Osteoclasts." *Journal of Ethnopharmacology* 297: 115565.

Peng, C. Y., J. Lu, J. Q. Liu, H. Huang, Y. Y. Zhu, and J. C. Shu. 2020. "Three Novel Pterosin Dimers from *Pteris obtusiloba*." *Fitoterapia* 146: 104713.

Petard, P., and T. Raau. 1972. The Use of Polynesia Medicinal Plants in Tahitian Medicine. Tech Paper No. 167. Noumea, New Caledonia: South Pacific Commission.

Petkov, V., T. Batsalova, P. Stoyanov, T. Mladenova, D. Kolchakova, M. Argirova, T. Raycheva, and B. Dzhambazov. 2021a. "Selective Anticancer Properties, Proapoptotic and Antibacterial Potential of Three *Asplenium* Species." *Plants* 10 (6): 1053.

Petkov, V. H., R. G. Ardasheva, N. A. Prissadova, A. D. Kristev, P. S. Stoyanov, and M. D. Argirova. 2021b. "Receptor-Mediated Biological Effects of Extracts Obtained from three *Asplenium* species." *Zeitschrift für Naturforschung C Journal of Biosciences* 76 (9–10): 367–73.

Phong, N. V., D. Gao, J. A. Kim, and S. Y. Yang. 2023. "Optimization of Ultrasonic-Assisted Extraction of *a*-Glucosidase Inhibitors from *Dryopteris crassirhizoma* Using Artificial Neural Network and Response Surface Methodology." *Metabolites* 13 (4): 557.

Phong, N. V., V. T. Oanh, S. Y. Yang, J. S. Choi, B. S. Min, and J. A. Kim. 2021. "PTP1B Inhibition Studies of Biological Active Phloroglucinols from the Rhizomes of *Dryopteris crassirhizoma:* Kinetic Properties and Molecular Docking Simulation." *International Journal of Biological Macromolecules* 188: 719–28.

Phong, N. V., Y. Zhao, B. S. Min, S. Y. Yang, and J. A. Kim. 2022. "Inhibitory Activity of Bioactive Phloroglucinols from the Rhizomes of *Dryopteris crassirhizoma* on Escherichia coli b-Glucuronidase: Kinetic Analysis and Molecular Docking Studies." *Metabolites* 12 (10): 938.

Piao, C. H., T. G. Kim, T. T. Bui, C. H. Song, D. U. Shin, J. E. Eom, S. Y. Lee, H. S. Shin, and O. H. Chai. 2019. "Ethanol Extract of *Dryopteris crassirhizoma* Alleviates Allergic Inflammation via Inhibition of Th2 Response and Mast Cell Activation in a Murine Model of Allergic Rhinitis." *Journal of Ethnopharmacology* 232: 21–29.

Pieroni, A., B. Dibra, G. Grishaj, I. Grishaj, and S. G. Macai. 2005. "Traditional Phytotherapy of the Albanians of Lepushe, Northern Albanian Alps." *Fitoterapia* 76 (3–4): 379–99.

Polasek, J., E. F. Queiroz, L. Marcourt, A. K. Meligova, M. Halabalaki, A. L. Skaltsounis, M. N. Alexis, B. Prajogo, J.-L. Wolfender, and K. Hostettmann. 2013. "Peltogynoids and 2-Phenoxychromones from *Peltophorum pterocarpum* and Evaluation of Their Estrogenic Activity." *Planta Medica* 79 (6): 480–86.

Ponnusamy, Y., N. J. Y. Chear, S. Ramanathan, and C. S. Lai. 2015. "Polyphenols Rich Fraction of *Dicranopteris linearis* Promotes Fibroblast Cell Migration and Proliferation in Vitro." *Journal of Ethnopharmacology* 168: 305–14.

Poór, M., Y. Li, S. Kunsági-Máté, Z. Varga, A. Hunyadi, B. Dankó, F. R. Chang, Y. C. Wu, and T. Kőszegi. 2013. "Protoapigenone Derivatives: Albumin Binding Properties and Effects on HepG2 cells." *Journal of Photochemistry and Photobiology* B 124: 20–26.

Portilla, M. 2022. "Huetar Etymology of the Word Toboba Venomous Snake." *Revista de Filología y Lingüística de la Universidad de Costa Rica* 48 (1): 48896.

Pouny, I., C. Etiévant, L. Marcourt, I. Huc-Dumas, M. Batut, F. Girard, M. Wright, and G. Massiot. 2011. "Protoflavonoids from Ferns Impair Centrosomal Integrity of Tumor Cells." *Planta Medica* 77 (5): 461–66.

Powell, C. 1979. *The Meaning of Flowers: A Garland of Plant Lore and Symbolism from Popular Custom and Literature*. Boulder, CO: Shambhala.

Prakash, A. O., V. Saxena, S. Shukla, R. K. Tewari, S. Mathur, A. Gupta, S. Sharma, and R. Mathur. 1985. "Anti-Implantation Activity of Some Indigenous Plants in Rats." *Acta Europaea Fertilitatis* 16 (6): 441–48.

Prasetyo, A., A. A. Rahardja, D. T. Azzahro, I. P. Miranti, I. Saraswati, and F. N. Kholis. 2019. "*Nephrolepis exaltata* Herbal Mask Increases Nasal IgA Levels and Pulmonary Function in Textile Factory Workers." *Advances in Preventative Medicine* 2019: 5687135.

Prata, M. N. L., I. Charlie-Silva, J. M. M. Gomes, A. Barra et al. 2020. "Anti-Inflammatory and Immune Properties of the Peltatoside, Isolated from the Leaves of *Annona crassiflora* Mart., in a New Experimental Model Zebrafish." *Fish and Shellfish Immunology* 101: 234–43.

Preethi, S., K. Arthiga, A. B. Patil, A. Spandana, and V. Jain. 2022. "Review of NAD(P) H Dehydrogenase Quinone 1 (NQO1) Pathway." *Molecular Biology Reports* 49: 8907–24.

Pukui, M. K., and S. Elbert. 1986. *Hawaiian-English Dictionary*. Honolulu, HI: University of Hawai'i Press. 248.

Punzón, C., A. Alcaide, and M. Fresno. 2003. "In Vitro Anti-Inflammatory Activity of *Phlebodium decumanum*. Modulation of Tumor Necrosis Factor and Soluble TNF Receptors." *International Immunopharmacology* 3 (9): 1293–99.

Purgato, G. A., S. Lima, J. V. P. B. Baeta, V. R. Pizziolo, G. N. de Souza, G. Diaz-Muñoz, and M. A. N. Diaz. 2021. "*Salvinia auriculata*: Chemical Profile and Biological Activity against *Staphylococcus aureus* Isolated from Bovine Mastitis." *Brazilian Journal of Microbiology* 52 (4): 2401–11.

Qi, G., Z. Liu, R. Fan, Z. Yin, Y. Mi, B. Ren, and X. Liu. 2017. "*Athyrium multidentatum* (Doll.) Ching Extract Induce Apoptosis via Mitochondrial Dysfunction and Oxidative Stress in HepG2 Cells." *Scientific Reports* 7 (1): 2275.

Qi, G. Y., L. Q. Yang, C. X. Xiao, J. Shi, Y. Mi, and X. B. Liu. 2015. "Nutrient Values and Bioactivities of the Extracts from Three Fern Species in China: A Comparative Assessment." *Food and Function* 6 (9): 2918–29.

Qi, W., Y. Chen, S. Sun, X. Xu, J. Zhan, Z. Yan, P. Shang, X. Pan, and H. Liu. 2021. "Inhibiting TLR4 Signaling by Linarin for Preventing Inflammatory Response in Osteoarthritis." *Aging* 13 (4): 5369–82.

Qian, W., W. Wu, Y. Kang, Y. Wang, P. Yang, Y. Deng, C. Ni, and J. Huang. 2020. "Comprehensive Identification of Minor Components and Bioassay-Guided Isolation of an Unusual Antioxidant from *Azolla imbricata* Using Ultra-High Performance Liquid Chromatography-Quadrupole Time-of-Flight Mass Spectrometry Combined with Multicomponent Knockout and Bioactivity Evaluation." *Journal of Chromatography A*. 1609: 460435.

Qiu, S., X. Wu, H. Liao, X. Zeng et al. 2017. "Pteisolic Acid G, a Novel *ent*-Kaurane Diterpenoid, Inhibits Viability and Induces Apoptosis in Human Colorectal Carcinoma Cells." *Oncology Letters* 14 (5): 5540–48.

Quadri-Spinelli, T., J. Heilmann, T. Rali, and O. Sticher. 2000. "Bioactive Coumarin Derivatives from the Fern *Cyclosorus interruptus*." *Planta Medica* 66 (8): 728–33.

Quincey, J. 1736. *Pharmacopoeia Officinalis & Extemporanea Or, A Complete English Dispensatory in Four Parts*. London: Longman Thomas.

Quisumbing, E. 1951. *Medicinal Plants of the Philippines*. Manila Department of Agriculture and Natural Resources Bulletin 16. Manila Bureau of Printing.

Rabiei, Z., and M. Setorki. 2019. "Effect of Ethanol *Adiantum capillus-veneris* Extract in Experimental Models of Anxiety and Depression." *Brazilian Journal of Pharmaceutical Sciences* 55: e18099.

Rachmi, E., B. B. Purnomo, A. T. Endharti, and L. E. Fitri. 2020. "Identification of Afzelin Potential Targets in Inhibiting Triple-Negative Breast Cancer Cell Migration Using Reverse Docking." *Porto Biomedical Journal* 5 (6) e095.

Radhika, N. K., P. S. Sreejith, and V. V. Asha. 2010. "Cytotoxic and Apoptotic Activity of *Cheilanthes farinosa* (Forsk.) Knaulf. against Human Hepatoma Hep3B Cells." *Journal of Ethnopharmacology* 128 (1): 166–71.

Rahayu, I., and K. H. Timotius. 2022. "Phytochemical Analysis, Antimutagenic and Antiviral Activity of *Moringa oleifera* L. Leaf Infusion: In Vitro and in Silico Studies." *Molecules* 27 (13): 4017.

Rahayu, S., R. Annisa, I. Anzila, Y. I. Christina, A. Soewondo, A. P. Warih Marhendra, and M. S. Djati. 2021. "*Marsilea crenata* Ethanol Extract Prevents Monosodium Glutamate Adverse Effects on the Serum Levels of Reproductive Hormones, Sperm Quality and Testis Histology in Male Rats." *Veterinary World* 14 (6): 1529–36.

Rahman, S. M. A., M. A. Kamel., and M. A. Ali et al. 2023. "Comparative Study on the Phytochemical Characterization and Biological Activities of *Azolla caroliniana* and *Azolla filiculoides*: In Vitro Study." *Plants* 12 (18): 3229.

Rajasekaran, M., A. G. Nair, W. J. Hellstrom, and S. C. Sikka. 1993. "Spermicidal Activity of an Antifungal Saponin Obtained from the Tropical Herb *Mollogo pentaphylla*." *Contraception* 47 (4): 401–12.

Rajesh, K. D., V. Subramani, P. Annamalai, R. Nakulan V., J. Narayanaperumal, and J. Solomon. 2016. "In Vitro Study of Trematodicidal Action of *Dicranopteris linearis* (Burm. f.) Underw. Extracts against Gastrothylax Crumenifer." *Biomedicine and Pharmacotherapy* 84: 2042–53.

Ramesha, K. P., N. C. Mohana, B. R. Nuthan, D. Rakshith, and S. Satish. 2020. "Antimicrobial Metabolite Profiling of *Nigrospora sphaerica* from *Adiantum philippense* L." *Journal Genetic Engineering and Biotechnology* 18 (1): 66.

Ramirez, M. S., R. A. Bonomo, and M. E. Tolmasky. 2020. "Carbapenemases: Transforming *Acinetobacter baumanii* into a Yet More Dangerous Menace." *Biomolecules* 10 (5): 720.

Rani, A., M. Uzair, S. Ali, M. Qamar, N. Ahmad, M. W. Abbas, and T. Esatbeyoglu. 2022. "*Dryopteris juxtapostia* Root and Shoot: Determination of Phytochemicals; Antioxidant, Anti-Inflammatory, and Hepatoprotective Effects: and Toxicity Assessment." *Antioxidants* 11 (9): 1670.

Rani, D., P. B. Khare, and P. K. Dantu. 2010. "In Vitro Antibacterial and Antifungal Properties of Aqueous and Non-Aqueous Frond Extracts of *Psilotum nudum, Nephrolepis biserrata* and

Nephrolepis cordifolia." *Indian Journal of Pharmaceutical Sciences* 72 (6): 818–22.

Rasmussen, L. H. 2021. "Presence of the Carcinogen Ptaquiloside in Fern-Based Food Products and Traditional Medicine: Four Cases of Human Exposure." *Current Research in Food Science* 4: 557–64.

Rastogi, S., M. M. Pandey, and A. K. S. Rawat. 2018. "Ethnopharmacological Uses, Phytochemistry and Pharmacology of Genus *Adiantum*: A Comprehensive Review." *Journal of Ethnopharmacology* 215: 101–9.

Rautray, S., S. Panikar, T. Amutha, and A. U. Rajananthini. 2018. "Anticancer Activity of *Adiantum capillus veneris* and *Pteris quadriureta* L. in Human Breast Cancer Cell Lines." *Molecular Biology Reports* 45 (6): 1897–1911.

Read, E. D. (ed.) 1946. *Plants Listed in the Chui Huang Pen T'sao*. Shanghai: Henry Lester Institute of Medicine.

Reddy, M. N., M. Adnan, M. M. Alreshidi, M. Saeed, and M. Patel. 2020. "Evaluation of Anticancer, Antibacterial and Antioxidant Properties of a Medicinally Treasured Fern *Tectaria coadunata* with its Phytoconstituents Analysis by HR-LCMS." *Anticancer Agents in Medicinal Chemistry* 20 (15): 1845–56.

Rehman, Z. U., H. M. Rasheed, K. Bashir, A. Gurgul, F. Wahid, C. T. Che, I. Shahzadi, and T. Khan. 2022. "UHPLC-MS-GNPS Based Phytochemical Investigation of *Dryopteris ramose* (Hope) C. Chr. and Evaluation of Cytotoxicity against Liver and Prostate Cell Lines." *Heliyon* 8 (11): e11286.

Remigio, A. C., H. H. Harris, D. J. Paterson, M. Edraki, A. van der Ent. 2023. "Chemical Transformations of Arsenic in the Rhizosphere-Root Interface of *Pityrogramma calomelanos* and *Pteris vittata*." *Metallomics* 15(8): mfad047.

Ren, Z., C. He, Y. Fan, H. Si, Y. Wang, Z. Shi, X. Zhao, Y. Zheng, Q. Liu, and H. Zhang. 2014a. "Immune-Enhancing Activity of Polysaccharides from *Cyrtomium macrophyllum*." *International Journal of Biological Macromolecules* 70: 590–95.

Ren, Z., C. He, Y. Fan, L. Guo, H. Si, Y. Wang, Z. Shi, and H. Zhang. 2014b. "Immuno-Enhancement Effects of Ethanol Extract from *Cyrtomium macrophyllum* (Makino) Tagawa on Cyclophosphamide-Induced Immunosuppression in BALB/c Mice." *Journal of Ethnopharmacology* 155 (1): 769–75.

Rhee, J. K., K. J. Woo, B. K. Baek, and B. J. Ahn. 1981. "Screening of the Wormicidal Chinese Raw Drugs on *Clonorchis sinensis*." *American Journal of Chinese Medicine* 9 (4): 277–84.

Riaz, A., A. Rasul, G. Hussain, M. K. Zahoor, F. Jabeen, Z. Subhani, T. Younis, M. Ali, I. Sarfraz, and Z. Selamoglu. 2018. "Astragalin: A Bioactive Phytochemical with Potential Therapeutic Activities." *Advances in Pharmacological Sciences* 2018: 9794625.

Ribeiro, D. da Silva, K. M. Keller, and B. Soto-Blanco. 2020. "Ptaquiloside and Pterosin B Levels in Mature Green Fronds and Sprouts of *Pteridium arachnoideum*." *Toxins* 12 (5): 288.

Riley, M. 1994. *Māori Healing and Herbal*. Paraparaumu: Viking Sevenseas N.Z. Ltd.

Rinehart, K. L., T. G. Holt, N. L. Fregeau, P. A. Keifer et al. 1990. "Bioactive Compounds from Aquatic and Terrestrial Sources." *Journal of Natural Products* 53 (4): 771–92.

Rodgers, A. L., D. Webber, R. Ramsout, and M. D. I. Gohel. 2015. "*Folium pyrrosiae* Ingestion Has No Effect on the Thermodynamic or Kinetic Urinary Risk Factors for Calcium Oxalate Urolithiasis in Healthy Subjects: A Poor Prognosis for Alternative Treatment in This Type of Stone Former." *Urolithiasis* 43 (1): 21–27.

Rogers, R. D. 2014a. *Sacred Snake Medicine Plants and Venom*. Edmonton, AB, Canada: Prairie Deva Press.

Rogers, R. D. 2014b. *Ancient Medicinal Remedies: Horsetail, Ferns, Lichens and More*. Edmonton, AB, Canada: Prairie Deva Press.

Rogers, R. 2016. *Mushroom Essences: Vibrational Healing from the Kingdom Fungi*. Berkeley, CA: North Atlantic Books.

Rogers, R. 2017. *Herbal Allies: My Journey with Plant Medicine*. Berkeley, CA: North Atlantic Books.

Rogers, R. D. 2019. *Rejuvenate Your Brain Naturally*. Edmonton, AB, Canada: Prairie Deva Press.

Roi, J. 1955. *Traites des plantes médicinales Chinoises*. Paris: Encylopediae Biologique XLVII.

Romero, J. B. 1954. *The Botanical Lore of the California Indians*. New York: Vantage Press.

Rotimi, D. E., T. C. Elebiyo, and O. A. Ojo. 2023. "Therapeutic Potential of Rutin in Male Infertility: A Mini Review." *Journal of Integrative Medicine* 21 (2): 130–35.

Roudsari, M. T., A. R. Bahrami, and H. Dehghani. 2012. "Bracken-Fern Extracts Induce Cell Cycle Arrest and Apoptosis in Certain Cancer Cell Lines." *Asian Pacific Journal of Cancer Prevention* 13 (12): 6047–53.

Rout, S. D., T. Panda, and N. Mishra. 2009. "Ethnomedicinal Studies of Some Pteridophytes of Similipal Biosphere Reserve, Orissa, India." *International Journal of Medicine and Medical Sciences* 1 (5): 192–97.

Roy, S., S. Dutta, and T. K. Chaudhuri. 2015a. "In Vitro Assessment of Anticholinesterase and NADH Oxidase Inhibitory Activities of an Edible Fern, *Diplazium esculentum*." *Journal of Basic and Clinical Physiology and Pharmacology* 26 (4): 395–401.

Roy, S., S. Tamang, P. Dey, and T. K. Chaudhuri. 2013. "Assessment of the Immunosuppressive and Hemolytic Activities of an Edible Fern, *Diplazium esculentum*." *Immunopharmacology and Immunotoxicology* 35 (3): 365–72.

Roy, S., and T. K. Chaudhuri. 2015b. "Assessment of Th1 and Th2 Cytokine Modulatory Activity of an Edible Fern, *Diplazium esculentum*." *Food and Agricultural Immunology* 26 (5): 690–702.

Roy, S., and T. K. Chaudhuri. 2017. "Toxicological Assessment of *Diplazium esculentum* on the Reproductive Functions of Male Swiss Albino Mouse." *Drug and Chemical Toxicology* 40 (2): 171–82.

Russo, E. B. 1992. "Headache Treatments by Native Peoples of the Ecuadorian Amazon. A Preliminary Cross-Disciplinary Assessment." *Journal of Ethnopharmacology* 36: 193–206.

Safar, H. F., A. H. Ali, N. H. Zakaria, N. Kamal, N. I. Hassan, H. K. Agustar, N. Talip, and J. Latip. 2022. "Steroids from *Diplazium esculentum*: Antiplasmodial Activity and Molecular Docking Studies to Investigate Their Binding Modes." *Tropical Biomedicine* 39 (4): 552–58.

Sahu, S., G. Dutta, N. Mandal, A. R. Goswami, and T. Ghosh. 2012. "Anticonvulsant Effect of *Marsilea quadrifolia* Linn. on Pentylenetetrazole Induced Seizure: A Behavioral and EEG Study in Rats." *Journal of Ethnopharmacology* 141 (1): 537–41.

Saleem, A., A. Mubeen, M. F. Akhtar, and A. Zeb. 2022. "*Polystichum braunii* Ameliorates Airway Inflammation by Attenuation of Inflammatory and Oxidative Stress Biomarkers, and Pulmonary Edema by Elevation of Aquaporins in Ovalbumin-Induced Allergic Asthmatic Mice." *Inflammopharmacology* 30 (2): 639–53.

Saleem, A., M. Saleem, M. F. Akhtar, A. Sharif, Z. Javaid, and K. Sohail. 2019. "In Vitro and in Vivo Anti-Arthritic Evaluation of *Polystichum braunii* to Validate Its Folkloric Claim." *Pakistan Journal of Pharmaceutical Sciences* 32 (3 suppl.): 1157–73.

Saleem, F., M. T. J. Khan, H. Saleem, M. Azeem et al. 2016. "Phytochemical, Antimicrobial and Antioxidant Activities of *Pteris cretica* L. (Pteridaceae) Extracts." *Acta Poloniae Pharmaceutica* 73 (5): 1397–403.

Salehi, B., S. M. Ezzat, P. V. T. Fokou, S. Albayrak et al. 2018. "*Athyrium* plants—Review on Phytopharmacy Properties." *Journal of Traditional and Complementary Medicine* 9 (3): 201–5.

Salmon, W. 1710. *Botanologia. The English Herbal, or, History of Plants.* London: I. Dawkes Publishers.

Samson, D. M., W. A. Qualls, D. Roque, D. P. Naranjo, T. Alimi, K. L. Arheart, G. C. Müller, J. C. Beier, and R. D. Xue. 2013. "Resting and Energy Reserves of *Ades albopictus* Collected in Common Landscaping Vegetation in St. Augustine, Florida." *Journal of the American Mosquito Control Association* 29 (3): 231–36.

Santhosh, K. S., P. Samydurai, and N. Nagarajan. 2014. "Indigenous Knowledge of Some Medicinal Pteriophytic Plant Species among the Malasar Tribes in Valparai Hills, Western Ghats of Tamil Nadu." *American Journal of Ethnomedicine* 1 (3): 164–73.

Santhosh, P., M. Kamaraj, M. Saravanan, and T. G. Nithya. 2023. "Dietary Supplementation of *Salvinia cucullata* in White Shrimp *Litopenaeus vannamei* to Enhance the Growth, Nonspecific Immune Responses, and Disease Resistance to *Vibrio parahaemolyticus*." *Fish and Shellfish Immunology* 132: 108465.

Saravanan, S., S. Mutheeswaran, M. Saravanan, M. Chellappandian, M. Gabriel Paulraj, M. Karunai Raj, S. Ignacimuthu, and V. Duraipandiyan. 2013. "Ameliorative Effect of *Drynaria quercifolia* (L.) J. Sm., an Ethnomedicinal Plant, in Arthritic Animals." *Food and Chemical Toxicology* 51: 356–63.

Sareen, B., A. Bhattacharya, and V. Srivatsan. 2021. "Nutritional Characterization and Chemical Composition of *Diplazium maximum* (D. Don) C. Chr." *Journal of Food Science and Technology* 58 (3): 844–54.

Sasaki-Hamada, S., M. Hoshi, Y. Niwa, Y. Ueda, A. Kokaji, S. Kamisuki, K. Kuramochi, F. Sugawara, and J.-I. Oka. 2016. "Neoechinulin A Induced Memory Improvements and Antidepressant-Like Effects in Mice." *Progress in Neuropsychopharmacology and Biological Psychiatry* 71: 155–61.

Ščevková, J., Z. Vašková, J. Dušička, M. Hrabovský. 2022. "Fern Spores: Neglected Airborne

Bioparticles Threatening Human Health in Urban Environments." *Urban Ecosystems* 25 (6).: 1825–38.

Schmidt, M., J. Skaf, G. Gavril, C. Polednik, J. Roller, M. Kessler, and U. Holzgrabe. 2017. "The Influence of *Osmunda regalis* Root Extract on Head and Neck Cancer Cell Proliferation, Invasion and Gene Expression." *BMC Complementary and Alternative Medicine* 17 (1): 518.

Scholz, T., J. M. Rogers, A. Krichevsky, S. Dhar, and G. R. D. Evans. 2010. "Inducible Nerve Growth Factor Delivery for Peripheral Nerve Regeneration in Vivo." *Plastic and Reconstructive Surgery* 126 (6): 1874–89.

Schultz, F., G. Anywar, B. Wack, C. L. Quave, and L. A. Garbe. 2020. "Ethnobotanical Study of Selected Medicinal Plants Traditionally Used in the Rural Greater Mpigi Region of Uganda." *Journal of Ethnopharmacology* 256: 112742.

Schultz, F., O. F. Osuji, B. Wack, G. Anywar, and L. A. Garbe. 2021. "Antiinflammatory Medicinal Plants from the Ugandan Greater Mpigi Region Act as Potent Inhibitors in the COX-2/PGH_2 Pathway." *Plants* 10 (2): 351.

Schwantes, D., A. C. Gonçalves Jr., A. da Paz Schiller, J. Manfrin, M. A. Campagnolo, and T. G. Veiga. 2019. "*Salvinia auriculata* in Post-Treatment of Dairy Industry Wastewater." *International Journal of Phytoremediation* 21 (13): 1368–74.

Segars, K., V. McCarver, R. A. Miller. 2021. "Dermatologic Applications of *Polypodium leucotomos*: A Literature Review." *Journal of Clinical and Aesthetic Dermatology* 14 (2) 50–60.

Seif, M., H. Aati, M. Amer, A. J. Ragauskas, A. Seif, A. H. El-Sappah, A. Aati, A. E. A. Madboli, and M. Emam. 2023. "Mitigation of Hepatotoxicity via Boosting Antioxidants and Reducing Oxidative Stress and Inflammation in Carbendazim-Treated Rats Using *Adiantum Capillus-Veneris* L. Extract." *Molecules* 28 (12): 4720.

Selim, K. A., A. A. El-Beih, T. M. Abdel-Rahman, and A. I. El-Diwany. 2014. "Biological Evaluation of Endophytic Fungus, *Chaetomium globosum* JN711454, as Potential Candidate for Improving Drug Discovery." *Cell Biochemistry and Biophysics* 68 (1): 67–82.

Selim, K. A., A. A. El-Beih, T. M. Abdel-Rahman, and A. I. El-Diwany. 2016. "High Expression Level of Antioxidants and Pharmaceutical Bioactivities of Endophytic Fungus *Chaetomium globosum* JN711454." *Preparative Biochemistry and Biotechnology* 46 (2): 131–40.

Semwal, P., S. Painuli, K. M. Painuli, G. Antika et al. 2021. "*Diplazium esculentum* (Retz.) Sw.: Ethnomedicinal, Phytochemical and Pharmacological Overview of the Himalayan Ferns." *Oxidative Medicine and Cellular Longevity*. (September): 1917890.

Seo, C., H. W. An, W. Han, J. W. Lee, K. K. Shrestha, W.-K. Jung, J. H. Shin, and S. G. Lee. 2022. "Screening of Antioxidant Capacity of Nepali Medicinal Plants with a Novel Singlet Oxygen Scavenging Assay." *Food Science and Biotechnology* 32 (2): 221–28.

Seong, J. Y., J. Y. Lee, Y. K. Lim, W. J. Yoon, S. Jung, J. K. Kook, and T. H. Lee. 2020. "*Osmunda japonica* Extract Suppresses Pro-Inflammatory Cytokines by Downregulating NF-kB Activation in Peridontal Ligament Fibroblasts Infected with Oral Pathogenic Bacteria." *International Journal of Molecular Sciences* 21 (7): 2453.

Serini, S., R. Guarino, R. O. Vasconcelos, L. Celleno, and G. Calviello. 2020. "The Combination of Sulforaphane and Fernblock® XP Improves Individual Beneficial Effects in Normal and Neoplastic Human Skin Cell Lines." *Nutrients* 12 (6): 1608.

Sessa, E. B., E. A. Zimmer, and T. J. Givnish. 2012. "Unraveling Reticulate Evolution in North American *Dryopteris* (Dryopteridaceae)." *BMC Evolutionary Biology* 12: 104.

Shah, A. B., A. Baiseitova, J. H. Kim, Y. H. Lee, and K. H. Park. 2022. "Inhibition of Bacterial Neuraminidase and Biofilm Formation by Ugonins Isolated from *Helminthostachys zeylanica* (L.) Hook." *Frontiers in Pharmacology* 12: 890649.

Shah, A. B., S. Yoon, J. H. Kim, K. Zhumanova, Y. J. Ban, K. W. Lee, and K. H. Park. 2020a. "Effectiveness of Cyclohexyl Functionality in Ugonins from *Helminthostachys zeylanica* to PTP1B and *a*-Glucosidase Inhibitions." *International Journal of Biological Macromolecules* 165 (Pt B): 1822–31.

Shah, M. D., B. A. Venmathi Maran, F. K. Haron, J. Ransangan, F. F. Ching, S. R. Muhamad Shaleh, R. Shapawi, Y. S. Yong, and S. Ohtsuka. 2020b. "Antiparasitic Potential of *Nephrolepis biserrate* Methanol Extract against the Parasitic Leech *Zeylanicobdella arugamensis* (Hirudinea) and LC-QTOF Analysis." *Scientific Reports* 10 (1): 22091.

Shah, M. D., C. Gnanaraj, A. T. M. E. Haque, and M. Iqbal. 2015. "Antioxidative and Chemopreventative Effects of *Nephrolepis biserrate* against Carbon Tetrachloride (CCl_4)-Induced Oxidative Stress and Hepatic Dysfunction in Rats." *Pharmaceutical Biology* 53 (1): 31–39.

Sharifi-Rad, J., A. Bahukhandi, P. Dhyani, P. Sati, E. Capanoglu, A. O. Docea, A. Al-Harrasi, A. Dey, and D. Calina. 2019. "Therapeutic Potential of Neoechinulins and Their Derivatives: An Overview of the Molecular Mechanisms behind Pharmacological Activities." *Frontiers in Nutrition* 8: 664197.

Shen B., S. Chen, Q. Zhou, Y. Jian et al. 2020. "Flavonoid Glycosides from the Rhizomes of *Pronephrium penangianum*." *Phytochemistry* 179: 112500.

Shen, Z. Y., and Y. F. Hsu. 2023. "Rediscovering a Species Not Seen for a Hundred Years, *Stathmopodaticata* (Meyrick, 1913) (Lepidoptera, Stathmopodidae), with Its Unusual Fern-Spore-Feeding Life History." *Biodiversity Data Journal* 11: e101468.

Sheng, J. W., D. M. Liu, L. Jing, G. X. Xia, W. F. Zhang, J. R. Jiang, and J. B. Tang. 2019. "Striatisporolide A, a Butanolide Metabolite from *Athyrium multidentatum* (Doll.) Ching, as a Potential Antibacterial Agent." *Molecular Medicine Reports* 20 (1): 198–204.

Sher, J., G. Jan, M. Israr, M. Irfan, N. Yousuf, F. Ullah, A. Rauf, A. Alshammari, and M. Alharbi. 2023. "Biological Characterization of *Polystichum lonchitis* L. for Phytochemical and Pharmacological Activities in Swiss Albino Mice Model." *Plants* 12 (7): 1455.

Shi, Y., X. Wang, N. Wang, F. F. Li, Y. L. You, and S. Q. Wang. 2020. "The Effect of Polysaccharides from *Cibotium barometz* on Enhancing Temozolomide-Induced Glutathione Exhausted in Human Glioblastoma U87 Cells, as Revealed by ^{1}H NMR Metabolomics Analysis." *International Journal of Biological Macromolecules* 56: 471–84.

Shi, Y. S., J. C. Chen, B. H. Lin, R. N. Wang, J. Zhao, S. Li, Y. Zhang, and X. F. Zhang. 2023. "*Pteris laeta* Wall. and Its New Phytochemical, Pterosinsade A, Promote Hippocampal

Neurogenesis *via* Activating the Wnt Signaling Pathway." *Journal of Agricultural and Food Chemistry* 71 (11): 4586–98.

Shi, Y. S., Y. Zhang, W. Z. Hu, X. F. Zhang, X. Fu, and X. Lv. 2017. "Dihydrochalones and Diterpenoids from *Pteris ensiformis* and Their Bioactivities." *Molecules* 22 (9): 1413.

Shih, C. C., J. B. Wu, J. Y. Jian, C. H. Lin, and H. Y. Ho. 2015. "(-)-Epicatechin-3-O-b-D-allopyranoside from *Davallia formosana*, Prevents Diabetes and Hyperlipidemia by Regulation of Glucose Transporter 4 and AMP-Activated Protein Kinase Phosphorylation in High-Fat-Fed Mice." *International Journal of Molecular Sciences* 16 (10): 24983–5001.

Shin, H. J., H. S. Lee, and D. S. Lee. 2010. "The Synergistic Antibacterial Activity of 1-Acetyl-beta-carboline and Beta-lactams against Methicillin-Resistant *Staphylococcus aureus* (MRSA)." *Journal of Microbiology and Biotechnology* 20 (3): 501–5.

Shoaib, A., L. Azmi, I. Shukla, S. S. Alqahtani, I. A. Alsarra, and F. Shakeel. 2021. "Properties of Ethnomedicinal Plants and Their Bioactive Compounds: Possible Use for COVID-19 Prevention and Treatment." *Current Pharmaceutical Design* 27 (13): 1579–87.

Shokeen, P., K. Ray, M. Bala, and V. Tandon. 2005. "Preliminary Studies on Activity of *Ocimum sanctum*, *Drynaria quercifolia*, and *Annona squamosa* against *Neisseria gonorrhoeae*." *Sexually Transmitted Diseases* 32 (2): 106–11.

Shrestha, S. S., S. Sut, S. B. Di Marco, G. Zengin, V. Gandin, M. De Franco, D. R. Pant, M. F. Mahomoodally, S. Dall'Acqua, and S. Rajbhandary. 2019. "Phytochemical Fingerprinting and in Vitro Bioassays of the Ethnomedicinal Fern *Tectaria coadunata* (J. Smith) C. Christensen from Central Nepal." *Molecules* 24 (24): 4457.

Siegfried, E. V. 1994. "Ethnobotany of the Northern Cree of Wabasca/Desmarais." M.A. thesis, Department of Archaeology, University of Calgary, Alberta.

Silva, A. G., V. A. O. Silva, R. J. S. Oliveira, A. R. de Rezende et al. 2020a. "Matteucinol, Isolated from *Miconia chamissois*, Induces Apoptosis in Human Glioblastoma Lines via the Intrinsic Pathway and Inhibits Angiogenesis and Tumor Growth in Vivo." *Investigational New Drugs* 38 (4): 1044–55.

Silva, H. A. M. F., A. L. Aires, C. L. R. Soares, J. L. F. Sá et al. 2020b. "Barbatic Acid from *Cladia aggregata* (Lichen): Cytotoxicity and in Vitro Schistosomicidal Evaluation and Ultrastructural Analysis against Adult Worms of *Schistosoma mansoni*." *Toxicology In Vitro* 65: 104771.

Sim, M. O., H. J. Lee, D. E. Jeong, J. H. Jang, H. K. Jung, and H. W. Cho. 2019. "6'-O-Acetyl Mangiferin from *Iris rossii* Baker Inhibits Lipid Accumulation Partly via AMPK Activation in Adipogenesis." *Chemico-Biological Interactions* 311: 108755.

Simán, S. E., A. C. Povey, T. H. Ward, G. P. Margison, and E. Sheffield. 2000. "Fern Spore Extracts Can Damage DNA." *British Journal of Cancer* 83 (1): 69–73.

Singh et al. 1989. "Ethnomedicinal Uses of Ferns." *Indian Fern Journal* 6 (1–2): 63–67.

Singh, B. P., and R. Upadhyay. 2012. "Ethnobotanical Importance of Pteridophytes Used by the Tribe of Pachmarhi, Central India." *Journal of Medicinal Plants Research* 6 (1): 14–18.

Singh, D., M. Gupta, M. Sarwat, and H. R. Siddique. 2022. "Apigenin in Cancer Prevention and Therapy: A Systematic Review and Meta-Analysis of Animal Models." *Critical Reviews in Oncology/Hematology* 176: 103751.

Singh, H. B. 1999. "Potential Medicinal Pteridophytes of India and Their Chemical Constituents." *Journal of Economic and Taxonomic Botany* 23 (1): 63–78.

Singh, H., K. C. Murall, S. Kumar, and A. K. Mangal. 2016. "Pharmacognostic and Preliminary Phytochemical Analysis of *Actiniopteris dichotoma* Bedd." *International Journal of Ayurvedic Medicine* 7 (3): 160–64.

Singh, M., N. Singh, P. B. Khare, and A. K. S. Rawat. 2008. "Antimicrobial Activity of Some Important *Adiantum* Species Used Traditionally in Indigenous Systems of Medicine." *Journal of Ethnopharmacology* 115 (2): 327–29.

Singh, P., M. Yasir, R. Khare, and R. Shrivastava. 2020a. "Green Synthesis of Silver Nanoparticles Using Indian Male Fern (*Dryopteris cochleata*), Operational Parameters, Characterization and Bioactivity on *Naja naja* Venom Neutralization." *Toxicology Research* (Cambridge) 9 (5): 706–13.

Singh, S., P. Gupta, A. Meena, and S. Luqman. 2020b. "Acacetin, a Flavone with Diverse Therapeutic Potential in Cancer, Inflammation, Infections and Other Metabolic Disorders." *Food and Chemical Toxicology* 145: 111708.

Singh, S., R. D. Dixit, and T. R. Sahu. 2005. "Ethnobotanical Use of Pteridophytes of Amarkantak (MP)." *Indian Journal of Traditional Knowledge* 4 (4): 392–95.

Singh, S., and R. Singh. 2012. "Ethnomedicinal Use of Pteridophytes in Reproductive Health in Tribal Women of Pachmarhi Biosphere Reserve, Madhya Pradesh, India." *International Journal of Pharmaceutical Sciences and Research* 3 (12): 4780–90.

Sirichai, P., S. Kittibunchakul, S. Thangsiri, N. On-Nom et al. 2022. "Impact of Drying Processes on Phenolics and in Vitro Health-Related Activities of Indigenous Plants in Thailand." *Plants* 11 (3): 294.

Smith, H. H. 1924. "Ethnobotany of Menomini Indians." *Bulletin of Public Museum of the City of Milwaukee 4*. Westport: Greenwood Press.

Snehunsu, A., C. Ghosal, M. Kandwal, P. K. Yadav et al. 2015. "1-Tricantanol Cerotate; Isolated from *Marsilea quadrifolia* Linn. Ameliorates Reactive Oxidative Damage in the Frontal Cortex and Hippocampus of Chronic Epileptic Rats." *Journal of Ethnopharmacology* 172: 80–84.

Snogan, E., I. Vahirua-Lechat, R. Ho, G. Bertho, J. P. Girault, S. Ortiga, A. Maria, and R. Lafont. 2007. "Ecdysteroids from the Medicinal Fern *Microsorum scolopendria* (Burm. f.)." *Phytochemical Analysis* 18 (5): 441–50.

Socolsky, C., E. Salamanca, A. Giménez, S. A. Borosky, and A. Bardón. 2016. "Prenylated Acylphloroglucinols with Leishmanicidal Activity from the Fern *Elaphoglossum lindbergii*." *Journal of Natural Products* 79 (1): 98–105.

Socolsky, C., L. Dominguez, Y. Asakawa, and A. Bardón. 2012a. "Unusual Terpenylated Acylphloroglucinols from *Dryopteris wallichiana*." *Phytochemistry* 80: 115–22.

Socolsky, C., M. E. Arena, Y. Asakawa, and A. Bardón. 2010a. "Antibacterial Prenylated

Acylphloroglucinols from the Fern *Elaphoglossum yungense*." *Journal of Natural Products* 73 (11): 1751–55.

Socolsky, C., S. Borkosky, and A. Bardón. 2011. "Structure-Molluscicidal Activity Relationships of Acylphloroglucinols from Ferns." *Natural Product Communications* 6 (3): 387–91.

Socolsky, C., S. A. Borkosky, M. H. de Terán, Y. Asakawa, and A. Bardón. 2010b. "Phloroglucinols from the Argentine Ferns *Elaphoglossum gayanum* and *E. piloselloides*." *Journal of Natural Products* 73 (5): 901–4.

Socolsky, C., S. M. K. Rates, A. C. Stein, Y. Asakawa, and A. Bardón. 2012b. "Acylphloroglucinols from *Elaphoglossum crassipes*: Antidepressant-Like Activity of Crassipin A." *Journal of Natural Products* 75 (6): 1007–17.

Somchit, M. N., H. Hassan, A. Zuraini, L. C. Chong, Z. Mohamed, Z. A. Zakaria. 2019. "*In vitro* Anti-Fungal and Anti-Bacterial Activity of *Drymoglossum piloselloides* L. Presl. against Several Fungi Responsible for Athlete's Foot and Common Pathogenic Bacteria." *Advanced Journal of Microbiology Research* 13 (5): 1–5.

Song, J., M. Chen, F. Meng, J. Chen, Z. Wang, Y. Zhang, J. Cui, J. Wang, and D. Shi. 2023. "Studies on the Interaction Mechanism between Xanthine Oxidase and Osmundacetone: Molecular Docking, Multi-Spectroscopy and Dynamical Simulation." *Spectrochimica Act Part A Molecular and Biomolecular Spectroscopy* 299: 122861.

Song, L., M. Cao, C. Chen, P. Qi et al. 2017. "Antibacterial Activity of *Pyrrosia petiolosa* Ethyl Acetate Extract against *Staphylococcus aureus* by Decreasing hla and sea Virulence Genes." *Natural Product Research* 31 (11): 1347–50.

Song, R. G., G. F. Li, and S. R. Li. 2015. "Aspidin PB, a Novel Natural Anti-Fibrotic Compound, Inhibited Fibrogenesis in TGF-b1-Stimulated Keloid Fibroblasts via PI-3K/Akt and Smad Signaling Pathways." *Chemico-Biological Interactions* 238: 66–73.

Songtrai, S., W. Pratchayasakul, B. Arunsak, T. Chunchai, A. Kongkaew, N. Chattipakorn, S. C. Chattipakorn, and S. Kaewsuwan. 2022. "*Cyclosorus terminans* Extract Ameliorates Insulin Resistance and Non-Alcoholic Fatty Liver Disease (NAFLD) in High-Fat Diet (HFD)-Induced Obese Rats." *Nutrients* 14 (22): 4895.

Souza, T. M., M. F. B. Morais-Braga, A. Á. F. Saraiva, M. Rolón, C. Vega, A. Rojas de Arias, J. G. M. Costa, I. R. A. Menezes, and H. D. M. Coutinho. 2013a. "Evaluation of the Anti-Leishmania Activity of Ethanol Extract and Fractions of the Leaves from *Pityrogramma calomelanos* (L.) Link." *Natural Product Research* 27 (11): 992–96.

Souza, T. M., M. F. B. Morais-Braga, J. G. M. Costa, A. A. F. Saraiva, M. A. Lima, and H. D. M. Coutinho. 2013b. "Herbs in Association with Drugs: Enhancement of the Aminoglycoside-Antibiotic Activity of *Pityrogramma calomelanos* (L.) Link." *Journal of Young Pharmacists* 5 (4): 188–90.

Srilaxmi, P., G. R. Sareddy, P. B. K. Kishor, O. H. Setty, and P. P. Babu. 2010. "Protective Efficacy of Natansnin, a Dibenzoyl Glycoside from *Salvinia natans* against CCl_4 Induced Oxidative Stress and Cellular Degeneration in Rat Liver." *BMC Pharmacology* 10: 13.

Srivastava, M., L. Q. Ma, and J. A. Cotruvo. 2005. "Uptake and Distribution of Selenium in Different Fern Species." *International Journal of Phytoremediation* 7 (1): 33–42.

Stainer, A. R., P. Sasikumar, A. P. Bye, A. J. Unsworth, L. M. Holbrook, M. Tindall, J. A. Lovegrove, and J. M. Gibbins. 2019. "The Metabolites of the Dietary Flavonoid Quercitin Possess Potent Antithrombotic Activity and Interact with Aspirin to Enhance Anti-platelet Effects." *TH Open* (*Companion Journal to Thrombosis and Haemostasis*) 3 (3): e244–58.

Stetsenko, N., and L. Tabachyi. 1984. "Content and Distribution of Ash Elements of p- and f-Families in Ferns." *Ukrains'kyi botanichnyi zhurnal* 1 (4): 45–49.

Stroppa, N., E. Onelli, M. Hejna, L. Rossi, A. Gagliardi, L. Bini, A. Baldi, and A. Moscatelli. 2020. "*Typha latifolia* and *Thelypteris palustris* Behavior in a Pilot System for the Refinement of Livestock Wastewaters: A Case of Study." *Chemosphere* 240: 124915.

Stuhr, E. T. 1933. *Manual of Pacific Coast Drug Plants*. Lancaster, PA: The Science Printing Company.

Stump, M., H. Dhinsa, J. Powers, and M. Stone. 2022. "Attenuation of Actinic Prurigo Eruptions with *Polypodium leucotomos* Supplementation." *Pediatric Dermatology* 39 (1): 145–46.

Su, C. H., Y. C. Chen, Y. H. Yang, C. Y. Wang et al. 2022. "Effect of the Traditional Chinese Herb *Helminthostachys zeylanica* on Postsurgical Recovery in Patients with Ankle Fracture: A Double-Blinded Randomized Controlled Clinical Trial." *Journal of Ethnopharmacology* 295: 115435.

Su, F., S. L. Zhu, J. L. Ruan, Y. Muftuoglu, L. B. Zhang, and Q. Y. Yuan. 2016a. "Combination Therapy of RY10-4 with the y-Secretase Inhibitor DAPT Shows Promise in Treating HER2-Amplified Breast Cancer." *Oncotarget* 7 (4): 4142–54.

Su, Y., D. Q. Wan, and W. Q. Song. 2016b. "Dryofragin Inhibits the Migration and Invasion of Human Osteosarcoma U2OS Cells by Suppressing MMP-2/9 and Elevating TIMP-1/2 through PI3K/AKT and p38 MAPK Signaling Pathways." *Anticancer Drugs* 27 (7): 660–68.

Suffredini, I. B., E. M. Bacchi, and J. A. Sertié. 1999. "Antiulcer Action of *Microgramma squamlosa* (Kaulf.) Sota." *Journal of Ethnopharmacology* 65 (3): 217–23.

Suhaini, S., S. Z. Liew, J. Norhaniza, P. C. Lee, G. Jualang, N. Embi, and M. S. Hasidah. 2015. "Anti-Malarial and Anti-Inflammatory Effects of *Gleichenia truncata* Mediated through Inhibition of GSK3b." *Tropical Biomedicine* 32 (3): 419–33.

Sukumaran, K., and R. Kuttan. 1991. "Screening of 11 Ferns for Cytotoxic and Antitumor Potential with Special Reference to *Pityrogramma calomelanos*." *Journal of Ethnopharmacology* 34 (1): 93–96.

Sul'ain, M. D., F. Zakaria, and M. F. Johan. 2019. "Anti-Proliferative Effects of Methanol and Water Extracts of *Pyrrosia piloselloides* on the HeLa Human Cervical Carcinoma Cell Line." *Asian Pacific Journal of Cancer Prevention* 20 (1): 185–92.

Sultana, S., J. K. Nandi, S. Rahman, R. Jahan, and M. Rahmatullah. 2014. "Preliminary Antihyperglycemic and Analgesic Activity Studies with *Angiopteris evecta* Leaves in Swiss Albino Mice." *World Journal of Pharmacy and Pharmaceutical Sciences* 3 (10): 1–12.

Sumathy, V., S. Jothy Lachumy, Z. Zuraini, and S. Sasidharan. 2010. "Effects of *Stenochianea palustris* Leaf Extract on Growth and Morphogenesis of Food Borne Pathogen, *Aspergillus niger*." *Malaysian Journal of Nutrition* 16: 439–46.

Sun, Y., F. S. Mu, C. Y. Li, W. Wang, M. Luo, Y. J. Fu, and Y. G. Zu. 2013. "Aspidin BB, a Phloroglucinol Derivative, Induces Cell Cycle Arrest and Apoptosis in Human Ovarian HO-8910 Cells." *Chemico-Biological Interactions* 204 (2): 88–97.

Sundarraj, S., R. Thangam, V. Sreevani, K. Kaveri, P. Gunasekaran, S. Achiraman, and S. Kannan. 2012. "g-Sitosterol from *Acacia nilotica* L. Induces G2/M Cell Cycle Arrest and Apoptosis through c-Myc Suppression in MCF-7 and A549 Cells." *Journal of Ethnopharmacology* 141 (3): 803–9.

Suriyachadkun, C., W. Ngaemthao, T. Pujchakarn, and S. Chunhametha. 2019. "*Gordonia asplenii* sp. nov., Isolated from umic Soil on Bird's Nest Fern (*Asplenium nidus* L.)." *International Journal of Systematic and Evolutionary Microbiology* 71 (3): 004746.

Swanton, J. R. 1905. *Haida Texts and Myths, Skidegate Dialect*. Bureau of American Ethnology Bulletin No. 29. Washington, DC: Smithsonian Institution.

Swanton, J .R. 1909. *Tlingit Myths and Texts*. Bureau of American Ethnology Bulletin No. 39. Washington, DC: Smithsonian Institution.

Swanton, J. R. 1911. "Haida." *In Handbook of American Indian Languages*, edited by F. Boas. Bureau of American Ethnology Bulletin No. 40., Washington, DC: Smithsonian Institution.

Szoka, L., J. Nazaruk, M. Stocki, and V. Isidorov. 2021. "Santin and Cirsimaritin from *Betula pubescens* and *Betula pendula* Buds Induce Apoptosis in Human Digestive System Cancer Cells." *Journal of Cellular and Molecular Medicine* 25 (24): 11085–96.

Szott-Rogers, L., and R. D. Rogers. 1997. *Prairie Deva Flower Essences*. Edmonton, AB, Canada: Prairie Deva Press.

Tabassum-Abbasi, N. Hussain, C. Khamrang, P. Patnaik, T. Abbasi, and S. A. Abbasi. 2023. "Different Species of Epigeic and Anecic Earthworms Cause Similarly Effective and Beneficial Biocomposting–A Case Study Involving the Pernicious Aquatic Weed Salvinia (*Salvinia molesta*, Mitchell)." *Life* 13 (3): 720.

Tabeshpour, J., D. Shakiban, A. Qobadi, E. Aghazadeh, and B. S. Yousefsani. 2023. "Cytotoxic Effects of Ethanolic Extract of *Polypodium vulgare* on Human Malignant Melanoma Cell Line." *Asian Pacific Journal of Cancer Prevention* 24 (1): 275–81.

Takomthong, P., P. Waiwut, C. Yenjai, B. Sripanidkulchai, P. Reubroycharoen, R. Lai, P. Kamau, and C. Boonyarat. 2020. "Structure-Activity Analysis and Molecular Docking Studies of Coumarins from *Toddalia asiatica* as Multifunctional Agents for Alzheimer's Disease." *Biomedicines* 8 (5): 107.

Takuli, P., K. Khulbe, P. Kumar, A. Parki, A. Syed, and A. M. Elgorban. 2020. "Phytochemical Profiling, Antioxidant and Antibacterial Efficacy of a Native Himalayan Fern: *Woodwardia unigemmata* (Makino) Nakai." *Saudi Journal of Biological Sciences* 27 (8): 1961–67.

'Tam, J. B. L., and Y. Y. Lim. 2015. "Antioxidant and Tyrosinase Inhibition Activity of the Fertile Fronds and Rhizomes of Three Different *Drynaria* Species." *BMC Research Notes* 8: 468.

Tan, K. C., T. X. Pham, Y. J. Lee, J. Y. Lee, and M. J. Balunas. 2021. "Identification of Apocarotenoids as Chemical Markers of In Vitro Anti-Inflammatory Activity for Spirulina Supplements." *Journal of Agricultural and Food Chemistry* 69 (43): 12674–85.

Tan, S. T., H. C. Ong, T. T. Chai, and F. C. Wong. 2018. "Identification of Potential Anticancer Protein Targets in Cytotoxicity Mediated by Tropical Medicinal Fern Extracts." *Pharmacognosy Magazine* 14 (54): 227–30.

Tanyeli, A., F. N. E. Akdemir, E. Eraslan, M. C. Güler, and T. Nacar. 2019. "Anti-Oxidant and Anti-Flamatuar (sic) Effectiveness of Caftaric Acid on Gastric Ulcer Induced by Indomethacin in Rats." *General Physiology and Biophysics* 38 (2): 175–81.

Tanzin, R., S. Rahman, Md. S. Hossain, B. Agarwala, Z. Khatun, S. Jahan, Md. M. Rahman, S. M. Mou, and M. Rahmatullah. 2013. "Medicinal Potential of Pteridophytes–an Antihyperglycemic and Antinociceptive Activity Evaluation of Methanolic Extracts of Whole Plants of *Christella dentata*." *Advances in Natural and Applied Sciences* 7 (1): 67–73.

Tao, J., Z. Huang, Y. Wang, Y. Liu, T. Zhao, Y. Wang, L. Tian, and G. Cheng. 2022. "Ethanolic Extract from *Pteris wallichiana* Alleviates DSS-Induced Intestinal Inflammation and Intestinal Barrier Dysfunction by Inhibiting the TLR4/NF-kB Pathway and Regulating Tight Junction Proteins." *Molecules* 27 (10): 3093.

Taveepanich, S., N. Kamthong, N. Sawasdipuksa, and S. Roengsumran. 2005. "Inhibitory Activities of Angiopteroside for HIV-1 Reverse Transcriptase and Lung Cancer Cell-Line." *Journal of Scientific Research of Chulalongkorn University* 30: 187–192.

Taylor, B. S., N. P. Manandhar, J. B. Hudson, and G. H. Towers. 1996. "Antiviral Activities of Nepalese Medicinal Plants." *Journal of Ethnopharmacology* 52 (3): 157–63.

Taylor, L. 2005. *The Healing Power of Rainforest Herbs*. Garden City Park: Square One Publishers.

Teiri, H., H. Pourzamzni, and Y. Hajizadeh. 2018. "Phytoremediation of Formaldehyde from Indoor Environment by Ornamental Plants: An Approach to Promote Occupants Health." *International Journal of Preventative Medicine* 9: 70.

Telagari, M., and K. Hullatti. 2015. "In-Vitro *a*-Amylase and *a*-Glucosidase Inhibitory Activity of *Adiantum caudatum* Linn. and *Celosia argentea* Linn. Extracts and Fractions." *Indian Journal of Pharmacology* 47 (4): 425–29.

Tewari, D., A. Mocan, E. D. Parvanov, A. N. Sah, S. M. Nabavi, L. Huminiecki, Z. F. Ma, Y. Y. Lee, J. O. Horbańczuk, and A. G. Atanasov. 2017. "Ethnopharmacological Approaches for Therapy of Jaundice: Part 1." *Frontiers in Pharmacology* 8: 518.

Throop, P. 1998. *Hiledgard von Bingen's Physica*. Rochester, VT: Healing Arts Press.

Tichaczek-Goska, D., M. Glensk, and D. Wojnicz. 2021. "The Enhancement of the Photodynamic Therapy and Ciprofloxacin Activity against Uropathogenic *Escherichia coli* Strains by *Polypodium vulgare* Rhizome Aqueous Extract." *Pathogens* 10 (12): 1544.

Tidow, H., and P. Nissen. 2013. "Structural Diversity of Calmodulin Binding to its Target Sites." *The FEBS Journal* 280 (21): 5551–65.

Tiwari, M. K., D. K. Yadav, and S. Chaudhary. 2019. "Recent Developments in Natural Product Inspired Synthetic 1,2,4-Trioxolanes (Ozonides): An Unusual Entry into Antimalarial Chemotherapy." *Current Topics in Medicinal Chemistry* 19 (10): 831–46.

Tiwari, O. P., S. K. Bhattamisra, P. K. Tripathi, and P. N. Singh. 2010. "Anti-Aggressive Activity of a Standardized Extract of *Marsilea minuta* Linn. in Rodent Models of Aggression." *Bioscience Trends* 4 (4): 190–94.

Tompkins, P., and C. Bird. 1973. *The Secret Life of Plants*. New York: Harper & Row.

Torres-Benítez, A., J. E. Ortega-Valencia, M. Flores-González, M. Sánchez, M. J. Simirgiotis, and M. P. Gómez-Serranillos. 2023. "Phytochemical Characterization and in Vitro and in Silico Biological Studies from Ferns of Genus *Blechnum* (Blechnacease, Polypodiales)." *Antioxidants* 12 (3): 540.

Tricini, O., T. Terencio, N. M. Pugno, F. Greco, B. Mazzolai, and V. Mattoli. 2017. "Air Trapping Mechanism in Artificial *Salvinia*-Like Micro-Hairs Fabricated via Direct Laser Lithography." *Micromachines* 8 (12): 366.

Trinh, P. T. N., M. D. Tri, D. C. Hien, N. H. An, P. N. Minh, P. N. An, and L. T. Dung. 2016. "A New Flavan from the *Drynaria bonii* H. Christ Rhizomes." *Natural Products Research* 30 (7): 761–67.

Trinh, T. A., Y. H. Seo, S. Y. Choi, J. Lee, and K. S. Kang. 2021. "Protective Effect of Osmundacetone against Neurological Cell Death Caused by Oxidative Glutamate Toxicity." *Biomolecules* 11 (2): 328.

Trinh, T. K., T. Tsubota, S. Takahashi, N. T. Mai, M. N. Nguyen, and N. H. Nguyen. 2020. "Carbonization and H_3PO_4 Activation of Fern *Dicranopteris linearis* and Electrochemical Properties for Electric Double Layer Capacitor Electrode." *Scientific Reports* 10 (1): 19974.

Tripathi, P., S. Dwivedi, A. Mishra, A. Kumar et al. 2012. "Arsenic Accumulation in Native Plants of West Bengal, India: Prospects for Phytoremediation but Concerns with the Use of Medicinal Plants." *Environmental Monitoring and Assessment* 184 (5): 2617–31.

Tryon, A. F. 1959. "Ferns of the Incas." *American Fern Journal* 49 (1): 10–24.

Tsai, M. M., H. C. Lin, M. C. Yu, W. J. Lin, M. Y. Chu, C. C. Tsai, and C. Y. Cheng. 2021. "Anticancer Effects of *Helminthostachys zeylanica* Ethyl Acetate Extracts on Human Gastric Cancer Cells through Downregulation of the TNF-*α*-Activated COX-2-cPLA$_2$ Pathway." *Journal of Cancer* 12 (23): 7052–68.

Tsang, S. W., H. J. Zhang, Y. G. Chen, K. K. W Auyeung, and Z. X. Bian. 2015. "Eruberin A, a Natural Flavanol Glycoside, Exerts Anti-Fibrotic Action on Pancreatic Stellate Cells." *Cellular Physiology and Biochemistry* 36 (6): 2433–46.

Tuan, H. N., B. H. Minh, P. T. Tran, J. H. Lee, H. V. Oanh, Q. M. T. Ngo, Y. N. Nguyen, P. T. K. Lien, and M. H. Tran. 2019. "The Effects of 2',4'-dihydroxy-6'-methoxy-3',5'-dimethylchalcone from *Cleistocalyx operculatus* Buds on Human Pancreatic Cancer Cell Lines." *Molecules* 24 (14): 2538.

Tung, C. P., F. R. Chang, Y. C. Wu, D. W. Chuang, A. Hunyadi, and S. T. Liu. 2011. "Inhibition of the Epstein-Barr Virus Lytic Cycle by Protoapigenone." *The Journal of General Virology* 92 (pt 8): 1760–68.

Tuo, Q. H., C. Wang, F. X. Yan, and D. F. Liao. 2004. "MAPK Pathway Mediates the Protective Effects of Onychin on Oxidative Stress-Induced Apoptosis in ECV304 Endothelial Cells." *Life Sciences* 76 (5): 487–97.

Tuominen, M., L. Bohlin, and W. Rolfsen. 1992. "Effects of Calaguala and an Active Principle, Adenosine, on Platelet Activating Factor." *Planta Medica* 58 (4): 306–10.

Turner, N. C., and M. A. M. Bell. 1971. "The Ethnobotany of the Coast Salish Indians of Vancouver Islands." *Economic Botany* 25: 63–69.

Turner, N. J. 1973. "Ethnobotany of the Bella Coola Indians of British Columbia." *Syesis* 6: 193–220.

Turner, N. J., L.C. Thompson, M.T. Thompson, A.Z. York. 1990. *Thompson Ethnobotany.* Memoir #3. Victoria, BC, Canada. Royal British Columbia Museum.

Turner, N. J. 1998. *Plant Technology of First Peoples in British Columbia*. Vancouver, BC: Royal British Columbia Museum Handbook. UBC Press.

Turner, N. J. 2004. *Plants of Haida Gwaii*. Winlaw, BC, Canada: Sononis Press.

Turner, N. J. 2014. *Ancient Pathways, Ancestral Knowledge: Ethnobotany and Ecological Wisdom of Indigenous Peoples of Northwestern North America*. Montreal and Kingston: McGill-Queen's University Press.

Turner, N. J., and R. J. Hebda. 2012. *Saanich Ethnobotany*. Victoria, BC, Canada: Royal BC Museum Publications.

Uddin, S. J., D. Grice, and E. Tiralongo. 2012. "Evaluation of Cytotoxic Activity of Patriscabratine, Tetracosane and Various Flavonoids Isolated from the Bangladeshi Medicinal Plant *Acrostichum aureum*." *Pharmaceutical Biology* 50 (10): 1276–80.

Uddin, S. J., I. D. Grice, and E. Tiralongo. 2011a. "Cytotoxic Effects of Bangladeshi Medicinal Plant Extracts." *Evidence-Based Complementary and Alternative Medicine* 2011 (1): 578092.

Uddin, S. J., T. L. H. Jason, K. D. Beattie, I. D. Grice, and E. Tiralongo. 2011b. "(2S,3S)-Sulfated Pterosin C, a Cytotoxic Sesquiterpene from the Bangladeshi Mangrove Fern *Acrostichum aureum*." *Journal of Natural Products* 74 (9): 2010–13.

Uhe, G. 1974. "Medicinal Plants of Samoa." *Economic Botany* 28: 1–30.

Ukwatta, K. M., J. L. Lawrence, and C. D. Wijayarathna. 2019. "The Study of Antimicrobial, Anti-Cancer, Anti-Inflammatory and *a*-Glucosidase Inhibitory Activities of Nigronapthaphenyl, Isolated from an Extract of *Nigrospora sphaerica*." *Mycology* 10 (4): 222–28.

Uma, R., and B. Pravin. 2013. "In Vitro Cytotoxic Activity of *Marsilea quadrifolia* Linn. of MCF-7 Cells of Human Breast Cancer." *International Research Journal of Medicine and Medical Sciences* 1 (1): 10–13.

Uphof, J. C. Rh. 1968. *Dictionary of Economic Plants*. New York: Stechert Hafner.

Usha, V., A. J. Lloyd, A. L. Lovering, and G. S. Besra. 2012. "Structure and Function of *Mycobacterium tuberculosis* Meso-Diaminopimelic Acid (DAP) Biosynthetic Enzymes." *FEMS Microbiology Letters* 330 (1): 10–16.

Usher, G. 1971. *A Dictionary of Plants Used by Man*. New York: Hafner Press.

Vadnere, G. P., A. R. Pathan, A. K. Singhai, B. U. Kulkarni, and J. C. Hundiwale. 2013. "Anti-Stress and Anti-Allergic Effect of *Antiniopteris radiata* in Some Aspects of Asthma." *Pakistan Journal of Pharmaceutical Sciences* 26 (1): 195–98.

Vasänge, M., W. Rolfsen, and L. Bohlin. 1997. "A Sulphonoglycolipid from the Fern *Polypodium decumanum* and Its Effect on the Platelet Activating-Factor Receptor in Human Neutrophils." *Journal of Pharmacy and Pharmacology* 49 (5): 562–66.

Vasänge-Tuominen, M., P. Perera-Ivarsson, J. Shen, L. Bohlin, and W. Rolfsen. 1994. "The Fern *Polypodium decumanum*, Used in the Treatment of Psoriasis, and Its Fatty Acid Constituents as Inhibitors of Leukotriene B4 Formation." *Prostaglandins Leukotrienes and Essential Fatty Acids* 50 (5): 279–84.

Vasudeva, S. M. 1999. "Economic Importance of Pteridophytes." *Indian Fern Journal* 16: 130–52.

Veiga-Malta, I., M. Duarte, M. Dinis, D. Tavares, A. Videira, and P. Ferreira. 2004. "Enolase from *Streptococcus sobrinus* is an Immunosuppressive Protein." *Cellular Microbiology* 6 (1): 79–88.

Verazaluce, J. J. G., V. Corzo, M. del C., A. Cordero, M. J., Ocaña Peinado, F., Sarmiento Ramírez, Á., and Guisado Barrilao, R. 2014. "Effect of *Phlebodium decumanum* and Coenzyme Q10 on Sports Performance in Professional Volleyball Players." *Nutricion Hospitalaria* 31 (1): 401–14.

Vickery, R. 1995. *Oxford Dictionary of Plant-Lore*. Oxford University Press.

Viral, D., P. Shivanand, and N. Jivani. 2011. "Anticancer Evaluation of *Adiantum venustum* Don." *Journal of Young Pharmacists* 3 (1): 48–54.

Wada, H., Y. Shimizu, N. Tanaka, R. C. Cambie, and J. E. Braggins. 1995. "Chemical and Chemotaxonomical Studies of Ferns. LXXXVII. Constituents of *Trichomanes reniforme*." *Chemical and Pharmaceutical Bulletin* (Tokyo) 43 (3): 461–65.

Wadaan, M. A., A. Baabbad, M. F. Khan, M. Saravanan, and A. Anderson. 2023. "Phytochemical Profiling, Anti-Hyperglycemic, Antifungal and Radicals Scavenging Potential of Crude Extracts of *Athyrium asplenioides*–an in Vitro Approach." *Environmental Research* 213 (Pt 1): 116129.

Wajant, H., S. Forster, D. Selmar, F. Effenberger, and K. Pfizenmaier. 1995. "Purification and Characterization of a Novel (R)-Mandelonitrile Lyase from the Fern *Phlebodium aureum*." *Plant Physiology* 109 (4): 1231–38.

Wan, C. X., P. H. Zhang, J. G. Luo, and L. Y. Kong. 2011. "Homoflavonoid Glucosides from *Ophioglossum pedunculosum* and Their Anti-HBV Activity." *Journal of Natural Products* 74 (4): 683–89.

Wan, D. Q., C. Y. Jiang, X. Hua, T. Wang, and Y. M. Chai. 2015. "Cell Cycle Arrest and Apoptosis Induced by Aspidin PB through P53/P21 and Mitochrondia-Dependent Pathways in Human Osteosarcoma Cells." *Anticancer Drugs* 26 (9): 931–41.

Wang, B. H., J. Shen, Z. X. Wang, J. X. Liu, Z. F. Ning, and M. C. Hu. 2018a. "Isomangiferin, a Novel Potent Vascular Endothelial Growth Factor Receptor 2 Kinase Inhibitor, Suppresses Breast Cancer Growth, Metastasis and Angiogenesis." *Journal of Breast Cancer* 21 (1): 11–20.

Wang, F., Z. B. Jiang, X. L. Wu, D. L. Liang, N. Zhang, M. Li, L. Shi, C. G. Duan, X. L. Ma, and D.-Z. Zhang. 2020. "Structural Determination and In Vitro Tumor Cytotoxicity Evaluation of Five New Cycloartane Glycosides from *Asplenium ruprechtii* Sa. Kurata." *Bioorganic Chemistry* 102: 104085.

Wang, J., Y. T. Yan, S. Z. Fu, B. Peng, L. L. Bao, Y. L. Zhang, J. H. Hu, Z. P. Zeng, D. H. Geng, and Z. P. Gao. 2017a. "Anti-Influenza Virus (H5N1) Activity Screening on the Phloroglucinols from Rhizomes of *Dryopteris crassirhizoma*." *Molecules* 22 (3): 431.

Wang, J. N., Y. Zhang, L. Y. Song, Y. B. Peng, and W. J. Li. 2017b. "Chemical Constituents from *Pteris dispar* and Their Anti-Tumor Activity in Vitro." *Zhongguo Zhong Yao Za Zhi* 42 (21): 4159–64.

Wang, K., X. Lu, X. Li, Y. Zhang, R. Xu, Y. Lou, Y. Wang, T. Zhang, and Y. Qian. 2022a. "Dual Protective Role of Velutin against Articular Cartilage Degeneration and Subchondral Bone Loss via the p38 Signaling Pathway in Murine Osteoarthritis." *Frontiers in Endocrinology* (Lausanne) 12: 926934.

Wang, M., K. Zhao, and R. Wang. 2012. "Textual Research on Original Plant of Chinese Herbal Medicine *Cyrtomium* Rhizome." *Zhongguo Zhong Yao Za Zhi* 37 (9): 1337–40.

Wang, Q., H.-C. Wei, S.-J. Zhou, Y. Li, T.-T. Zheng, C.-Z. Zhou, and X.-H. Wan. 2022b. "Hyperoside: A Review of its Sources, Biological Activities, and Molecular Mechanisms." *Phytotherapy Research* 36 (7): 2779–802.

Wang, T. C., C. C. Lin, H. I. Lee, C. Yang, and C. C. Yang. 2010a. "Anti-Hyperlipidemic Activity of Spider Brake (*Pteris multifida*) with Rats Fed a High Cholesterol Diet." *Pharmaceutical Biology* 48 (2): 221–26.

Wang, W., H. Li, J. Yu, M. Hong et al. 2015. "Protective Effects of Chinese Herbal Medicine *Rhizoma drynariae* in Rats after Traumatic Brain Injury and Identification of Active Compound." *Molecular Neurobiology* 53 (7): 4809–20.

Wang, W., and Z. Renquan. 2023. "Acacetin Restrains the Malignancy of Esophageal Squamous Carcinoma Cells via Regulating JAK2/STAT3 Pathway. *Chemical Biology and Drug Design* 102 (3): 564–573.

Wang, X., J. G. Cao, L. Tian, B. D. Liu, Y. W. Fan, and Q. X. Wang. 2023. "Elucidating Flavonoid and Antioxidant Activity in Edible and Medicinal Herbs *Woodwardia japonica* (L.f.) Sm. Based on HPLC-ESI-TOF-MS and Artificial Neural Network Model: Response to Climatic Factors." *Molecules* 28 (4): 1985.

Wang, X., J. T. Guo, S. Q. Zang, B. D. Liu, and Y. H. Wu. 2024. "Comparison of Flavonoid Content, Antioxidant Potential, Acetylcholinesterase Inhibition Activity and Volatile Components Based on HS-SPME-GC-MS of Different Parts from *Matteuccia struthiopteris* (L.) Todaro." *Molecules* 29 (5): 1142.

Wang, X., S. G. Tang, H. Y. Zhai, and H. Q. Duan. 2011. "Studies on Anti-Tumor Metastatic Constituents from *Ardisia crenata*." *Zhongguo Zhong Yao Za Zhi* 36 (7): 881–85.

Wang, Y., X. Shen, K. Yin, C. Miao, Y. Sun, S. Mao, D. Liu, and J. Sheng. 2022c. "Structural Characteristics and Immune Enhancing Activity of Fractionated Polysaccharides from *Athyrium multidentatum* (Doll.) Ching." *International Journal of Biological Macromolecules* 205: 76–89.

Wang, Y. J., B. D. Liu, X. Wang, and Y. Fan. 2022d. "Comparison of Constituents and Antioxidant Activity of Above-Ground and Underground Parts of *Dryopteris crassirhizoma* Nakai Based on HS-SPME-GC-MS and UPLC/Q-TOF-MS." *Molecules* 27 (15): 4991.

Wang, Y. J., J. Su, J. J. Yu, M. Q. Yan, and M. L. Shi. 2021. "Buddleoside-Rich *Chrysanthemum indicum* L. Extract Has a Beneficial Effect on Metabolic Hypertensive Rats by Inhibiting the Enteric-Origin LPS/TLR4 Pathway." *Frontiers in Pharmacology* 23: 755140.

Wang, Y. R., and W. D. Yang. 2018b. "Lithagogue effects of *Pyrrosia lingua* from Guizhou Province on Experimental Renal Calculus in Rats." *Zhongguo Zhong Yao Za Zhi* 43 (16): 3291–300.

Wang, Z., J. Y. Xie, H. Xu, X. Q. Cheng, X. L. Yue, H. Li, Y. Y. Zhang, Y. Lu, and D. F. Chen. 2010b. "Effect of *Matteuccia struthiopteris* Polysaccharides on Systemic Lupus Erythematosus-Like Syndrome Induced by *Campylobacter jejuni* in BALB/c Mice." *Yao Xue Xue Bao* 45 (6): 711–17.

Ward, N. B. 1842. *On the Growth of Plants in Closely Glazed Cases*. Cambridge Library Collection.

Watt, J. M., and M. G. Breyer-Brandwijk. 1962. *The Medicinal and Poisonous Plants of South and Eastern Africa*. Second edition. Edinburgh: E. & S. Livingstone.

Weaver, W. W. 2001. *Sauer's Herbal Cures: America's First Book of Botanic Healing 1762–1778*. Translated. New York and London: Routledge.

Wei, A., G. H. Wu, C. M. Xiong, D. N. Zhou, Y. L. Cai, and J. L. Ruan. 2011a. "Flavonoids with Special B-Ring from *Macrothelypteris viridifrons* and their Anti-Proliferative Effects on Tumor Cell." *Zhongguo Zhong Yao Za Zhi*. 36 (5): 582–84.

Wei, A. H., D. N. Zhou, C. M. Xiong, Y. L. Cai, J. L. and Ruan. 2011b. "A Novel Non-Aromatic B-Ring Flavonoid: Isolation, Structure Elucidation and Its Induction of Apoptosis in Human Colon HT-29 Tumor Cell via the Reactive Oxygen Species-Mitochondrial Dysfunction and MAPK Activation." *Food and Chemical Toxicology* 49 (9): 2445–52.

Wei, A. H., D. N. Zhou, J. L. Ruan, Y. L. Cai, C. M. Xiong, and G. H. Wu. 2012. "Anti-Tumor and Anti-Angiogenic Effects of *Macrothelypteris viridifrons* and Its Constituents by HPLC-DAD/MS Analysis." *Journal of Ethnopharmacology* 139 (2): 373–80.

Wei, A. H., D. N. Zhou, Z. C. Gu, and D. Liu. 2019. "HPLC Analysis, Optimization of Extraction and Purification Conditions, Biological Evaluation of Total Protoflavones from *Macrothelypteris viridifrons*." *Natural Product Research* 33 (21): 3167–3170.

Wei, A. H., L. Zeng, J. L. Ruan, and D. N. Zhou. 2022a. "Apoptosis Induced by DICO, a Novel Non-Aromatic B-Ring Flavonoid *via* a ROS-Dependent Mechanism in Human Colon Cancer Cells." *Natural Product Research* 36 (23): 6050–55.

Wei, H., G. Wu, J. Chen, X. Zhang, C. Xiong, Y. Lei, W. Chen, and J. Ruan. 2013a. "(2S)-5,2',5'-trihydroxy-7-methoxyflavanone, a Natural Product from *Abacopteris penangiana*, Presents Neuroprotective Effects in Vitro and in Vivo." *Neurochemical Research* 38 (8): 1686–94.

Wei, H., G. H. Wu, Y. F. Lei, C. M. Xiong, and J. L. Ruan. 2011c. "Neuroprotective Constituents from the Rhizomes of *Abacopteris penangiana*." *Journal of Asian Natural Products Research* 13 (8): 707–13.

Wei, T., L. Wang, J. Tang, T. J. Ashaolu, and O. J. Olatunji. 2022b. "Protective Effect of Juglanin against Doxorubicin-Induced Cognitive Impairment in Rats: Effect of Oxidative, Inflammatory and Apoptotic Machineries." *Metabolic Brain Disease* 37 (4): 1185–95.

Wei, H. A., T. W. Lian, Y. C. Tu, J. T. Hong, M. C. Kou, and M. J. Wu. 2007. "Inhibition of Low-Density Lipoprotein Oxidation and Oxidative Burst in Polymorphonuclear

Neutrophils by Caffeic Acid and Hispidin Derivatives Isolated from Sword Brake Fern (*Pteris ensiformis* Burm.)." *Journal of Agricultural and Food Chemistry* 55 (26): 10579–84.

Wei, H., X. N. Zhang, G. H. Wu, X. Yang, S. W. Pan, Y. Y. Wang, and J. L. Ruan. 2013b. "Chalcone Derivatives from the Fern *Cyclosorus parasiticus* and Their Anti-Proliferative Activity." *Food and Chemical Toxicology* 60: 147–52.

Weinstein, M. 2020. *The Complete Book of Ferns*. Beverly, MA: Cool Springs Press, Quarto Publishing Group USA.

Wen, C. C., L. F. Shyur, J. T. Jan, P. H. Liang, C. J. Kuo, P. Arulselvan, J. B. Wu, S. C. Kuo, and N. S. Yang. 2011. "Traditional Chinese Medicine Herbal Extracts of *Cibotium barometz*, *Gentiana scabra*, *Dioscorea batatas*, *Cassia tora*, and *Taxillus chinensis* Inhibit SARS-CoV Replication." *Journal of Traditional and Complementary Medicine* 1: 41–50.

Wen, F., J. Yu, and Y. Cheng. 2022. "Network Pharmacology-Based Dissection of the Mechanism of Drynariae Rhizoma for Lower Back Pain." *BioMed Research International* 2022: 6092424.

Wen, S., M. Hu, and Y. Xiong. 2021. "Effect of Eriodictyol on Retinoblastoma via the PI3K/Akt Pathway." *Journal of Healthcare Engineering* 2021: 6091585.

Wills, P. J., and V. V. Asha. 2006. "Protective Effect of *Lygodium flexuosum* (L.) Sw. (Lygodiaceae) against D-Galactosamine Induced Liver Injury in Rats." *Journal of Ethnopharmacology* 108 (1): 116–23.

Wills, P. J., and V. V. Asha. 2009. "Chemopreventative Action of *Lygodium flexuosum* Extract in Human Hepatoma PLC/PRF/5 and Hep 3B Cells." *Journal of Ethnopharmacology* 122 (2): 294–303.

Windham, M. D., L. Huiet, J. S. Metzgar, T. A. Ranker, G. Yatskievych, C. H. Haufler, and K. M. Pryer. 2022. "Once More Unto the Breach, Dear Friends: Resolving the Origins and Relationships of the *Pellaea wrightiana* Hybrid Complex." *American Journal of Botany* 109 (5): 821–50.

Woerdenbag, H. J., L. R. Lutke, R. Bos, J. F. Stevens et al. 1996. "Isolation of two Cytotoxic Diterpenes from the Fern *Pteris multifida*." *Zeitschrift für Naturforschung C* 51 (9–10): 635–38.

Wong, W. 1976. "Some Folk Medicinal Plants from Trinidad." *Economic Botany* 30 (2): 103–42.

Woo, E. R., H. J. Kim, J. H. Kwak, Y. K. Lim, S. K. Park, H. S. Kim, C. K. Lee, and H. Park. 1997. "Anti-Herpetic Activity of Various Medicinal Plant Extracts." *Archives of Pharmacal Research* 20 (1): 58–67.

Wood, M. 2021. *Holistic Medicine and the Extracellular Matrix: The Science of Healing at the Cellular Level*. Rochester, VT: Healing Arts Press.

Wu, B. Y., and J. C. Shih. 2023. "In Vitro and in Vivo Assays Characterizing MAO A Function in Cancers." *Methods in Molecular Biology* 2558: 171–82.

Wu, C. R., H. C. Chang, Y. D. Cheng, W. C. Lan, S. E. Yang, and H. Ching. 2018a. "Aqueous Extract of *Davallia mariesii* Attentuates 6-hydroxydopamine-Induced Oxidative Damage and Apoptosis in B35 Cells through Inhibition of Caspase and Activation of PI3K/AKT/GSK-3b Pathway." *Nutrients* 10 (10): 1449.

Wu, G. H., Y. L. Cai, H. Wei. A. H. Wei, C. M. Xiong, W. Fu, and J. L. Ruan. 2012. "Nephroprotective Activity of *Macrothelypteris oligophlebia* Rhizomes Ethanol Extract." *Pharmaceutical Biology* 50 (6): 773–77.

Wu, H., Y. Cao, J. Wang, R. Liu, Y. Sun, C. Zhang, and Y. Sun. 2022. "Pharmacokinetic and Metabolic Profiling Studies of Osmundacetone in Rats with UPLC-MS/MS and UPLC-QE-Orbitrap-HRMS." *Biomedical Chromatography* 36 (1): e5251.

Wu, J. K., L. Meng, M. J. Long, Y. Ruan, X. Li, Y. Huang, and W. S. Qiu. 2017a. "Inhibition of Breast Cancer Cell Growth by the *Pteris semipinnata* Extract *ent*-11alpha-hydroxy-15-oxo-kaur-16-en-19-oic-acid." *Oncology Letters* 14 (6): 6809–14.

Wu, K. C., S. S. Huang, Y. H. Kuo, Y. L. Ho, C. S. Yang, Y. S. Chang, and G. J. Huang. 2017b. "Ugonin M, a *Helminthostachys zeylanica* Constituent, Prevent LPS-Induced Acute Lung Injury through TLR4-Mediated MAPK and NF-kB Signaling Pathways." *Molecules* 22 (4): 573.

Wu, K. C., Y. L. Ho, Y. H. Kuo, S. S. Huang, G. J. Huang, and Y. S. Chang. 2018b. "Hepatoprotective Effect of Ugonin M, A *Helminthostachys zeylanica* Constituent, on Acetaminophen-Induced Acute Liver Injury in Mice." *Molecules* 23 (10): 2420.

Wu, M. J., C. Y. Weng, L. Wang, and T. W. Lian. 2005a. "Immunomodulatory Mechanism of the Aqueous Extract of Sword Brake Fern (*Pteris ensiformis* Burm.)" *Journal of Ethnopharmacology* 98 (1–2): 73–81.

Wu, P. L., Y. L. Hsu, C. W. Zao, A. G. Damu, and T. S. Wu. 2005b. "Constituents of *Vittaria anguste-elongata* and Their Biological Activities." *Journal of Natural Products* 68 (8): 1180–84.

Wu, S. Q., J. Li, Q. X. Wang, H. Cao, J. G. Cao, and J. B. Xiao. 2017c. "Seasonal Dynamics of the Phytochemical Constituents and Bioactivities of Extracts from *Stenoloma chusanum* (L.) Ching." *Food and Chemical Toxicology* 108 (pt B): 458–66.

Wu, X., Q. Huang, N. Xu, J. Cai, D. Luo, Q. Zhang, Z. Su, C. Gao, and Y. Liu. 2018c. "Antioxidative and Anti-Inflammatory Effects of Water Extract of *Acrostichum aureum* Linn. against Ethanol-Induced Gastric Ulcer in Rats." *Evidence Based Complementary and Alternative Medicine* 2018: 3585394.

Wufuer, H., Y. C. Xu, D. Wu, W. W. He, D. Y. Wang, W. M. Zhu, and L. P. Wang. 2022. "Liglaurates A-E, Cytotoxic Bis (Lauric Acid-12yl) Lignanoates from the Rhizomes of *Drynaria roosii* Nakaike." *Phytochemistry* 198: 113143.

Wyman, L. C., and S. K. Harris. 1951. *The Ethnobotany of the Kayenta Navaho: An Analysis of the John and Louisa Wetherill Ethnobotanical Collection*. Albuquerque, NM: The University of New Mexico Press.

Xiang, L., C. R. Werth, S. N. Emery, and D. E. McCauley. 2000. "Population-Specific Gender-Biased Hybridization between *Dryopteris intermedia* and *D. carthusiana*: Evidence from Chloroplast DNA." *American Journal of Botany* 87 (8): 1175–80.

Xiao, W., Y. Peng, Z. Tan, Q. Y. Lv, C.O. Chan, J. Y. Yang, S. B Chen. 2017. "Comparative Evaluation of Chemical Profiles of Pyrrosiae Folium Originating from Three *Pyrrosia*

Species by HPLC-DAD Combined with Multivariate Statistical Analysis." *Molecules* 22 (12): 2122.

Xie, M. P., L. Li, H. Sun, A. Q. Lu, B. Zhang, J. G. Shi, D. Zhang, and S. J. Wang. 2017. "Hepatoprotective Hemiterpene Glycosides from the Rhizome of *Cibotium barometz* (L.) J. Sim." *Phytochemistry* 138: 128–33.

Xie, Y. H., Y. X. Zheng, X. L. Dai, Q. W. Wang, J. G. Cao, and J. B. Xiao. 2015. "Seasonal Dynamics of Total Flavonoid Contents and Antioxidant Activity of *Dryopteris erythrosora*." *Food Chemistry* 186: 113–18.

Xin, X. W., Q. S. Liu, Y. Y. Zhang, and D. G. M. Gao. 2016. "Chemical Composition and Antibacterial Activity of the Essential Oil from *Pyrrosia tonkinensis* (Giesenhagen) Ching." *Natural Product Research* 30(7): 853–56.

Xiong, C. Q., B. B. Yan, S. H. Xia, F. Yu, J. J. Zhao, and H. Bai. 2021. "Tilianin Inhibits the Human Ovarian Cancer (PA-1) Cell Proliferation via Blocking Cell Cycle, Inducing Apoptosis and Inhibiting JAK2/STAT3 Signaling Pathway." *Saudi Journal of Biological Sciences* 28 (9): 4900–7.

Xiong, Z. W., Y. S. Cui, J. H. Wu, L. Y. Shi, Q. Wen, S. L. Yang, and Y. L. Feng 2022. "Luteolin-7-O-rutinoside from *Pteris cretica* L. var. *nervosa* Attenuates LPS/D-gal-Induced Liver Injury by Inhibiting PI3K/AKT/AMPK/NF-kB Signaling Pathway." *Naunyn-Schmiedeberg's Archives of Pharmacology* 395 (10): 1283–95.

Xu, G., M. J. Zhao, N. Sun, C. G. Ju, and T. Z. Jia. 2014. "Effect of the RW-Cb and Its Active Ingredient Like P-Acid and P-Aldehyde on Primary Rat Osteoblasts." *Journal of Ethnopharmacology* 151 (1): 237–41.

Xu, H. X, S. Kadota, M. Kurokawa, K. Shiraki, T. Matsumoto, and T. Namba. 1993. "Isolation and Structure of Woodorien, a New Glucoside Having Antiviral Activity, from *Woodwardia orientalis*." *Chemical and Pharmaceutical Bulletin* (Tokyo) 41 (10): 1803–6.

Xu, X. W., J. Chen, H. Lv, Y. Y. Xi, A. Y. Ying, and X. Hu. 2022. "Molecular Mechanism of *Pyrrosia lingua* in the Treatment of Nephrolithiasis: Network Pharmacology Analysis and in Vivo Experimental Verification." *Phytomedicine* 98: 153929.

Xu, Y., Y. Y. Tong, Z. M. Lei, J. Y. Zhu, and L. J. Wan. 2023. "Abietic Acid Induces Ferroptosis via the Activation of the HO-1 Pathway in Bladder Cancer Cells." *Biomedicine and Pharmacotherapy* 158: 114154.

Xue, B. X., Y. X. Shan, and G. Xiang. 2008. "Clinical Evaluation on Fengweicao Granule in Treating Benign Prostatic Hyperplasia." *Zhongguo Zhong Xi Yi Yie He Za Zhi* 28 (5): 456–58.

Xun, Y., L. Feng, Y. D. Li, and H. C. Dong. 2017. "Mercury Accumulation Plant *Cyrtomium macrophyllum* and Its Potential for Phytoremediation of Mercury Polluted Sites." *Chemosphere* 189: 161–70.

Yadav, S. K., Archana, R. Singh, P. K. Singh, and P. G. Vasudev. 2019. "Insecticidal Fern Protein Tma12 is Possibly a Lytic Polysaccharide Monooxygenase." *Planta* 249 (6): 1987–96.

Yadegari, M., S. Riahy, S. Mirdar, G. Hamidian, S. M. Afkhami, A. Saeidi, F. Rhibi, A. Ben Abderrahman, A. C. Hackney, and H. Zouhal. 2019. "The TNF-*a*, P53 Protein Response and Lung Respiratory Changes to Exercise, Chronic Hypoxia and *Adiantum capillus-veneris* Supplementation." *Advances in Respiratory Medicine* 87 (4): 226–34.

Yamahara, J., H. Matsuda, H. Shimoda, N. Wariishi, N. Yagi, N. Murakami, and M. Yoshikawa. 1995. "Effects of Thunberginol A Contained in *Hydrangeae dulcis* Forium on Types I-IV Allergies." *Nihon Yakurigaku Zasshi* 105 (5): 365–79.

Yamasaki, K., R. Hishki, E. Kato, and J. Kawabata. 2010. "Study of Kaempferol Glycoside as an Insulin Mimic Reveals Glycon to Be the Key Active Structure." *ACS Medicinal Chemistry Letters* 2 (1): 17–21.

Yamauchi, K., T. Mitsunaga, and I. Batubara. 2013. "Novel Quercetin Glucosides from *Helminthostachys zeylanica* Root and Acceleratory Activity of Melanin Biosynthesis." *Journal of Natural Medicines* 67 (2): 369–74.

Yamauchi, K., T. Mitsunaga, Y. Itakura, and I. Batubara. 2015. "Extracellular Melanogenesis Inhibitory Activity and the Structure-Activity Relationships of Ugonins from *Helminthostachys zeylanica* roots." *Fitoterapia* 104: 69–74.

Yan, H., H. Wang, L. Ma, X. Ma, J. Yin, S. Wu, H. Huang, and Y. Li. 2018. "Cirsimaritin Inhibits Influenza A Virus Replication by Downregulating the NF-kB Signal Transduction Pathway." *Virology Journal* 15 (1): 88.

Yang, J., J. Fa, and B. X. Li. 2017. "Apoptosis Induction of Epifriedelinol on Human Cervical Cancer Cell Line." *African Journal of Traditional Complementary and Alternative Medicines* 14 (4): 80–86.

Yang, J. H., T. P. Kondratyuk, K . C. Jermihov, L. E. Marler et al. 2011. "Bioactive Compounds from the Fern *Lepisorus contortus*." *Journal of Natural Products* 74 (2): 129–36.

Yang, J. H., T. P. Kondratyuk, L. E. Marler, X. Qiu et al. 2010. "Isolation and Evaluation of Kaempferol Glycosides from the Fern *Neocheiropteris palmatopedata*." *Phytochemistry* 71 (5–6): 641–47.

Yang, L. L., K. Y. Yen, Y. Kiso, and H. Hikino. 1987. "Antihepatotoxic Actions of Formosan Plant Drugs." *Journal of Ethnopharmacology* 19 (1): 103–10.

Yang, M., H. L. Huang, B. Y. Zhu, Q. H. Tuo, and D. F. Liao. 2005. "Onychin Inhibits Proliferation of Vascular Smooth Muscle Cells by Regulating Cell Cycle." *Acta Pharmacologica Sinica* 26 (2): 205–11.

Yang, Q., L. Gao, J. Y. Si, Y. P. Sun, J. H. Liu, L. Cao, and W. H. Feng. 2013a. "Inhibition of Porcine Reproductive and Respiratory Virus Replication by Flavaspidic Acid AB." *Antiviral Research* 97 (1): 66–73.

Yang, R. C., C. C. Chang, J. M. Sheen, H. T. Wu, J. H. S. Pang, and S. T. Huang. 2014a. "*Davallia bilabiate* Inhibits TNF-*a*-induced Adhesion Molecules and Chemokines by Suppressing IKK/NF-kappa B Pathway in Vascular Endothelial Cells." *The American Journal of Chinese Medicine* 42 (6): 1411–29.

Yang, S., M. Liu, N. Liang, Q. Zhao, Y. Zhang, W. Xue, and S. Yang. 2013b. "Discovery and Antitumor Activities of Constituents from *Cyrtomium fortunei* (J.) Smith Rhizomes." *Chemistry Central Journal* 7 (1): 24.

Yang, S. J., M. C. Liu, N. Liang, H. M. Xiang, and S. Yang. 2013c. "Chemical Constituents of *Cyrtomium fortunei* (J.) Smith." *Natural Product Research* 27 (21): 2066–68.

Yang, S. J., M. C. Liu, Q. Zhao, H. G. Zhao, W. Xue, and S. Yang. 2015a. "Antiproliferative and Apoptosis Inducing Effect of Essential Oil Extracted from *Cyrtomium fortunei* (J.) Smith Leaves." *Medicinal Chemistry Research* 24 (4): 1644–52.

Yang, X., L. L. Yuan, C. M. Xiong, C. P. Yin, and J. L. Ruan. 2014b. "*Abacopteris penangiana* Exerts Testosterone-Induced Benign Prostatic Hyperplasia Protective Effect through Regulating Inflammatory Responses, Reducing Oxidative Stress and Anti-Proliferative." *Journal of Ethnopharmacology* 157: 105–13.

Yang, X., L. L. Yuan, J. L. Chen, C. M. Xiong, and J. N. Ruan. 2014c. "Multitargeted Protective Effect of *Abacopteris penangiana* against Carrageenan-Induced Chronic Prostatitis in Rats." *Journal of Ethnopharmacology* 151 (1): 343–51.

Yang, X. L., P. Wu, J. H. Xue, H. X. Li, and X. Y. Wei. 2023. "Seco-Pimarane Diterpenoids and Androstane Steroids from an Endophytic *Nodulisporium* Fungus Derived from *Cyclosorus parasiticus*." *Phytochemistry* 210: 113679.

Yang, Y., P. Y. He, Y. H. Hou, Z. C. Liu, X. P. Zhang, and N. Li. 2022. "Osmundacetone Modulates Mitochondrial Metabolism in Non-Small Cell Lung Cancer Cells by Hijacking the Glutamine/Glutamate/*a*-KG Metabolic Axis." *Phytomedicine* 100: 154075.

Yang, Z. Y., T. Kuboyama, K. Kazuma, K. Konno, and C. Todha. 2015b. "Active Constituents from *Drynaria fortunei* Rhizomes on the Attenuation of Ab(25-35)-Induced Axonal Atrophy." *Journal of Natural Products* 78 (9): 2297–2300.

Yokouchi, Y., T. Saito, C. Ishigaki, and M. Aramoto. 2007. "Identification of Methyl Chloride-Emitting Plants and Atmospheric Measurements on a Subtropical Island." *Chemosphere* 69 (4): 549–53.

Yonathan, M., K. Asres, A. Assefa, and F. Bucar. 2006. "In Vivo Anti-Inflammatory and Anti-Nociceptive Activities of *Cheilanthes farinosa*." *Journal of Ethnopharmacology* 108 (3): 462–70.

Yoo, G., S. J. Park, H. Yang, X. N. Nguyen, N. Kim, J. H. Park, and S. H. Kim. 2017. "Two New Phenolic Glycosides from the Aerial Part of *Dryopteris erythrosora*." *Pharmacognosy Magazine* 13 (52): 673–76.

Yoshikawa, M., H. Matsuda, H. Shimoda, H. Shimada, E. Harada, Y. Naitho, A. Miki, J. Yamahara, N. Murakami. 1996. "Development of Bioactive Functions in *Hydrangea dulcis* Folium. V. On the Antiallergic and Antimicrobial Principles of *Hydrangea dulcis* Folium. (2). Thunberginols C, D, and E, Thunberginol G 3'-O-glucoside, (-)-Hydrangenol 4'-O-glucoside, and (+)-Hydrangenol 4'-O-Glucoside." *Chemical and Pharmaceutical Bulletin* 44 (8): 1440—47.

You, Y. X., S. Shahar, H. Haron, H. M. Yahya, and N. C. Din. 2020. "Relationship between Traditional Malaysian Vegetables (Ulam) Intake and Cognitive Status among Middle-Aged Adults from Low Cost Residential Areas." *Malaysian Journal of Health Sciences* 17.

Young, D. 2014. *The Mouse Woman of Gabriola*. British Columbia: Coastal Tides Press.

Young, D., R. Rogers, and R. Willier. 2015. *A Cree Healer and His Medicine Bundle*. Berkeley, CA: North Atlantic Books.

Yu, C. Q., J. W. Chen, and L. Huang. 2013. "A Study on the Antitumour Effect of Total Flavonoids from *Pteris multifida* Poir in H22 Tumour-Bearing Mice." *African Journal of Traditional, Complementary, and Alternative Medicines* 10 (6): 459–63.

Yu, W. M., W. L. Hu, X. M. Ke, X. F. Zhou, C. C. Yin, and M. Yin. 2020. "Different Effects of Total Flavonoids from *Arachniodes exilis* on Human Umbilical Cord Mesenchymal Stem Cells in Vitro." *Medicine* (Baltimore) 99(25): e20628.

Yu, Y. M., J. S. Yang, C. Z. Peng, V. Caer, P. Z. Cong, Z. M. Zou, Y. Lu, S. Y. Yang, and Y. C. Gu. 2009. "Lactones from *Angiopteris caudatiformis*." *Journal of Natural Products* 72 (5): 921–24.

Yuk, H. J., J. Y. Kim, Y. Y. Sung, and D. S. Kim. 2020. "Phloroglucinol Derivatives from *Dryopteris crassirhizoma* as Potent Xanthine Oxidase Inhibitors." *Molecules* 26 (1): 122.

Yurdakok, B., G. Kismali, and D. Ozen. 2014. "Ptaquiloside-Induced Cytotoxicity in Crandall Feline Kidney and HGC-27 Cells." *Onocology Letters* 8 (4): 1839–43.

Zakaria, Z. A., A. M. Mohamed, N. S. Mohd Jamil, M. S. Rofiee, M. N. Somchit, A. Zuraini, A. K. Arifah, and M. R. Sulaiman. 2011. "*In Vitro* Cytotoxic and Antioxidant Properties of the Aqueous, Chloroform and Methanol Extracts of *Dicranopteris linearis* Leaves." *African Journal of Biotechnology* 10 (2): 273–82.

Zakaria, Z. A., F. H. Kamisan, N. M. Nasir, L. K. The, and M. Z. Salleh. 2019. "Aqueous Partition of Methanolic Extract of *Dicranopteris linearis* Leaves Protects against Liver Damage Induced by Paracetamol." *Nutrients* 11 (12): 2945.

Zakaria, Z. A., F. H. Kamisan, T. L. Kek, and M. Z. Salleh. 2020a. "Hepatoprotective and Antioxidant Activities of *Dicranopteris linearis* Leaf Extract against Paracetamol-Induced Liver Intoxication in Rats." *Pharmaceutical Biology* 58 (1): 478–89.

Zakaria, Z. A., R. A. J. Roosli, N. H. Marmaya, M. H. Omar, R. Basir, and M. N. Somchit. 2020b. "Methanol Extract of *Dicranopteris linearis* Leaves Attenuate Pain via the Modulation of Opioid/NO-Mediated Pathway." *Biomolecules* 10 (2): 280.

Zakaria, Z. A., Z. D. Ghani, R. N. Nor, H. K. Gopalan, M. R. Sulaiman, and F. C. Abdullah. 2006. "Antinociceptive and Anti-Inflammatory Activities of *Dicranopteris linearis* Leaves Chloroform Extract in Experimental Animals." *Yakugaku Zasshi* 126 (11): 1197–203.

Zeb, A., and F. Ullah. 2017. "Reversed Phase HPLC-DAD Profiling of Carotenoids, Chlorophylls and Phenolic Compounds in *Adiantum capillus-veneris* Leaves." *Frontiers in Chemistry* 5: 29.

Zeng, W. W., and L. S. Lai. 2019a. "Multiple-Physiological Benefits of Bird's Nest Fern (*Asplenium australasicum*) Frond Extract for Dermatological Applications." *Natural Product Research* 33 (5): 736–41.

Zeng, W. W., and L. S. Lai. 2019b. "Anti-Melanization Effects and Inhibitory Kinetics of Tyrosinase of Bird's Nest Fern (*Asplenium australasicum*) Frond Extracts on Melanoma and Human Skin." *Journal of Bioscience and Bioengineering* 127 (6): 738–43.

Zhang, F., Q. Li, J. Wu, H. Ruan, C. Sun, J. Zhu, Q. Song, X. Wei, Y. Shi, and L. Zhu. 2022a. "Total Flavonoids of Drynariae Rhizoma Improve Glucocorticoid-Induced Osteoporosis of Rats: UHPLC-MS-Based Qualitative Analysis, Network Pharmacology Strategy and Pharmacodynamic Validation." *Frontiers in Endocrinology* (Lausanne) 13: 020931.

Zhang, F. X., and R. S. Xu. 2018. "Juglanin Ameliorates LPS-Induced Neuroinflammation in Animal Models of Parkinson's Disease and Cell Culture via Inactivating TLR4/NF-kB Pathway." *Biomedicine & Pharmacotherapy* 97: 1011–19.

Zhang, J., Y. He, Y. Zhou, L. Hong et al. 2022b. "Epifriedelinol Ameliorates DMBA-Induced Breast Cancer in Albino Rats by Regulating the PI3K/AKT Pathway." *The Tohoku Journal of Experimental Medicine* 257 (4): 283–89.

Zhang, J. H., J. L. Chen, W. B. Xu, Y. P. Xia, H. Y. Zhu, J. H. Wang, Y. L. Li, G. C. Wang, Y. B. Zhang, and N. H. Chen. 2023. "Undescribed Phloroglucinol Derivatives with Antiviral Activities from *Dryopteris atrata* (Wall. ex Kunze) Ching." *Phytochemistry* 208: 113585.

Zhang, M., J. G. Cao, X. L. Dai, X. F. Chen, and Q. X. Wang. 2012a. "Flavonoid Contents and Free Radical Scavenging Activity of Extracts from Leaves, Stems, Rachis and Roots of *Dryopteris erythrosora*." *Iranian Journal of Pharmaceutical Research* 11 (3): 991–97.

Zhang, P., Y. Y. Cheng, and Z. J. Ma. 2008. "New Cycloartane Glycosides from *Camptosorus sibiricus* Rupr." *Journal of Asian Natural Products Research* 10 (11–12): 1069–74.

Zhang, S., N. Feng, J. Huang, M. Wang, L. Zhang, J. Yu, X. Dai, J. Cao, and G. Huang. 2020. "Incorporation of Amino Moiety to Alepterolic Acid Improve Activity against Cancer Cell Lines: Synthesis and Biological Evaluation." *Bioorganic Chemistry* 98: 103756.

Zhang, S. J., W. T. Xia, X. H. Yang, and T. T. Zhang. 2016a. "Inhibition Effect of Aquaculture Water of *Salvinia natans* (L.) All. on *Microcystis aeruginosa* PCC7806." *Wei Sheng Yan Jiu* 45 (1): 81–86.

Zhang, T., L. Wang, D. H. Duan, Y. H. Zhang, S. X. Huang, and Y. Chang. 2018. "Cytotoxicity-Guided Isolation of Two New Phenolic Derivatives from *Dryopteris fragrans* (L.) Schott." *Molecules* 23 (7): 1652.

Zhang, X., H. Wei, Z. Liu, Q. Yuan, A. Wei, D. Shi, X. Yang, and J. Ruan. 2013. "A Novel Protoapigenone Analog RY10-4 Induces Breast Cancer MCF-7 Cell Death through Autophagy via the Akt/mTOR Pathway." *Toxicology and Applied Pharmacology* 270 (2): 122–28.

Zhang, X. Q., J. H. Kim, G. S. Lee, H. B. Pyo, E. Y. Shin, E. G. Kim, and Y. H. Zhang. 2012b. "In Vitro Antioxidant and in Vivo Anti-Inflammatory Activities of *Ophioglossum thermale*." *American Journal of Chinese Medicine* 40 (2): 279–93.

Zhang, X. X., X. Wang, M. L. Wang, J. G. Cao, J. B. Xiao, and Q. X. Wang. 2019. "Effects of Different Pretreatments on Flavonoids and Antioxidant Activity of *Dryopteris erythrosora* leave." *PLoS One* 14 (1): e0200174.

Zhang, Y., H. Y. Tian, Y. F. Tan, and Y. L. Wong. 2016b. "Isolation and Identification of Polyphenols from *Marsilea quadrifolia* with Antioxidant Properties in Vitro and in Vivo." *Natural Product Research* 30 (12): 1404–10.

Zhang, Y., M. Luo, Y. G. Zu, Y. J. Fu, C. B. Gu, W. Wang, L. P. Yao, and T. Efferth. 2012c. "Dryofragin, a Phloroglucinol Derivative, Induces Apoptosis in Human Breast Cancer MCF-7 Cells through ROS-Mediated Mitochondrial Pathway." *Chemico-Biological Interactions* 199 (2): 129–36.

Zhang, Y., Y. Hu, B. Xu, and J. Fan. 2022c. "Robust Underwater Air Layer Retention and Restoration on *Salvinia*-Inspired Self-Grown Heterogeneous Architectures." *ACS Nano* 16 (2): 2730–40.

Zhang, Y., Y. S. Shi, W. Z. Hu, L. Y. Song, and X. Z. Chen. 2016c. "Chemical Constituents from *Pteris multifida* and Cytotoxic Activity." *Zhongguo Zhong Yao Za Zhi* 41 (24): 4610–14.

Zhang, Y. S., J. H. He, S. J. Luo, Y. Y. Li, and M. Liang. 2007. "Effects of 5F from *Pteris semipinnate* (sic) L on Growth of Human Pathological Scars in Nude Mice." *Nan Fang Yi Ke Da Xue Xue Bao* 27 (11): 1677–80.

Zhao, D. D., Q. S. Zhao, L. Liu, Z. Q. Chen, W. M. Zeng, H. Lei, and Y. L. Zhang. 2014. "Compounds from *Dryopteris fragrans* (L.) Schott with Cytotoxic Activity." *Molecules* 19 (3): 3345–55.

Zhao, K., M. Chen, T. Liu, P. Zhang, S. Wang, X. Liu, Q. Wang, and J. Sheng. 2021a. "Rhizoma Drynariae Total Flavonoids Inhibit the Inflammatory Response and Matrix Degeneration via MAPK Pathway in a Rat Degenerative Cervical Intervertebral Disc Model." *Biomedicine and Pharmacotherapy* 138: 111466.

Zhao, L., X. Jin, Y. B. Li, Y. Yu, L. Z. He, and R. Liu 2022a. "Effects of A-Type Oligomer Procyanidins on Protein Glycation Using Two Glycation Models Coupled with Spectroscopy, Chromatography, and Molecular Docking." *Food Research International* (Ottawa) 155: 111068.

Zhao, S., C. Liu, W. Zheng, Z. Ma, T. Cao, J. Zhao, K. Yan, W. Xiang, and X. Wang. 2017a. "*Micromonospora parathelypteridis* sp. nov., an Endophytic Actinomycete with Antifungal Activity Isolated from the Root of *Parathelypteris beddomei* (Bak.) Ching." *International Journal of Systematic and Evolutionary Microbiology* 67 (2): 268–74.

Zhao, X., Z. X. Wu, Y. Zhang, Y. B. Yan, Q. He, P. C. Cao, and W. Lei. 2011. "Anti-Osteoporosis Activity of *Cibotium barometz* Extract on Ovariectomy-Induced Bone Loss in Rats." *Journal of Ethnopharmacology* 137 (3): 1083–88.

Zhao, X. F., J. Liu, A. Q. Fang, Y. Duan, S. J. He, J. Li, and S. X. Li. 2022b. "A New Sesquiterpene Lactone from Biological Transformation of *Hericium erinaceus* and Artemisiae Annuae Herba." *Zhongguo Zhong Yao Za Zhi* 47 (24): 6647–54.

Zhao, X. Y., J. Y. Li, Y. Q. Liu, D. T. Wu, P. F. Cai, and Y. J. Pan. 2017b. "Structural Characterization and Immunomodulatory Activity of a Water Soluble Polysaccharide Isolated from *Botrychium ternatum*." *Carbohydrate Polymers* 171: 136–42.

Zhao, Y., W. Hu, H. Zhang, C. Ding, Y. Huang, J. Liao, Z. Zhang, S. Yuan, Y. Chen, and M. Yuan. 2019. "Antioxidant and Immunomodulatory Activities of Polysaccharides from the Rhizome of *Dryopteris crassirhizoma* Nakai." *International Journal of Biological Macromolecules* 130: 238–44.

Zhao, Y. H. 1985. "Analysis of the Therapeutic Effect of 1,148 cases of Bacillary Dysentery Treated with *Pyrrosia sheareri*." *Zhong Xi Yi Jie He Za Zhi* 5 (9): 530–33, 514.

Zhao, Y. Y., Q. M. Yu, Z. H. Qiao, J. Li, H. X. Tang, G. Y. Chen, and Y. H. Fu. 2021b. "Chemical Constituents from *Morinda citrifolia* and Their Inhibitory Activities on Proliferation of Synoviocytes in Vitro." *Zhongguo Zhong Yao Za Zhi* 46 (10): 2519–26.

Zhao, Z. G., J. L. Ruan, J. Jin, J. Zou, D. N. Zhou, W. Fang, and F. B. Zeng. 2006. "Flavan-4-ol Glycosides from the Rhizomes of *Abacopteris penangiana*." *Journal of Natural Products* 69 (2): 265–68.

Zhao, Z. H., X. Y. Ju, K. W. Wang, X. J. Chen, H. X. Sun, and K. J. Cheng. 2022c. "Structure Characterization, Antioxidant and Immunomodulatory Activities of Polysaccharide from *Pteridium aquilinum* (L.) Kuhn." *Foods* 11 (13): 1834.

Zhao, Z. X., J. Ruan, J. Jin, C. C. Zhu, and Y. X. Liu. 2010. "A novel Anthocyanidin Glycoside from the Rhizomes of *Abacopteris penangiana*." *Fitoterapia* 81 (8): 1171–75.

Zhen, Z. G., S. H. Ren, H. M. Ji, J. H. Ma, X. M. Ding, F. Q. Feng, S. L. Chen, P. Zou, J. R. Ren, and L. Jia. 2017. "Linarin Suppresses Glioma through Inhibition of NF-kB/p65 and Upregulating p53 Expression in Vitro and in Vivo." *Biomedicine and Pharmacotherapy* 95: 363–74.

Zheng, M. 1990. "Experimental Study of 472 Herbs with Antiviral Action against the Herpes Simplex Virus." *Zhong Xi Yi Jie He Za Zhi* 10 (1): 39–41.

Zheng, S. Q., G. Q. Song, C. P. Yin, Y. F. Chen, S. S. Wang, and Z. B. Shen. 2022. "A New Phloroglucinol from *Dryopteris fragrans* and Its Antibacterial Activity in Vitro." *Zhongguo Zhong Yao Za Zhi* 47 (9): 2474–79.

Zheng, X. M., L. Huang, Y. Xiao, H. Su, G. L. Xu, F. Fu, J. T. Li, and S. G. Sun. 2012. "A Dicranopteris Like Fe-Sn-Sb-P Alloy as a Promising Anode for Lithium Ion Batteries." *Chemical Communications* (Cambridge) 48 (54): 6854–56.

Zhong, Z. C., D. D. Zhao, Z. D. Liu, S. Jiang, and Y. L. Zhang. 2017. "A New Human Cancer Cell Proliferation Inhibition Sesquiterpene, Dryofraterpene A, from Medicinal Plant *Dryopteris fragrans* (L.) Schott." *Molecules* 22 (1): 180.

Zhou, D. N., A. H. Wei, C. Cao, and J. N. Ruan. 2013. "DICO, a Novel Nonaromatic B-Ring Flavonoid, Induces G2/M Cell Cycle Arrest and Apoptosis in Human Hepatoma Cells." *Food and Chemical Toxicology* 57: 322–29.

Zhou, D. N., J. L. Ruan, Y. L. Cai, Z. M. Xiong, W. Fu, and A. H. Wei. 2010. "Antioxidant and Hepatoprotective Activity of Ethanol Extract of *Arachniodes exilis* (Hance) Ching." *Journal of Ethnopharmacology* 129 (2): 232–37.

Zhou, F. M., and X. S. Wang. 2022. "*Pyrrosia petiolosa* Extract Ameliorates Ethylene Glycol-Induced Uroliathiasis in Rats by Inhibiting Oxidative Stress and Inflammatory Response." *Disease Markers* 2022: 1913067.

Zhou, J., L. Chan, and S. Zhou. 2012. "Trigonelline: A Plant Alkaloid with Therapeutic Potential for Diabetes and Central Nervous System Disease." *Current Medicinal Chemistry* 19 (21): 3523–31.

Zhou, L., K. Y. Wong, C. C. W. Poon, W. Yu, H. Xiao, C. O. Chan, D. K. W. Mok, and M. S. Wong. 2022. "Water Extract of Rhizome Drynaria Selectively Exerts Estrogenic Activities in Ovariectomized Rats and Estrogen Receptor-Positive Cells." *Frontiers in Endocrinology* 13: 817146.

Zhou, Q., J. Yuping, P. Yi, J. Sun, X. L. Zhou, S. H. Chen, and W. Wang. 2019. "A Comprehensive Review on *Pronephrium penangianum*." *Israel Journal of Chemistry* 59 (5): 371–77.

Zhou, X. H. 1987. "Therapeutic Effect of *Drynaria baronii* Diels on Experimental Osteoarthritis." *Zhong Yao Tong Bao* 12 (10): 41–44.

Zhu, X. M., Y. W. Kuang, D. Xi, L. Jiong, and F. G. Wang. 2013a. "Absorption of Hazardous Pollutants by a Medicinal Fern *Blechnum orientale* L." *BioMed Research International* 2013: 192986.

Zhu, X. X., Y. J. Li, L. Yang, D. Zhang, Y. Chen, E. Kmonickova, X. G. Weng, Q. Yang, and Z. Zídek. 2013b. "Divergent Immunomodulatory Effects of Extracts and Phenolic Compounds from the Fern *Osmunda japonica* Thunb." *Chinese Journal of Integrative Medicine* 19 (10): 761–70.

Živković, S., M. Skorić, M. Ristić, B. Filipović, M. Milutinović, M. Perišić, and N. Puač. 2021. "Rehydration Process in Rustyback Fern (*Asplenium ceterach* L.): Profiling of Volatile Organic Compounds." *Biology* 10 (7): 574.

Zou, J., Y. Duan, Y. Wang, A. Liu et al. 2022. "Phellopterin Cream Exerts an Anti-Inflammatory Effect that Facilitates Diabetes-Associated Cutaneous Wound Healing via SIRT1." *Phytomedicine* 107: 154447.

Zuloaga, F. O., O. Morrone, and D. Rodriguez. "*Análisisde la biodiversidad en plantas vasculares de la Argentina*." *Kurtziana* 27: 17–167.

Zuo, G. Y., C. J. Wang, J. Han, Y. Q. Li, and G. C. Wang. 2016. "Synergism of Coumarins from the Chinese Drug Zanthoxylum Nitidum with Antibacterial Agents against Methicillin-resistant *Staphylococcus aureus* (MRSA)." *Phytomedicine* 23 (14): 1814–20.

Index of Ferns and Medicinal Applications

Ferns listed under medical conditions represent the most relevant genus entries for that condition. Other passing references to these conditions can be found in the text.